PHYSICAL FITNESS

A Wellness Approach

SECOND EDITION

Jerrold S. Greenberg

University of Maryland

David Pargman

Florida State University

PRENTICE HALL, ENGLEWOOD CLIFFS, NEW JERSEY 07632

Library of Congress Cataloging-in-Publication Data

Greenberg, Jerrold S.
   Physical fitness: a wellness approach/Jerrold S. Greenberg,
David Pargman.—2nd ed.
      p. cm.
   Bibliography.
   Includes index.
   1. Health. 2. Physical fitness. 3. Exercise. 4. Mental health.
I. Pargman, David. II. Title.
RA776.G789 1989   88-6894
613.7—dc19   CIP
ISBN 0-13-668872-1

Editorial/production supervision: **Marjorie Shustak**
Cover art: **Steve Kuzma**
Manufacturing buyer: **Peter Havens**

Photo credits
Chapter openings: Ch.1: The Library of Congress; Chs. 2,14b: Jim McCauler, Florida Flambeau Newspaper; Chs. 3, 4, 6, 7, 9, 10, 12, 13, 14a: The Diamondback, University of Maryland; Ch. 5: Randall Roberts; Ch. 8: The 52 Association, Inc.; Ch. 11: Florida State University Photo Lab. All interior photos, Ch. 9: Universal Gym Equipment, Inc.

 © 1989 by Prentice-Hall, Inc.
A Division of Simon & Schuster
Englewood Cliffs, New Jersey 07632

Printed in the United States of America
10 9 8 7 6 5 4 3 2 1

ISBN 0-13-668872-1

Prentice-Hall International (UK) Limited, *London*
Prentice-Hall of Australia Pty. Limited, *Sydney*
Prentice-Hall Canada Inc., *Toronto*
Prentice-Hall Hispanoamericana, S.A., *Mexico*
Prentice-Hall of India Private Limited, *New Delhi*
Prentice-Hall of Japan, Inc., *Tokyo*
Simon & Schuster Asia Pte. Ltd., *Singapore*
Editora Prentice-Hall do Brasil, Ltda., *Rio de Janeiro*

A book on physical fitness should be dedicated to someone who is fit. This book is dedicated to two women who are fit in mind, body, and spirit; two people who contribute immeasurably to *our own* fitness as well as that of our children; two women whose support, encouragement, and confidence enables *our* wellness to attain higher and higher levels. This book is dedicated to our wives, Karen Ann Greenberg and Marsha Pargman.

Contents

3

Training: Your Body's Response,   38

4

Assessment: Medical Evaluation and Fitness Appraisal,   63

5

How to Get to Where You Want to Be: Choices, 87

6

Planning Your Individualized Program and Keeping It Going, 99

8

9

10

11

Nutrition and Weight Control,   211

12

Stress Management and Physical Fitness, 235

13

Common Fitness Injuries, 261

Appendix D: The Recommended Quantity and Quality of Exercise for Developing and Maintaining Fitness in Healthy Adults, 320

Preface

Physical fitness has become popular—almost faddish. Some people believe it will prevent them from becoming ill, even though the evidence for this belief is sketchy. Others believe it will make them thin, even though exercise alone does not usually burn off enough calories fast enough to transform their bodies for the approaching bathing suit season. Still others believe physical fitness activities will rehabilitate them from conditions of ill health, even though they are unwilling to tolerate the commitment required in terms of time and energy.

This book considers these and other reasons for achieving and maintaining a satisfactory level of physical fitness. However, the emphasis within these pages is upon the *wellness* benefits—as distinct from the health benefits. We underline the importance of enjoyment while becoming fit, of improving your social life while becoming fit, and of becoming *spiritually* healthy at the same time you are becoming *physically* healthy.

We define wellness as a state of health—where your physical, social, mental, emotional, and spiritual healths are balanced, integrated, and coordinated. We show you how to achieve this state of high-level wellness and, once achieved, how to maintain it. We describe the psychology and sociology of physical fitness, as well as its physiology.

Here's how we do all of that. First, we present the changes that will occur within your body when you exercise. Then we get you started on a physical fitness program by helping you to determine 1) your motivation for exercising regularly, 2) some of your unique personality and character traits that relate to regular exercise, and 3) your present level of physical fitness. This information about yourself is obtained through various assessment devices presented within this book—for example, questionnaires, scales, and exercises. Next, we show you how to exercise in a healthy manner, which exercises serve which purposes, and how you can use results of research done by psychologists and sociologists to make it more likely that you will continue your fitness program. Lastly, we discuss other considerations that pertain to regular exercise: sex differences, age differences, environmental differences, nutrition and weight control, and stress management through exercise. We even discuss common athletic injuries—their causes, means of preventing their occurrence, and how to treat them should that be necessary.

This second edition of *Physical Fitness: A Wellness Approach* benefits from the experience of many fitness instructors and their students. After having used the first edition, they were able to advise us on which parts of the book should be expanded and which should remain unchanged. The result is an improved book—one that helps us to better help you become physically fit in a way in which your health and wellness goals are also met. The specific changes incorporated in this edition of *Physical Fitness: A Wellness Approach* include:

1. Chapter Objectives on the opening page of each chapter to guide the reader toward greater learning about the chapter's contents.
2. A Summary at the end of each chapter to highlight the more important content and to reinforce learning about that information.
3. An updating of the chapter content so that the most current information is presented; for example, the most current guidelines for exercise testing and prescription from the American College of Sports Medicine.
4. New information on such topics as phases of the workout, amenorrhea and participation in sports, longevity and exercise, static and ballistic flexibility exercises, dietary nutrients, time management, and low-impact aerobics.
5. Two appendices on the American College of Sports Medicine's position statements on "Prevention of Heat Injuries During Distance Running" and "The Recommended Quantity and Quality of Exercise for Developing and Maintaining Fitness in Healthy Adults."

Well, enough talk. This book is about activity. Come with us now on a journey toward better health, higher wellness, and an improved quality of life. Although it sounds like a tall order, we think you'll find it filled. Come, let us help you get fit.

ACKNOWLEDGMENTS

Any book requires a great deal of effort, and not just on the part of the authors. This book is no exception to that rule. We have been fortunate in having an editor, Joe Heider, who believed in this project and nurtured it along the way. Joe prodded us to make the book even better than the first edition, and our success, in good measure, is due to that prodding. We also had a production staff that was committed to publishing a book of high quality. The assistance of this Prentice Hall family was vital to the publication of this book and we thank them.

We are also grateful for the help of all the reviewers who made many worthwhile suggestions. To the extent that this book is a meaningful one, their contributions were vital, and very much appreciated.

Finally, we thank our families. The encouragement and nurturance they gave us were more important in the production of this book than the paper it was printed on or the cover that encloses it. We want them to know that we have not overlooked their contributions and that we appreciate them.

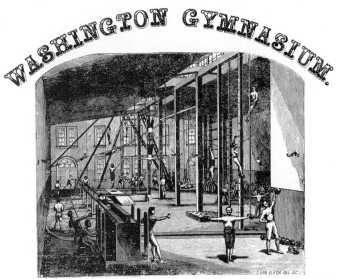

Personal Fitness:
Wellness

Over the years, physical fitness—the ability to do one's work and have energy remaining for basic recreational activities—has been advocated for two basic reasons: to prevent illness and disease and to help rehabilitation. Since the leading killers in our society are the cardiovascular diseases (heart disease and stroke), it is not surprising that the benefits of exercise in preventing these diseases are often cited.

Regular exercise conditions the heart to be more efficient by allowing it to pump out more blood per contraction (stroke volume) while at the same time decreasing the rate at which it beats. When more oxygen and energy sources are needed by the body during exercise, the fit heart meets these needs by pumping out more blood per heartbeat. In addition, regular exercise increases high-density lipoproteins, which are thought to provide some protection from atherosclerosis—clogging of the arteries supplying the heart—and also decreases the level of serum cholesterol.

Exercise can also be used to control blood pressure. Hypertension (high blood pressure) causes an inordinate amount of pressure on the walls of the arteries. This pressure can result in a rupture of these vessels. When a rupture of the arteries in the brain occurs, this is called a stroke. A hypertensive who exercises regularly is able to lower his or her blood pressure, thereby helping to prevent stroke, the third leading cause of death in the United States. Regular exercise helps prevent obesity, which is related to both coronary heart disease and hypertension, and improves muscle tone. And regular exercise can be an effective way of managing stress, since the stress response is really a preparedness of the body to do something physical (the "fight-or-flight" response). Blood pressure increases, heart rate speeds up, muscles tense, and blood glucose increases. Doing something physical "uses" this preparedness and results in better health.

Achieving and maintaining physical fitness helps prevent the premature occurrence of numerous illnesses and diseases. It also helps in rehabilitation after the illness or disease has happened. A friend of the authors had a triple bypass operation in which three of the blood vessels supplying his heart were found to be obstructed. The obstructed sections were bypassed with blood vessels grafted from his legs. A very short time after the operation, he was expected to get out of bed and walk around, and this had him somewhat alarmed. Anyone who knows about exercise and the rehabilitative process, however, would not be surprised. More and more, the aid exercise provides in healing is being recognized. Women are moving around shortly after delivering babies, and many surgical procedures are now done on an outpatient basis, with the patient returning to physical activity quickly.

Pain clinics are using exercise to help people manage pain of various kinds. As we will see later, the secretion of endorphins from the brain during exercise has an analgesic (pain-relieving) effect. Consequently, exercise is recommended for those suffering from pain, when it is not for some other reason contraindicated. Even with mental illness, the benefits of exercise are recognized. Many rehabilitative programs for the mentally ill include exercise programs of one sort or another, with jogging one of the favorites.

In addition to the prevention of illness and disease, or the rehabilitation from them, regular exercise enhances health and adds to our wellness. These new goals of physical fitness are now recognized as significant outcomes of regular exercise. We turn next to a consideration of these goals, and of the unique opportunity they provide for developing personal fitness.

PERSONAL FITNESS

We need first to differentiate among illness, health, and wellness. Health consists of five components: social, mental, emotional, spiritual, and physical. When these components are in balance, a high level of wellness is achieved. Physical fitness programs should be designed to achieve this balance and to improve each component of health. In this way, fitness programs will result in high-level wellness.

The Health-Illness Continuum

It is important that we consider health as separate from illness. You may wonder about the need to do that, for many people define illness as ill health, and health as lack of illness. These people might depict health and illness as a straight line and call that a health continuum. This conceptualization is depicted in Figure 1.1, with ill health at one end and perfect health at the other.

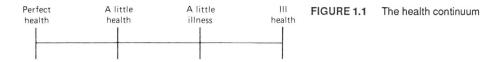

FIGURE 1.1   The health continuum

However, when we consider them as separate, the continuum must not show illness and health overlapping. That is, at some point one must stop and the other must begin. The model for this conceptualization appears in Figure 1.2. Illness occupies the right half of the continuum, ending at the midpoint, and health begins there and occupies the left half of the continuum (Dintiman and Greenberg, 1986, p. 8).

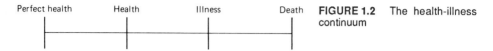

FIGURE 1.2   The health-illness continuum

Of course, one may argue that even if someone is ill, that person may have some degree of health. For example, a physically handicapped person who exercises regularly and participates in the Special Olympics may be healthier than a person who is outwardly "normal" but not physically fit. For now, though, let's withhold objection until we can explain how we intend to use the continuum.

The Components of Health

In the space provided, list five ways you could improve your health.

1. _eating right_
2. _exercising regularly_
3. _sleeping right_
4. _feeling happier_
5. _drinking more water_

We're willing to bet that most of you listed ways to improve your *physical* health. At least this is what we've found when we've asked groups of people to do what you just did. When most people think of health, they think of the body; and they usually think of preventing illness rather than being healthy. But physical health is not the total health picture; there are other components.

1. *Social health.* Ability to interact well with people and the environment. Having satisfying interpersonal relationships.
2. *Mental health.* Ability to learn; intellectual capabilities.
3. *Emotional health.* Ability to control emotions so that one feels comfortable expressing them when appropriate and does express them appropriately. Ability not to express emotions when it is inappropriate to do so.
4. *Spiritual health.* Belief in some unifying force. For some people that will be nature, for others it will be scientific laws, and for others it will be a Godlike force.

So health is more than just caring for the body. It concerns your social interactions, mind, feelings, and spirituality. And often we decide, though perhaps not in these terms, to give up health in one area to gain greater health in another. Walter Greene describes a man willing to sacrifice some of his physical health so he can achieve greater social and mental health. See if this doesn't make sense to you (Greene, 1974, p. 114):

> A businessman might be 15 pounds overweight for no apparent reason other than careless eating habits, or an unawareness of the advantages of trim physique, and ignorance of the basic principles of weight control. This should be classed as a remedial health defect and one important indicator of reduced health status. However, let us compare this case with the case of another businessman, equally overweight, who happens to be a well-informed and enthusiastic amateur gourmet. His library of cookbooks includes directions for preparing many of the most popular dishes of other cultures. He spends many interesting hours in offbeat markets shopping for hard-to-get food items. The meals he prepares constitute focal points of an interesting, satisfying social life. This man realizes he is overweight; he knows how to reduce and control his weight; and he may even suspect that his coronary may arrive a year or two ahead of schedule. But he does not care. His overweight condition constitutes a health defect only in the absolute sense. When viewed in relation to his value system, it represents a logical concomitant to his particular pattern of good health.

Think of the decisions you make about *your* health. Do you sacrifice greater health in one area to achieve greater health in another? Of course you do. And this is your right. How can any person decide for another person which health area should be sacrificed to achieve health in some other area? That decision should be left to the individual. No one should tell you how much time to spend on fitness activities, since that means taking time from another health component. Only you can juggle these components based upon your valuing of them.

Evaluate your health status by completing Figure 1.3. In each health area, list your strong and your weak points. See if you can choose one or two weak points to work on, and one or two strong points to work on to gain even greater strength. As we shall soon see, the result will be greater wellness.

FIGURE 1.3   Health status awareness chart

	Mental health	Physical health	Social health	Spiritual health	Emotional health
Strong points:	1. quick to learn 2. strong capacity 3. good base 4. focused	not overweight exercise some conscious of diet high metabolism	self-esteem tend to be happy interesting intelligent	God nature intellect	try to be happy optimistic learning expression strong
Weak points:	1. not creative 2. not motivated 3. not always open-minded 4. focused	improper diet improper sleep exercise irregular	not outgoing picky insecure high expectations	doubting faith misanthrope	poor control don't know when appropriate dependent fatigue strong

Wellness

We'd now like you to look at the health-illness continuum under a microscope. Notice that the line isn't a line at all, but a series of dots. The continuum would then look like Figure 1.4.

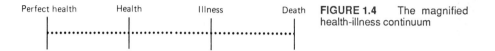

Perfect health   Health   Illness   Death   **FIGURE 1.4**   The magnified
health-illness continuum

If we could get an even more powerful microscope and focus it on just one of the dots on the continuum, we suggest you might see something like Figure 1.5.

FIGURE 1.5   A single health-illness continuum dot

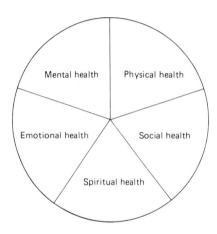

Each dot on the continuum, therefore, is composed of the five components of health. And now the puzzle can be completed: *wellness* is the integration of social, mental, emotional, spiritual, and physical health at any level of health or illness. Put another way, you can be *well* regardless of whether you are ill or healthy. Paraplegics, for example, may not be defined as healthy, but they can achieve high-level wellness by maximizing and integrating the five components of health so that, within their physical limitations, they are living a quality life. They may interact well with family and friends (social health), they may do well at school, on the job, or with a hobby (mental health), they may be able to express their feelings when appropriate (emotional health), they may have a sense of how they fit into the "grand scheme of things" either through a religious belief or a belief in the laws of nature (spiritual health), and they may exercise within the boundaries of their capabilities, such as finishing a marathon on crutches or in a wheelchair (physical health).

Each of us, then, has some degree of wellness. We may be ill, yet possess high-level wellness; or we may be healthy, but possess low-level wellness. Likewise, a person who is physically healthy may not have satisfying interpersonal relationships, may "fly off the handle" easily, and may even maintain a low level of physical *fitness*. And, of course, there are gradations between these two extremes, so that at any point on the continuum a person may have some components of health at high levels and other components at low levels.

The integration of these components is important. For example, someone may emphasize one component of health to such a degree that the other components suffer. We all know people who are so concerned with their physical health that they approach obsession; they jog, weight lift, or do calisthenics for so many hours a day they have no time for developing other sides of their total health—meaningful relationships, reading, and so forth. Others always want to have fun and socialize, so they sacrifice adequate physical fitness or success in school. The person possessing high-level wellness can integrate each component of health into a life-style that includes attention to the other components of health.

High-Level Wellness

We know regular exercise can improve health. Now let's look at how it can improve *wellness*. To do so, we have to recall that wellness is the integration of the five health components into any one life, so that one component isn't improved at a significant cost to the others.

Let's first look at poor attempts at wellness. Many of us can remember the tough, unsympathetic physical education teacher we've met somewhere during our schooling. We'll call that teacher A. Symmetrical. Now A believed that people—children, in particular—had to be pushed and threatened in order to tolerate the pain of strenuous physical activity. Without such pain, A believed, fitness was not being improved. Left to themselves, people would not get beyond the pain and therefore would not develop high levels of physical fitness. So A. Symmetrical pushed, and A. Symmetrical threatened. If we were young and sufficiently scared, we may even have become physically fit—while hating every minute of it. The world is full of sedentary people who were turned off to regular exercise by an A. Symmetrical. To them, physical activity is associated with "pain," "threat," and "scare." You see, A. Symmetrical exaggerated the physical component of health to the detriment of the others, creating an asymmetrical dot on the health-illness continuum. This dot is depicted in Figure 1.6.

As you can see, the dot is no longer round. If used as a tire, it would give a bumpy ride. When our health components are organized in this manner, we too get a bumpy ride—and eventually suffer for it. One typical reaction is to deflate the large portion of the tire—in this case, physical health—while inflating the others. That is what A. Symmetrical's students are doing when they are so turned off to physical activity that they become sedentary.

The physical education teacher concerned with wellness will attempt to create a well-rounded dot—and person. Physical fitness will be stressed, but not at the expense of the other health components. This is how regular exercise can help you attain greater wellness.

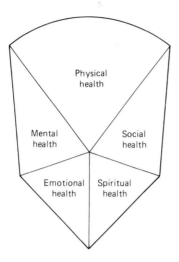

FIGURE 1.6   The asymmetrical dot on the health-illness continuum

Physical
health

Mental
health

Social
health

Emotional
health

Spiritual
health

THE STATE OF THE NATION

There are numerous problems related to health in our society. The obvious ones concern illness and diseases that kill and disable. There are also the not so obvious, those that pervade our society and wreak their havoc quietly over long periods of time. We divided these into two categories: health-specific problems and health-related problems.

Health-Specific Problems

Table 1.1 lists the major causes of death in 1900 and today. Heading the 1900 list are diseases that are passed from one person to another or are the result of unsanitary practices. The incidence of these diseases has, for the most part, been drastically reduced through legislation requiring proper disposal of waste, sewage systems, quarantines, and other community actions to prevent their spread.

The killers of today do not lend themselves to such remedies. These conditions are more a result of life-style than of some microorganism. In a democratic society, we cannot legislate life-style. To produce significant decreases in disease and illness caused by unhealthy life-style behaviors, such as cigarette smoking, large numbers of people themselves must decide to change their behavior. We're speaking, for example, of not smoking cigarettes, of getting enough sleep, of maintaining a favorable weight, of not abusing alcohol and other drugs, of eating nutritious foods, and of exercising regularly.

Besides causing premature death, unhealthy behaviors diminish the quality of our lives. We become less resistant to disease and consequently spend more time sick than is necessary. Furthermore, once ill, we do not recover as quickly. These behaviors affect us in many ways. Cigarette smoking may lead to emphysema. Excessive consumption of alcohol can lead to cirrhosis of the liver. A sedentary life style can lead to a general feeling of fatigue and malaise—aside from its effects on the body's organs.

Table 1.1
Leading Causes of Death

Rank in 1900 [*]	Today [†]
1. Tuberculosis	1. Diseases of the heart
2. Pneumonia and influenza	2. Cancer
3. Enteritis, gastritis, colitis	3. Stroke or apoplexy
4. Diseases of the heart	4. Accidents
5. Stroke or apoplexy	5. Influenza and pneumonia
6. Kidney diseases	6. Cirrhosis of the liver
7. Accidents	7. Suicide
8. Cancer	8. Diabetes mellitus
9. Diseases of early infancy	9. Homicide
10. Diphtheria	10. Tuberculosis

[*]Data from the National Vital Statistic Division, National Center for Health Statistics, 1976.

[†]Data from the U.S. Department of Health and Human Services, *Health—United States*, 1981 (Hyattsville, MD: National Center for Health Services Research, 1981), p. 117.

Recognizing the need to encourage the adoption of healthy life styles, the Surgeon General of the United States, in a report on the nation's health, included broad national goals for reducing death and disability (Office of the Assistant Secretary for Health and the Surgeon General, 1979a, 1979b). A second report made these goals more specific and measurable (Public Health Services, 1980). Although some of the health goals outlined in these reports appear at first glance unrelated to life style, closer examination shows how wrong that impression is. For example, one goal is to decrease infant mortality. One means to meet that goal is to develop better hospital facilities and equipment and better trained health care providers. However, the most significant impact upon infant mortality rates can be made by what pregnant women do, not by what their doctors do. If pregnant women eat properly, refrain from using alcohol, tobacco, and other drugs, and seek prenatal care early in their pregnancies, they will significantly and dramatically increase the chances of their babies being born alive and well. Likewise, regular exercise will have a greater effect on decreasing heart disease than the development of the artificial heart.

When the federal government evaluated the progress made toward the achievement of the national health objectives, it found that many had been achieved even before the target date (Office of Disease Prevention and Health Promotion, 1986). This is evidence of the ability of people to alter their behaviors and thereby achieve a greater status of health and wellness.

Health-Related Problems

Other things about our life-style affect our health. In his book *Future Shock*, Alvin Toffler (1970) describes our society as one which changes so rapidly that stress is the inevitable result. No sooner do we learn how to play games on our home computers, for instance, than we are expected to bank and shop with them. Just yesterday we waited in line at the movie theater; today we rent a film and play it at home on a videocassette recorder. Toffler pictures an even faster-changing future-oriented society in his book *The Third Wave* (1980), in which he predicts we will not only bank and shop at home but work at home as well. Since the definition of stress (discussed further in Chapter 12) entails adaptation to change—that is, we are going along fine when something happens to which we need to adjust—it is not surprising that our rapidly changing society is suspected of contributing to stress and thus to ill health.

Another sign of "progress" is technological advance. The quotation marks are necessary because some people argue that technological advances have been harmful, not progressive. For example, science has brought us useful synthetic materials, such as nylon. And nylon is used by fishermen to make sturdy, long-lasting nets with which to catch fish. Unfortunately, these nets are not biodegradable (as hemp nets were), and when they break or are left at seas, they contaminate the oceans. Most of us have heard about the fluorocarbons found, for example, in some hair sprays and the effect they have on the ozone layer. We learn about the pollution of water, land, and air after the fact through industrial waste. And then there are the psychological effects of the threat of nuclear war or the potential of disaster associated with nuclear power plants.

In addition, technological advances such as the automobile and the jet airplane have made us more mobile, desensitizing us to space and distance. As a result, more and more of us live some distance from our extended families. Parents, grandparents, aunts, uncles, and cousins do not see one another as often as in the past. And as we become alienated and isolated, the result is more ill health. Both suicide and homicide are related to alienation and isolation, as are a wide variety of mental illnesses.

In 1986, there were almost 1.2 million divorces in the United States (National Center for Health Statistics, April 1987). One in three marriages results in divorce. The annual divorce total has risen dramatically. For each divorce, on the average of one child under 18 years of age is involved—almost 1.25 million children each year. The impact of divorce on the physical and psychological health of spouses and children needs no description here: we are all aware of the toll it takes.

Three other characteristics of our society also have a major impact on health: sexism, racism, and ageism. People deprived of opportunity, of equality, of freedom of choice can become ill in a number of ways. Being deprived of equal opportunity at work, for example, can lead to low socioeconomic status, not enough money to eat properly or to pay for medical care, and lack of opportunity for education. An abundance of data reveals the relationship between low socioeconomic status and poor health and between low educational attainment and poor health.

The last health-related problem we will consider is unemployment. A rapidly changing, technologically advancing society endures cycles of high unemployment. They occur because today's workers are no longer needed for tomorrow's jobs. This kind of unemployment has serious health consequences. Harvey Brenner has conducted several studies of the effects of unemployment on the health of the unemployed and their families and has concluded that a one-quarter of 1 percent rise in the unemployment rate is directly associated with some 1,500 additional suicides; 1,700 additional homicides; 25,000 additional stroke, heart, and kidney deaths; 5,500 added mental admissions; and 800 additional deaths from cirrhosis of the liver—all within a five-year period (Brenner, 1982).

HEALTH BEHAVIOR ASSESSMENT

How does all this information affect you? We all know people who are physically unfit, people who smoke cigarettes or abuse alcohol or other drugs, people who overwork and are overstressed. What's more, we know how to advise these friends and relatives. We tell them to give up the cigarettes, learn how to deal with conflicts, exercise regularly, and so forth. But how about our own behavior? Can we advise ourselves?

How well are you doing at staying healthy? Are you willing to take your own advice and improve your health behavior? The Office of Health Information and Promotion of the Public Health Services (U.S. Department of Health and Human Services) has developed a health behavior scale to help you answer these questions.

You will find that the scale—see Figure 1.7—has six sections: smoking, alcohol and drugs, nutrition, exercise and fitness, stress control, and safety. Complete one section at a time by circling the number corresponding to the

FIGURE 1.7   The health behavior scale

Source: U.S. Department of Health and Human Services. *Health Style: A Self Test* (Washington, DC: Public Health Service, 1981).

Cigarette Smoking

	Almost Always	Sometimes	Almost Never

If you never smoke, enter a score of 10 for this section and go to the next section on *Alcohol and Drugs*.

	Almost Always	Sometimes	Almost Never
1. I avoid smoking cigarettes.	2	1	0
2. I smoke only low tar and nicotine cigarettes *or* I smoke a pipe or cigars.	2	1	0

Smoking Score: _____

Eating Habits

	Almost Always	Sometimes	Almost Never
1. I eat a variety of foods each day, such as fruits and vegetables, whole grain breads and cereals, lean meats, dairy products, dry peas and beans, and nuts and seeds.	4	1	0
2. I limit the amount of fat, saturated fat, and cholesterol I eat (including fat on meats, eggs, butter, cream, shortenings, and organ meats such as liver).	2	1	0
3. I limit the amount of salt I eat by cooking with only small amounts, not adding salt at the table, and avoiding salty snacks.	2	1	0
4. I avoid eating too much sugar (especially frequent snacks of sticky candy or soft drinks).	2	1	0

Eating Habits Score: _____

Figure 1.7 (continued)

Alcohol and Drugs

	Almost Always	Sometimes	Almost Never
1. I avoid drinking alcoholic beverages *or* I drink no more than 1 or 2 drinks a day.	4	1	0
2. I avoid using alcohol or other drugs (especially illegal drugs) as a way of handling stressful situations or the problems in my life.	2	1	0
3. I am careful not to drink alcohol when taking certain medicines (for example, medicine for sleeping, pain, colds, and allergies), or when pregnant.	2	1	0
4. I read and follow the label directions when using prescribed and over-the-counter drugs.	2	1	0

Alcohol and Drugs Score: _____

Exercise/Fitness

	Almost Always	Sometimes	Almost Never
1. I maintain a desired weight, avoiding overweight and underweight.	3	1	0
2. I do vigorous exercises for 15-30 minutes at least 3 times a week (examples include running, swimming, brisk walking).	3	1	0
3. I do exercises that enhance my muscle tone for 15-30 minutes at least 3 times a week (examples include yoga and calisthenics).	2	1	0
4. I use part of my leisure time participating in individual, family, or team activities that increase my level of fitness (such as gardening, bowling, golf, and baseball).	2	1	0

Exercise/Fitness Score: _____

Stress Control

	Almost Always	Sometimes	Almost Never
1. I have a job or do other work that I enjoy.	2	1	0
2. I find it easy to relax and express my feelings freely.	2	1	0
3. I recognize early, and prepare for, events or situations likely to be stressful for me.	2	1	0
4. I have close friends, relatives, or others whom I can talk to about personal matters and call on for help when needed.	2	1	0
5. I participate in group activities (such as church and community organizations) or hobbies that I enjoy.	2	1	0

Stress Control Score: _____

Safety

	Almost Always	Sometimes	Almost Never
1. I wear a seat belt while riding in a car.	2	1	0
2. I avoid driving while under the influence of alcohol and other drugs.	2	1	0
3. I obey traffic rules and the speed limit when driving.	2	1	0
4. I am careful when using potentially harmful products or substances (such as household cleaners, poisons, and electrical devices).	2	1	0
5. I avoid smoking in bed.	2	1	0

Safety Score: _____

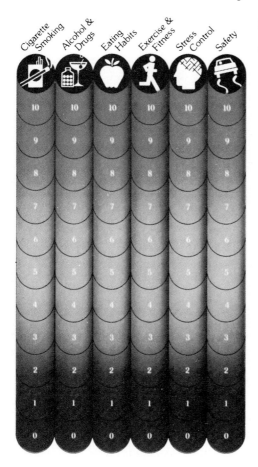

FIGURE 1.8   Your health-behavior score

Source: U.S. Department of Health and Human Services. *Health Style: A Self Test* (Washington, DC: Public Health Service, 1981)

answer that best describes your behavior. Then add the numbers you have circled to determine your score for that section. Write the score on the line provided at the end of each section. The highest score for each section is 10. Then see Figure 1.8 for how your scores can be interpreted.

Your Health-Behavior Scores

After you have figured your scores for each of the six sections, circle the number in each column in Figure 1.7 that matches your score for that section of the test.

Remember, there is no total score for this test. Consider each section separately. You are trying to identify aspects of your health behavior that you can improve in order to be healthier and to reduce the risk of illness. Let's see what your scores reveal.

What Your Scores Mean to You

SCORES OF 9 AND 10

- Excellent! Your answers show that you are aware of the importance of this area to your health. More important, you are putting your knowledge to work for you by practicing good health habits. As long as you continue to do so, this area should not pose a serious health risk. It's likely that you are setting an example for your family and friends to follow. Since you got a very high score on this part of the test, you may want to consider other areas where your scores indicate room for improvement.

SCORES OF 6 TO 8

- Your health practices in this area are good, but there is room for improvement. Look again at the items you answered with a "Sometimes" or "Almost Never." What changes can you make to improve your score? Even a small change can often help you achieve better health.

SCORES OF 3 TO 5

- Your health risks are showing! Would you like more information about the risks you are facing and why it is important for you to change these behaviors? Perhaps you need help in deciding how successfully to make the changes you desire. In either case, help is available.

SCORES OF 0 TO 2

- You may be taking serious and unnecessary risks with your health. Perhaps you are not aware of the risks and what to do about them. You can easily get the information and help you need to improve.

THIS BOOK

This book tells the physical fitness story. It describes the physiological and psychological effects of physical activity. It offers advice on starting a program of regular exercise. It outlines effective procedures for assuming greater control of behavior so that you can maintain your exercise program once you've started it. Other subjects include the relationship of sex, age, environment, and nutrition to physical training; the prevention and care of common fitness injuries, and ways to manage stress through physical activity. This book also introduces the more popular fitness activities—some of which you might consider incorporating into your own fitness program.

Two themes are basic to the overall approach. First, good health practices need not be boring and painful, be considered a chore. We will show you how to make good health practices an enjoyable part of your daily life—a part you look forward to. Second, there is evidence that certain health-related behaviors *do* result in a longer life. Other health-related behaviors, while not contributing to longevity, *do* affect the quality of our lives.

Before we start our story, however, it is important to place physical fitness in the proper perspective. That was the purpose of this chapter. We spoke of illness and disease, of health and of wellness, of traditional and nontraditional objectives of physical fitness, and of perhaps the most overlooked yet most important of considerations—*personal* fitness.

The aim of *Physical Fitness: A Wellness Approach* is to provide you with the necessary knowledge to develop your own program of physical fitness—to achieve personal fitness. Since each of you is unique, no one program can be prescribed. However, we present enough information so that you can select those activities which can improve the aspects of physical fitness you choose to work on and help you get your program started and stay with it—all the while having fun. Our goals, as we work with you, are to help you prevent illness and disease, achieve greater health, and experience high-level wellness.

SUMMARY

1. Physical fitness is the ability to do one's work and have energy remaining for recreational activities.
2. Physical fitness has been advocated to prevent illness and disease, to speed up rehabilitation from illness, to enhance health, and to add to wellness.
3. Health consists of five components: social, mental, emotional, spiritual, and physical. Health and illness are separate from one another; that is, they are on different ends of the health-illness continuum.
4. Wellness is the integration of social, mental, emotional, spiritual, and physical health at any level of health or illness. Put another way, you can be "well" regardless of whether you are ill or healthy.
5. High-level wellness is the integration of the five components of health and their balance so no one component suffers to exaggerate another.
6. The major causes of death today are the result of unhealthy life-styles. The three leading causes of death are heart disease, cancer, and stroke. Exercising regularly can help postpone the occurrence of these conditions.
7. Good health practices need not be boring, nor need they be considered a chore. They can become an enjoyable part of your daily life if selected and organized in an appropriate manner.
8. There is evidence that certain health-related behaviors—regular exercise among them—can result in a longer life and/or in an improved quality of life.

REFERENCES

BRENNER, M. HARVEY. "Assessing the Social Costs of National Unemployment Rates." Testimony presented before the Subcommittee on Domestic Monetary Policy of the Committee on Banking, Finance, and Urban Affairs, U.S. House of Representatives, Washington, DC, August 12, 1982.

DINTIMAN, GEORGE B. and JERROLD S. GREENBERG. *Health Through Discovery*. New York: Random House, 1986, p. 8.

GREENE, WALTER. "The Search for a Meaningful Definition of Health." In Donald A. Read (ed.), *New Directions in Health Education: Some Contemporary Issues for an Emerging Age*. New York: Macmillan, 1974, p. 114.

NATIONAL CENTER FOR HEALTH STATISTICS. "Births, Marriages, Divorces, and Deaths for 1986." *Monthly Vital Statistics Report,* 35 (April 1987), 1.

OFFICE OF DISEASE PREVENTION AND HEALTH PROMOTION. *The 1990 Health Objectives for the Nation: A Midcourse Review*. Washington, DC: Public Health Service, 1986.

OFFICE OF THE ASSISTANT SECRETARY FOR HEALTH AND THE SURGEON GENERAL. *Healthy People: The Surgeon General's Report on Health Promotion and Disease Prevention*, 1979. Washington, DC: Public Health Service, 1979a.

OFFICE OF THE ASSISTANT SECRETARY FOR HEALTH AND THE SURGEON GENERAL. Healthy People: *The Surgeon General's Report on Health Promotion and Disease Prevention, Background Papers*, 1979. Washington, DC: Public Health Service, 1979b.

TOFFLER, ALVIN. *Future Shock*. New York: Random House, 1970.

TOFFLER, ALVIN. *The Third Wave*. New York: William Morrow, 1980.

U.S. DEPARTMENT OF HEALTH AND HUMAN SERVICES. *Promoting Health/Preventing Disease: Objectives for the Nation*. Washington, DC: Public Health Services, 1980.

2

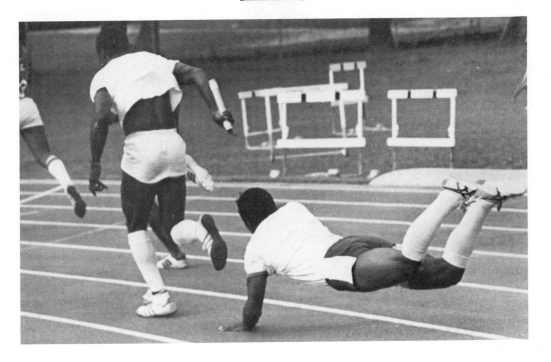

Exercise:
Your Body's Response

CHAPTER OBJECTIVES

1. To be able to define a motor unit.
2. To be able to define and describe the three types of muscle tissue.
3. To be able to differentiate between fast-twitch and slow-twitch muscle fibers.
4. To be able to identify parts of the autonomic nervous system and understand their function.
5. To be able to describe the course of blood circulation through the cardiovascular system.
6. To be able to discuss the psychological implications of participating in sport.

When we use the term *exercise* in this book, we refer to physical activity or work of a fairly rigorous nature. We all know that exercise involves muscles such as those of the shoulders, arms, and thighs. But exercise involves other body parts as well. Because the lungs, for example, must satisfy a greater demand for oxygen by millions upon millions of body cells, the respiratory rate increases during exercise. In fact, all the various functions of the body "rev up" during exercise.

Exercise is not always performed in a sport or training setting. When you shovel snow, paint your room, or change a flat tire, you are exercising. And when you exercise, a number of important bodily changes take place. Many of these changes influence physiological as well as psychological functioning in very striking ways. If you are eventually to organize a realistic personal program of exercise, it is important that you understand these changes.

In this chapter we will examine two broad categories of reactions to exercise: (1) *physiological responses*, which deal with the functioning of body parts, and (2) *psychological responses*, which deal with behavior and the ways in which we think and feel.

We look first at some of the important physiological reactions to exercise, expressed in the form of five concepts:

- *Concept 1*: Exercise involves physical work.
- *Concept 2*: To contract against resistance created by the body itself or externally imposed resistance (that is, the dirt you lift on your shovel as you dig in the yard), muscles must be stimulated.
- *Concept 3*: The nervous system typically provides the stimulation for muscular contraction.
- *Concept 4*: The cardiovascular system distributes nutrient and oxygen (fuel) necessary for muscular contraction.
- *Concept 5*: Exercise is physiologically arousing.

THE MUSCLES

Work is defined as the product of a force acting through a distance. It involves contraction of large muscles, which in turn produces limb movement. But limb movement doesn't necessarily imply *locomotion* (change of location of the body from one place to another). When you drive a golf ball, bench press a heavy weight, pass a football, dig in your yard, or shake sand from a beach blanket, you are performing exercise, but your body's relative position in space does not change; only some of its parts do.

Muscles must be physiologically ready to respond. Diseased or weakened muscle will not contract properly when stimulated. And the signal or stimulus triggering muscle contraction must be strong enough to do the job.

We will deal with the cardiovascular system a little later. Now let us become familiar with the muscles themselves, their structure and parts. Then we'll see how the nervous system communicates with muscles to stimulate contraction. We really do not fully understand what happens physically and chemically when a muscle contracts. But we know that a motor unit contracts (shortens) completely, or it doesn't contract at all. That is, when a motor unit contracts, all muscle fibers that are innervated contract.

Three Types of Muscle

Three types of muscle tissue are found in humans. (A *tissue* is a collection of cells pretty much alike in the ways they appear and perform.) *Smooth, striated* (or striped), and *cardiac* muscle differ according to the ways in which they are structured as well as the roles they perform. Let's begin by looking at the first two.

Smooth muscle tissue, for the most part, contracts involuntarily. That is, unless elaborate training procedures (such as biofeedback) are applied, smooth muscle will not respond to conscious messages. The digestive system is lined with smooth muscle, which, by contraction, moves food from the *esophagus* (food pipe leading from the back of the mouth) to the stomach and to the small and large intestines. Under ordinary circumstances, these muscles respond only to the presence of food and chemical stimuli. Since we are usually unable to command smooth muscle to contract, we also use the term *involuntary* when referring to such muscle. Most of the internal organs of the body contain smooth muscle.

Smooth muscle, although not under conscious command, plays an important role in physical activity. The following organs depend mostly upon smooth muscle function. Now think about the importance of this kind of tissue in exercise.

1. Alveoli in lungs
2. Urinary bladder
3. Opening through which food passes from stomach to small intestine (sphincter)

Skeletal or *striated muscles* are involved in movement in space, or locomotion. Figure 2.1 should be helpful in enabling you to understand how the skeletal and muscular systems interact. You are usually able to control skeletal muscle contraction through conscious mental processes. You think, "I will now move my right arm and press the doorbell with my finger." Seconds later the chime is heard, and shortly thereafter the door opens. Your friend says, "Please come in." And because you *decide* to enter and because you *anticipated* the invitation to enter (thinking), you step over the threshold and into the home of your host or hostess. Powerful skeletal muscles in your legs, abdominal area, feet, and lower back have contracted and moved you in accordance with your plan for movement.

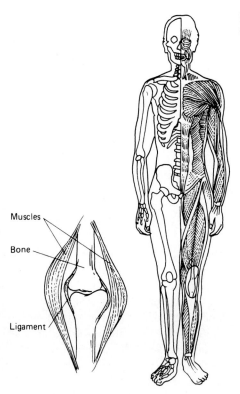

FIGURE 2.1   The skeletal and muscular systems of the body

Muscles

Bone

Ligament

Under the microscope, skeletal muscles appear striped. Alternating sections of fiber of varying shades of color produce this effect. Fibers of striped muscle are organized into *fascicula* or bundles. These, in turn, combine to form a variety of shapes that seem to fit the muscle's purpose and function. Some muscles are cigar shaped, some are arranged in thin sheets, some are very long, some are exceptionally short and small. The biceps and triceps muscles of the upper arm are examples of voluntary muscle. So are the calf and thigh muscles of the leg. Sometimes striated muscles can be made to contract involuntarily, as in the case of reflex movements like the knee jerk (Figure 2.2).

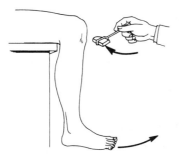

FIGURE 2.2   Method for eliciting the knee-jerk reflex

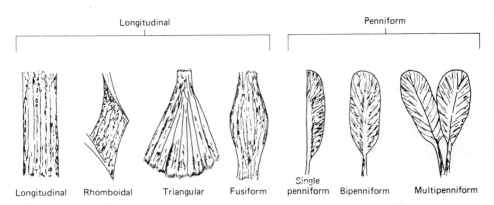

Longitudinal

Penniform

| Longitudinal | Rhomboidal | Triangular | Fusiform | Single penniform | Bipenniform | Multipenniform |

FIGURE 2.3   Striated muscle shapes

Examine Figure 2.3 and notice the different shapes striated muscles assume. Are you able to relate the shapes of these muscles to their functions?

Fast-Twitch and Slow-Twitch Muscle Fibers

Voluntary muscle fibers may be classified into fast-twitch (FT) and slow-twitch (ST) types. The two differ in coloring and also in the type of physical activity in which they are involved. ST fibers predominate in endurance activities and FT fibers in explosive, short-term exertion. Cycling, swimming, jogging, situps, pullups, and pushups are examples of *endurance activities*. Muscular contractions held over relatively long periods of time are also found in endurance activities (for example, holding a handstand).

ST fibers are of a darker color than FT fibers, which are used primarily for quick contractions (lifting a heavy suitcase, shot putting, sprinting). The chicken drumstick you love to eat is mostly dark meat, and the chicken breast is white. The drumstick is the chicken's thigh, which is used in walking (endurance), and the breast meat is muscle that moves the wings for very infrequent, short periods of time. The former is slow-twitch and the latter is fast-twitch fiber. It appears that heredity determines how many FT and ST fibers you have.

Most muscular actions in physical work have both fast-twitch and slow-twitch fiber contraction, but the emphasis may shift during exercise. For example, as the jogger proceeds up a hill, relatively more FT fibers become activated. Similarly, as the competitive swimmer makes a turn and pushes off the wall of the pool, a brief change occurs in kind of voluntary muscle contraction. If you have a higher percentage of ST fibers in your thigh and leg muscles, you have an advantage in endurance activities over those with a higher percentage of FT fibers. The opposite is true for those with FT fibers in sprintlike or power activities.

The Heart Muscle

Now let's look at the third of our three major muscle groups. *Cardiac muscle* (heart muscle) is intermediary between smooth and skeletal muscle tissue. Its fibers interlock to form a lattice of closely knit cells that permit a wavelike transmission of nervous impulses. Beginning in a location in the heart known as the *pacemaker* or sinoauricular node, the impulse spreads across all four chambers of the heart from one fiber to the next. Cardiac muscle contracts without stopping, at a rate of approximately 72 beats a minute, as a result of this contagious stimulation, which is called *intrinsic rhythmicity*. Although most smooth muscle fibers exhibit a similar rhythmicity, it is typically associated with the heart.

The heart is about the size of your fist and is located in the center of the chest. The two lower, more muscular chambers (the ventricles) pump blood out of the heart through a large artery known as the *aorta*, and the two upper chambers receive blood on its return trip from all parts of the body (Figure 2.4).

Common Muscle Characteristics

Although differences in appearance and function exist among the three kinds of muscle tissue, they all respond to heavy workloads in similar ways: (1) they all experience fatigue; (2) they all contain packets of energy known as *adenosine triphosphate* (ATP), which provide the fuel for contraction; (3) they all produce waste products; and (4) they all may be damaged if subjected to unusually high demands. All three kinds of muscle tissue regularly require rest and must be nourished by blood supplies, even cardiac muscle. When arteries carrying blood to the heart become clogged or damaged, pathological death may occur to cardiac muscle tissue. This condition is known as *myocardial infarction*.

THE NERVOUS SYSTEM

Although all parts of our bodies are marvelous in their design and the ways in which they contribute to our well-being, perhaps the most incredible organ of all is the human brain. Its complexity is astonishing, its responsibilities awesome, and its capabilities not yet entirely fathomed.

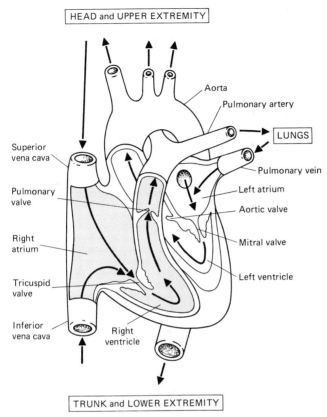

HEAD and UPPER EXTREMITY

FIGURE 2.4   The functional parts of the heart

Aorta

Pulmonary artery

LUNGS

Superior vena cava

Pulmonary vein

Pulmonary valve

Left atrium

Aortic valve

Right atrium

Mitral valve

Tricuspid valve

Left ventricle

Inferior vena cava

Right ventricle

TRUNK and LOWER EXTREMITY

Today, we marvel at the wonders the computer performs. But despite the tremendous technological advances by the computer industry and despite the many attractive comparisons drawn between the computer and the human brain, the computer's wizardry cannot hold a candle to the mass of convoluted gray matter housed in the skull. Probably, the computer will never be able to achieve certain brain functions. The human brain conceptualized the electronic computer; it created the design for its construction and built its command programs, which enable it to communicate with other machines, with itself, as well as with humans.

The Brain

If you are to understand the body's response to exercise, then at least a superficial understanding of brain function is necessary.

The brain is the control center for all human activity, although higher levels of consciousness do not always prevail in certain basic functions. For example, lower brain centers regulate breathing and heart rate during sleep without conscious awareness. These activities are known as *autonomic functions* because they happen automatically. Higher centers process stimuli necessary for the activity known as reasoning and enable recall of previously stored images and information.

The Spinal Cord

The brain sits atop a long cablelike structure that runs the length of the neck and upper and lower back and is known as the *spinal cord*. The cord is located within a series of 24 bony ringlike structures *(vertebrae)* which, when stacked one on top of the other, create a long tube known as the *vertebral column*. This column protects the spinal cord, which leads to or from the brain.

Functions of the various brain parts are related to their location within the brain. The lowermost parts correspond to basic functions and drives such as breathing, hunger, thirst, and sex. The highest brain centers (those farthest away from the base of the brain) control cognitive (reasoning and feeling) and intellectual processes (see Figure 2.5).

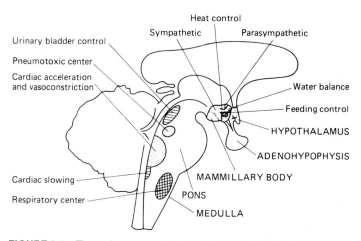

FIGURE 2.5   The major autonomic control centers of the brain stem

Arising from the spinal cord are many branching projections that carry messages from the brain to the body's organs. Information from special sense organs (eyes, nose, ears) is transmitted through these branches to the brain, where it is processed. In response to these stimuli, nervous impulses travel from the brain to the organ.

Use your imagination for a moment. As we follow the sequence of hypothetical events, you should be able to appreciate the role of the brain. A mosquito bites your hand. The skin is broken and irritated. Sensory organs in the skin relay a message (afferent message) through one of the branches to the spinal cord and then to the brain. The brain interprets the stimulus, attaches meaning to it (perception), and sends out a message (efferent message) to the other (nonbitten) hand: "Scratch the bite." You respond. Next, the brain's relatively higher centers consider the transaction and forward additional commands: (1) "Stop scratching, it's bad for you." (2) "Apply lotion to the area of the bite." Now you must deal consciously with the problem of locating the lotion. You *remember* where it is stored (bathroom cabinet). Now the brain instructs your legs to carry you to the bathroom and tells your arm to reach for the bottle. Finally, you apply the lotion and soothe the discomfort.

The Autonomic Nervous System

The brain, the spinal cord, and its branches are called the *central nervous system (CNS)*. The term *autonomic nervous system* refers to those parts of the nervous system that operate with very little direct brain control. Autonomic processes occur in rapid response to pressing stimuli that require immediate reaction. Some examples are the reflexes or contractions of certain smooth muscles in response to biochemical shifts necessary for involuntary actions.

Although the brain does not issue commands directly to all muscles and organs, it ultimately processes information about what is happening to, and in, the body. In this sense, it monitors all bodily activity. The autonomic nervous system controls increased blood flow to muscles during exercise and to tiny blood vessels near the skin which, when dilated, help cool the body. During exercise, more heat than usual is generated from muscular contraction. This heat must be released somehow. Capillary dilation and increased blood flow is handled autonomically. But through a complex exchange of messages, signals, and interaction of organic systems, the brain becomes aware of what is happening.

Nerve Pathways

Electrochemical messages travel rapidly throughout the body from one nerve cell to another. Nervous impulses travel along one cell's axons and are received by the dendrites of another nerve cell (see Figure 2.6) at junctions called *synapses*. Synapses are points where nerve cells are linked to one another, forming chains of nerves, some of which can be very long.

Sometimes messages are transmitted through special chemical agents called *neurotransmitters*. Small amounts of these substances are released by the little hairlike structures at the end of the long axon and received by the small tufts on the dendrites of another nerve cell. These deposits cause a chemical change in the material located in the receiving nerve cells, which is followed by a change in the biochemistry of the entire nerve cell. Changes in the electrical level of fluid inside the nerve cell are also transmitted along the length of the axon to other nerve cells through their dendrite tufts.

Long chains of nerve cells carry electrochemical stimulation to organs and muscles. Some of these messages originate in the brain or are processed by the brain; others are handled autonomically, since response is required so rapidly that time for conscious control is simply not available.

Exercise and the Nervous System

During exercise, and sometimes even in anticipation of exercise, stimulation of organs and muscles may occur. Great demands are placed on all systems as

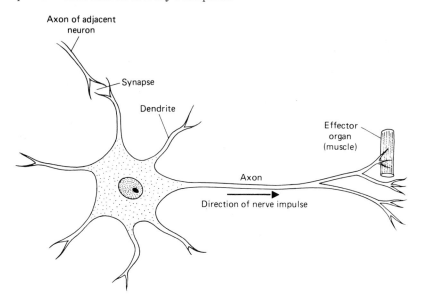

FIGURE 2.6   An idealized nerve cell

they prepare to perform physical work. Sometimes, anticipation of exercise can be arousing.

In this sequence, the brain's role is like that of the symphony conductor's. It controls, coordinates, and regulates. Certain large and powerful muscle groups must be in contraction if the force of gravity is to be overcome and an upright position maintained. When the brain is made ineffective because of a severe blow to the head or the administration of an anesthetizing drug, the large skeletal muscles lose their *tonus* (the condition of contraction which is always maintained by the muscles). As a result, the person falls to the ground unconscious. A *ganglion* (collection of nerve cells) in the jaw is particularly sensitive to physical force. When a boxer receives a severe blow to this area, the result may be a knockout. Only the basic (lower brain) functions remain operational when this happens. The boxer therefore lies on the canvas, unable to move. However, he still breathes, and his heart continues to pump blood.

Exercise relies on constant adjustment from the central nervous system. As you exercise or perform any physical activity, changes in movement patterns depend upon information reaching the CNS from various receptor organs located throughout the body. After stimuli (changes in the physical environment) are converted to electrochemical messages, they reach the brain and provide information that is processed in special centers. Communications are then dispatched to limbs and organs, and movement modifications follow.

As you walk vigorously down a crowded stadium ramp after the conclusion of a ball game, your brain makes numerous strategic decisions relating to a safe and efficient descent and exit. Your eyes and ears provide information about the environment to processing centers in the brain. In turn, messages are forwarded to the muscles that move your body. The messages reach the muscle at the myoneural junction (Figure 2.7), the point at which the nerve and muscle interact, and the muscle contracts, resulting in body movement: "Step over the beer can." "Check and see if your wallet is in your pocket or purse." "Turn left as you reach the parking lot and find Section C, where your car is located."

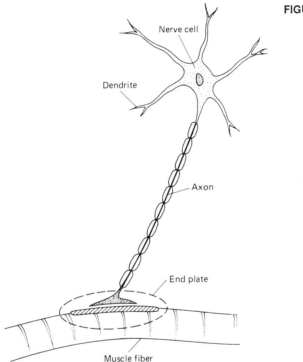

FIGURE 2.7   Myoneural junction

Nerve cell

Dendrite

Axon

End plate

Muscle fiber

Metabolism refers to the rate at which all chemical processes occur within the body. Some of these processes are said to be *aerobic* (they occur in the presence of oxygen), and some are *anaerobic* (they occur in the absence of oxygen). Metabolism, therefore, involves numerous and complex physiological adjustments. During exercise these modifications are especially important since many of them are involved in providing energy for muscular contractions. Therefore, we can also conceive of aerobic as well as anaerobic preparedness for exercise, each involving a respective source of energy release. Aerobic fitness is exemplified by cycling, walking, jogging, and swimming. Fitness of the heart and blood vessels as well as the respiratory mechanisms are emphasized in aerobic fitness, since oxygen must be distributed throughout the body. On the other hand, energy is released without using oxygen in anaerobic activities such as weight lifting and sprinting over short distances. An activity that occurs for approximately 2 or more minutes emphasizes aerobic fitness.

Biochemical shifts occur as the concentrations of *hormones* (chemical compounds secreted by endocrine glands directly into the bloodstream for rapid circulation throughout the body), and *enzymes* (protein substances that speed up chemical processes) are altered to meet the demands of physical activity. The nervous system plays many important roles in the regulation of metabolism. Many of the aforementioned physiological adjustments are under nervous system control or influence.

THE CARDIORESPIRATORY SYSTEM

Exercise makes all the individual "motors" that power the organs, tissues, and cells in the body operate at higher "revolutions per minute." We've already noted that greater quantities of blood and oxygen are required when you engage in physical activity. Since your blood supply remains fairly constant (except when the physical activity is particularly long and demanding, when blood volume may decrease somewhat), more of it has to reach the large working muscles when you perform physical work. Therefore the distribution system (heart and blood vessels) must handle a relatively greater volume of blood in any given time.

The heart may be thought of as a powerful pump connected to a complex network of tubes that beats approximately 100,000 times per day. These tubes are the blood vessels. They range in size from large, wide, and thick *arteries* to tiny, very thin-walled *capillaries*. Arteries, which carry blood away from the heart, are generally larger and more deeply located under the skin than are *veins*, which bring blood back to the heart after it has nourished the body's cells.

But the heart is really more than a pumping station attached to a maze of pipes. It also controls the rate of blood flow and hence the distribution of all its components. The heart receives nervous messages from the brain *(medulla oblongata)* that stimulate or retard heart rate. The heart's pacemaker in the right auricle receives these messages.

Although many substances are delivered to the body cells by the circulating blood (for example, nutrients and hormones), oxygen is the most essential. Your tissues can survive for a significant period of time with diminished supplies of nutrients and various biochemical substances. Without oxygen, they are usually irreparably damaged. Brain cells will die within minutes of being deprived of oxygen.

The circulatory and respiratory systems combine forces to carry out the vital responsibility of providing oxygen-bearing blood throughout the body. Thus the term *cardiorespiratory* refers to the cooperative efforts of the heart, the blood vessels, and the organs of respiration, which are responsible for bringing environmental air into the lungs and ultimately expelling waste gases.

The really critical structures are the tiny capillary vessels. It is through their thin walls that the circulating blood releases its valuable ingredients to the body cells. In addition, it takes on waste products which it carries back to the heart. It is only in the microscopic capillaries that such exchanges take place. Particles of these substances tend to move from areas of greater to lesser concentration through the capillary walls, in both directions. This process is known as *diffusion*. The heart and large blood vessels are essentially support structures for this vital capillary function.

Blood relinquishes to the lungs waste products it collects from body tissues. At the lungs it also takes on a fresh supply of oxygen for eventual distribution throughout your body. Figure 2.8 illustrates the path of blood circulation.

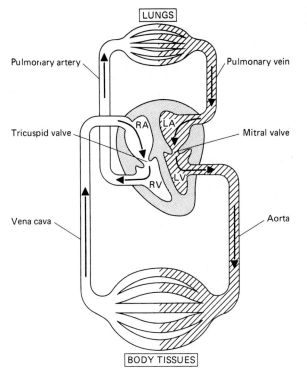

FIGURE 2.8   The course of blood circulation

When you exercise, all these processes accelerate. Your muscles produce increased amounts of metabolic waste materials. They also require additional supplies of fuel and oxygen. To satisfy these changing needs, your cardiorespiratory mechanisms must work more rapidly and/or more fully. Therefore you breathe more deeply and your heart beats faster.

The Course of Circulation

Each of the heart's four chambers connects with a large blood vessel. The *aorta* leaves the left ventricle and branches into smaller vessels that supply *arterial blood* (blood traveling away from the heart) to all parts of the body. *Venous blood*, returning from body tissues, flows through the *vena cava* into the right auricle. The right auricle is connected with the right ventricle by the *tricuspid valve*, an opening with three flaps that permit blood flow only in one direction: from auricle to ventricle. Venous blood collected in the right ventricle leaves through the *pulmonary artery*, which leads to the lungs. The blood is *oxygenated* (combined with oxygen) and returns through the *pulmonary vein* into the left auricle.

A *mitral valve* separates left auricle from left ventricle, permitting blood flow only into the ventricle. Valves are also located where the aorta and pulmonary artery leave the left and right ventricle, respectively.

The left and right chambers of the heart are not directly connected. Arterial blood is accommodated only by the left chambers and venous blood only by the right chambers.

The Breathing Process

A breathing center is located in the medulla (near the junction of skull and neck). When too much waste gas (*carbon dioxide*) is present in the blood, the activity of the brain's breathing center is accelerated. Exercise, of course, results in a relatively higher concentration of carbon dioxide (CO_2) in the blood. This causes nerve impulses to be sent to certain muscles that play important roles in breathing: the diaphragm and the rib muscles. When these so-called breathing muscles contract, the chest cavity enlarges and the small sacs of which the lungs are made (*alveoli*) are forced open. Environmental air then rushes in. Nerves located in the walls of the stretched alveolar walls send messages to the breathing center in the brain to stop the stimulating response caused by CO_2 in the blood. The breathing muscles then relax.

Alveoli, which are filled with air, release oxygen through the walls of the tiny blood capillaries surrounding them. As you've already noted, this oxygenated blood is carried back to the heart via the pulmonary vein. The heart then pumps the blood to all regions of the body.

PSYCHOLOGICAL RESPONSES

There's a psychic side to physical activity, and a very important side at that. So much so, that in today's world of international professional sport, team psychologists are often hired to help athletes and coaches grapple with interpersonal conflicts and problems in learning and performance. Clearly, it is necessary to go beyond the physical when studying behavior in sport and physical activity.

It is also necessary to go beyond the physical in evaluating yourself when considering an exercise program. Appendix A contains questionnaires to help you construct your own psychosocial profile. You should complete these questionnaires now, before reading further. The insights you gain into yourself will make the discussion here and in the next chapter more meaningful, and the results you obtain are part of the data you will use in Chapter 6 to plan your individualized fitness program and keep it going.

We ask you now to think about ways in which you might react psychologically to an episode of sustained, rigorous activity. First, we'd like you to consider the need to be psychologically ready or *motivated* for exercise. Sometimes your goals may center on having fun, or improving the skill or efficiency with which you execute a skill. Sometimes you may simply want to end the experience as fast as possible (for example, finish raking the leaves and get back to the ball game on TV). Occasionally you feel pressure to play, compete, or work because of peer or parental insistence.

Motivation

When we inquire about *why* a person behaves in a certain way, we are expressing interest in motivation. Two individuals may be engaged in the same activity, yet their reasons for involvement may differ.

One person may be cutting grass in the yard because she feels a need to do something physical on a glorious, bright and sunny day. She wishes to enjoy the scent of freshly cut grass, to hear the birds sing, and to feel her muscles respond against the resistance of the lawn mower. In contrast, a teenager who has been avoiding the activity may be doing it reluctantly and only after the following announcement by his father: "What! You haven't cut the grass yet? I asked you to finish that job three days ago. If that lawn is not cut today, you can forget about using the car tonight." Differences in motivation are likely to result in variations in performance. Which of the two lawn cutters do you believe would work with more speed, diligence, or care?

Imagine you are enjoying a sail on the open sea. A sudden squall overturns the boat and dumps you into the water two miles from shore. You head for land, battling the turbulence created by the storm. Your life is at stake, and you realize that only your own courage, strength, and swimming skill will save you. You finally reach safety and lie breathlessly on the beach, overwhelmed by your self-rescue. You are astonished at your own ability to overcome a formidable physical challenge.

As this anecdote suggests, there is a significant gap between psychological and physiological fatigue. When you narrow this gap, you may increase the duration and quality of your performance. In other words, you are usually able to continue physical activity long after the onset of psychological fatigue. But you have to learn this (although a life-threatening situation is not the recommended way). The point is that you can probably do more than you think you can, and motivation is the key.

Achievement in physical activity helps clarify self-concept. Your notion of who you are is sharpened by the transference of outcomes on the exercise mat or playing field to other areas. So psychological factors such as motivation, personality, self-concept, and emotion deserve attention as we consider the body's response to exercise.

Let's define and examine certain psychological conditions in relation to physical activity. See if you recognize the following common psychological states. Think about the ways in which you may recently have experienced them. Try and relate them to exercise. Do you believe that any of these conditions have been caused or relieved by participation in physical activity?

Anxiety

Imagine that the hour is very late, perhaps 2:30 AM. You find yourself walking in a narrow, dimly lit, deserted street in an inner city with a reputation for rampant and violent crime. You know you shouldn't be in this place, but your automobile engine has failed unexpectedly. Consequently, you walk quickly, seeking assistance, looking for a public telephone booth, for an all-night gas station. Suddenly, from out of the shadows step three large men: One wields a piece of lead pipe, the second brandishes a length of clanking chain, and the third flaunts a brick. With apparent intent and seriousness of purpose, they fan out across the street and block your way. In a flash, you understand the challenge facing you: You are confronted with a serious threat to your safety. You try to select an effective strategy for resolving the situation. You review your abilities and competences: How good a street fighter are you? How persuasive can you be in oral argument? How fast a runner are you? Underlying all your thoughts is an emotional reaction you also have to deal with. You experience a feeling that derives from the strong probability of physical harm. In a word, you are *afraid*!

Fear entails a clearly identifiable basis for harm (which need not be physical). It implies the existence of some thing or person that will eventually visit you in a destructive manner but a force on which you are able, so to speak, to put your finger, something real and recognizable (like the three men).

Anxiety is a related mood or feeling tone and may be viewed as a form of fear. It generates the same physiological responses as fear: for example, a gnawing sensation in the pit of the stomach; increases in perspiration, heart, and respiratory rates; and heightened blood pressure. But the source of fear is vague and elusive. Remember when, as a child, you sat in the dentist's waiting room, worried, apprehensive, wishing you could leave before the receptionist called your name? *You were anxious*!

You may have felt this way before tackling an important exam for which you had studied hard. You may have experienced anxiety before your first piano recital, or your entrance on stage in a class play. Your teachers have assured you of your readiness to perform, you have practiced and prepared well. Intellectually, you accept the high probability of a smooth, efficient, and accurate performance; however, the butterflies in your stomach will flutter. Your brow and palms remain wet with perspiration. *You are anxious*!

Can exercise be used to reduce anxiety? Does it have the potential for soothing the stomach rumblings of a frightened piano player, nervous actor, or anxious test taker?

Depression

The psychological state wherein an individual is convinced that all his or her efforts are to no avail is known as *depression*. Understandably, when this occurs frequently and for long periods of time, it becomes difficult to deal with daily responsibilities and to maintain social relations. One's attention becomes riveted on "all the things that are no good and everything that is going wrong."

Depression may be only temporary, and it need not be an indication of mental illness. On occasion, all of us become downtrodden and disappointed with the outcomes of certain events in our lives. But when this occurs often or for extended periods of time, the condition may indicate deep-seated conflict requiring the intervention of a professional helper (psychiatrist, psychologist, counselor). Another correlate of depression particularly relevant here is a marked decrease in physical activity. Deeply depressed individuals tend to mope around, to be lethargic.

What are the implications for exercise as a means of alleviating depression? What are the immediate effects of physical activity on this psychological condition?

Self-esteem

Self-esteem refers to the judgments you make about your own competence. Children often express this evaluation by declaring themselves to be a "good boy or good girl" or "bad boy or bad girl." Your individual experiences enable you to make these determinations. Sometimes you learn from others in your environment about your worth. Your attitudes about self are either denied or reinforced by those who react to your behavior and achievements. But you also process information about your competence that derives from self-testing experience. The stopwatch provides information about your mile run that influences judgments about your physical fitness. Sometimes your perceived esteem may not jibe with reality or with the ways in which others react to you.

Positive Psychological Responses

In the next chapter we deal with *training*, a planned program of physical activity maintained over a specified period of time. Here, we speak only of vigorous physical activity, conducted without regard to changing cardiorespiratory or neuromuscular status. The body's reactions to short-term or sporadic physical activity are not the same as in training. We need to keep this distinction in mind as we look at some of the psychological responses we experience in response to physical activity.

We admit to a biased point of view—that is, that exercise is essentially a positive and even necessary human experience.

Subjects in studies on the psychological response to physical activity usually report "feeling better." They maintain they are able to get rid of burdensome feelings and unwanted thoughts. Some people maintain they gain special insights into problems or are able to resolve certain personal problems while jogging or swimming.

The neurobiological mechanisms that account for these outcomes are not yet precisely known, but some interesting speculations are available. Consider some of the following points.

Exercise often requires a change of social as well as physical environment. When you retreat from a frustrating and heated argument to jog, lift weights, or cycle and return an hour later feeling calm, your change of attitude may be due to nothing more than your temporary physical withdrawal from the situation. You would probably attribute your anger and anxiety reduction to exercise. The shower you may have taken and the subsequent grooming done immediately prior to reappearing before your adversary may also have contributed to your feeling of relaxation and relative calm.

But exercise has also been observed to cause biochemical changes in the body that are known to be related to various psychological moods and states. Some researchers have reported that certain conditions, such as depression and anxiety, are related to a deficiency of norepinephrine at CNS synapses. Norepinephrine is a neurotransmitter that carries messages to the body's organs. Stimulation for activity of all kinds is inhibited when norepinephrine levels are substandard. Exercise (particularly running and cold-water swimming) has been shown to elevate the level of many neurotransmitting chemicals in the body.

Many undesirable psychological conditions are managed pharmacologically (with drugs), but *some* of the same biochemical effects may be achieved in safer ways through exercise. Endurance exercises, such as distance running or jogging, evidently stimulate production of brain secretions known collectively as *endorphins*. One kind of endorphin in particular, Beta endorphin, acts on the nervous system in a fashion identical to the drug opium. Without examining in detail the effects of opium and its derivatives on psychological processes such as reasoning, mood, and perception, we can say that high endorphin levels may very well influence some of these processes. In addition, the chemical *dopamine* has been reported to be present in elevated amounts in the bloodstreams of runners who had just completed a marathon. Dopamine is believed to be an antidepressant as well as an activator of erotic and sexual responses. Sexual activity is not a particularly high priority after struggling through a marathon run, but this fact does point up our theme, namely, that exercise has the potential to generate positive psychological effects.

Some forms of physical activity, such as hiking, weightlifting, racket sports, cycling, jogging, and, of course, all team sports, can be shared with other persons. Even more mundane physical activities such as yard work, car washing, and house painting may be done in small groups. Social relationships may therefore be fostered, explored, and improved. Often, the personalities of others are revealed during such activity; a participant may emerge in a different light. One's concept of the social as well as the physical self may thus be modified as a result of exercise.

The tenacity you display during exercise may surprise you. Your ability to finish a difficult physical task may encourage you to try and meet other physical or intellectual challenges (transference). Successful performance of a complex sports skill may contribute to modification of body image and self-concept, which happen to correlate very highly with one another. The ways in which you think about yourself, your abilities, your self-esteem, the value you place on your physical performance capabilities all may be modified by the positive information fed back to you as you perform, or after you perform, physical activity.

MANIPULATING CONDITIONS FOR EXERCISE

You can arrange your environment to optimize the physiological and psychological outcomes of physical activity.

Frame of Mind

Sometimes you may wish to avoid making a commitment to the length and intensity of your exercise bout. You may decide to play things "by ear." You may not have firmly established workout goals for the session. This is fine on occasion. Take it as it comes; if your performance feels comfortable, extend it. Perhaps you may feel like increasing the intensity of the movement by elevating effort or adding resistance. If things are not going well, slacking off may be wise.

But remember, if you proceed in this purely arbitrary way every time you exercise, some of your activity objectives may not be achieved. Try to select reasonable goals for the amount of work you wish to accomplish before stopping. Have a plan. Know approximately how long you intend to sustain your session.

On occasion, attempt to take your mind off your work performance: *dissociate*—let your mind follow its own preferred direction and see what bubbles up into your consciousness. You'll be surprised how time will fly. Then do just the opposite: Talk to yourself; try to imagine what you look like as you work. Think about the muscles you are using; try to identify them by name and location. Listen to your breath as it escapes your mouth. Determine if your breathing rate is increasing or decreasing as you work. *Associate* with the exercise performance. Permit your efforts to be relaxing and fun.

Time of Day

We seem to have personal ranges of peak productivity during the day. We learn that mentally and physically we function best during certain hours. This has a lot to do with our personal biochemical clocks, which establish patterns known as *circadian rhythms*. Many of our metabolic processes function in relation to time of day.

Determine the time of day in which it is best for you to exercise. Some of you are "morning persons." You like to be "up and at-em" bright and early. Exercise seems less difficult and more enjoyable at the day's beginning. Others are slow to get going in the morning. The thought of weight training, jogging, or a set of tennis at 6 or 7 A.M. is repugnant to them. What is your most productive time of day? When do you feel strongest, most able, most competent?

Think now of your favorite classes and teachers in school. When have your best class performances taken place? During which classes do you seem to be sharp, attentive, best able to follow what the instructor is saying? Now ask the same questions about your notable physical performances. What time of day was it when you were recently unconquerable on the tennis court or virtually infallible on the pitcher's mound? Answers to these questions relate, at least in part, to variations in the time of day.

Other Realities

It is important to identify your biologically preferred time of day for exercise. But there are also other realities to consider. For example, if you are a racketball player, you must find a partner whose available time is compatible with yours. If you must perform tedious work or labor (shoveling, painting, trimming bushes), give attention to the weather, your clothing, and the tools and utensils you use. Then there are professional, vocational, and school commitments that must be examined. Try to control these things as much as possible to enable your performance to be as safe, efficient, and enjoyable as possible. By raising a number of simple questions and making a few personal assessments, you should be able to determine the circumstances and time of day when your physical activity program can be pursued with maximum physical and psychological benefits.

If the exercise you are about to engage in is sport related, decide on the degree to which you want it to be competitive with the performance of others. Determine beforehand the kind of feedback you want to receive about your performance. Think about how you intend to use this kind of information, how it might bear on future performances. Above all, try to enjoy your exercise. Look for the positive effects it may produce; they are yours for the taking.

CONCLUSION

This chapter emphasized two categories of reactions to exercise. First, physiological responses involving the muscles were discussed. Three types of muscle tissues were identified: smooth, skeletal, and cardiac. Two kinds of skeletal muscle fibers were described—fast and slow twitch. The former predominate in explosive, short-term activities, such as sprinting or lifting heavy weights. Endurance-type activities, such as swimming and pullups, involve mostly slow twitch fibers. Both types of fiber contraction are part of most muscular actions. All three kinds of muscle tissue experience fatigue and contain energy packets known as *adenosine triphosphate*.

Another physiological category of responses to exercise included in this chapter was the nervous system. The central nervous system, comprising the brain and spinal cord, the autonomic nervous system and nerve pathways, were discussed in terms of their reaction to exercise.

The circulatory and respiratory systems' reactions to exercise were also reviewed in this chapter. When you are performing physical activity, the heart and lungs and the network of special tissues whose functions support these organs work harder than when you are resting.

A second category of reaction to exercise dealt with in this chapter were psychological responses. Among the topics discussed in this section were motivation, anxiety, depression, and self-esteem. Positive results of exercise were examined from these and other psychological perspectives.

Last, ways in which you can arrange your environment to improve overall chances for positive physiological and psychological reactions to exercise were discussed.

SUMMARY

1. A motor unit consists of individual motor nerves and all the muscle fibers it innervates.
2. Three types of muscle tissues are smooth, skeletal, and cardiac.
3. There are two kinds of skeletal muscle fibers: fast twitch and slow twitch. The former is predominantly used in explosive short-term activities while use of the latter is emphasized during endurance-type activites.
4. All three types of muscle tissue experience fatigue and rely on adenosine triphosphates (ATP) as an energy source.
5. The central nervous system consists of the brain, spinal cord, the autonomic nervous system and nerve pathways. Exercise participation stimulates integration between the central nervous system and the musculature system. For optimal physical performance, both have to be in good working order.
6. Since physical activity taxes the system to a greater extent than does inactivity or a sedentary lifestyle, the muscular, nervous, and circulatory systems must be able to adapt to increased demands.
7. There is evidence that one's psychological outlook improves with participation in physical activity. A part of the overall well-being may be due to the psychobiological adaptations brought about by vigorous physical activity involving the endorphins.

REFERENCES

AYRES, A. "Will Running Change the Kind of Person You Are?" *Running Times*, 9 (1982); 17-22.

GUYTON, A.C. *Function of the Human Body*. Philadelphia: W. B. Saunders, 1974.

NOBLE, B.J. *Physiology of Exercise and Sport*. St. Louis: Times Mirror, 1986.

NORTHRUP, J., G.A. LOGAN, and W.C. MCKINNEY. *Introduction to Biomechanic Analysis of Sport*, 2nd ed. Dubuque, IA: Wm. C. Brown, 1979.

3

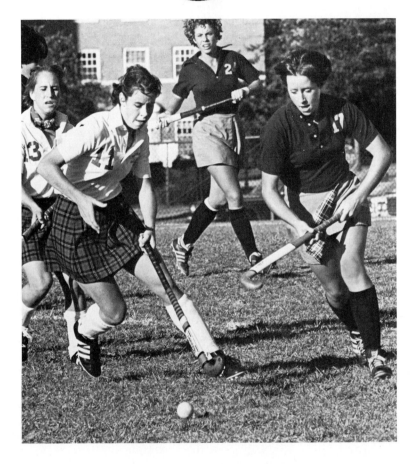

Training:
Your Body's Response

During one of his regular morning training runs, a middle-aged physician collapsed. He had been preparing for a marathon and had already completed 18 miles of his run when he dropped. Within minutes, he was dead. Soon thereafter, three of his former colleagues gathered to discuss the autopsy report. It revealed a blockage of more than 90 percent in two major arteries servicing the heart.

The first physician pointed out that his colleague's death was evidence that regular exercisers are also vulnerable to heart attack. Training, he suggested, even of the aerobic kind, doesn't necessarily confer immortality. Those who exercise regularly, he maintained, shouldn't believe they are immune from vascular disease. This, he felt, was the important lesson to be learned from this incident.

The second physician was quick to disagree. He argued that it was highly likely that had the deceased not been a regular runner and in such excellent shape, he would have succumbed to heart attack years before. Therefore, the important lesson here was that exercise prolonged the life of his colleague, who evidently had been afflicted by cardiovascular disease for a long time.

The third physician insisted that the most noteworthy outcome of the autopsy report related to the deceased's ability to run more than 18 miles with coronary arterial occlusion exceeding 90 percent. This, he felt, was astonishing and in conflict with what most physicians would have imagined to be possible.

What are the effects of training? How does exercise done regularly over an extended period of time influence health and wellness? These are the issues we address in this chapter. You need answers to these questions so that you can design an exercise program that will satisfy your personal health and wellness goals.

Remember, when thinking about training programs, bear in mind that they vary in length, intensity, and purpose. They come in all shapes and sizes. Some programs entail years of participation for preferred results to be achieved; others, weeks or months. A training program should be consistent with desired outcomes.

Regardless of the method you select for training, your workouts should include three essential parts: (1) the warmup, (2) the conditioning part per se, and (3) the cooldown. If these parts are incorporated properly and if your training method suits your needs and goals, you can anticipate certain physiological and psychological benefits. The next three sections of this chapter are devoted, therefore, to a discussion of the physiological and psychological responses to these dimensions of the workout.

In addition to these three essential parts of the workout, your training program, or the long-range plan you make for weeks and months of training, should be characterized by certain phases:

1. An *initial or preparatory phase*, in which you become familiar with elements and skills required in the program (for example, how to perform a certain exercise) and in which you adapt to the rigors of training. This may take weeks.

2. An *improvement phase*, in which you attempt to develop tolerance for increased intensity, duration, or frequency of exercise. The American College of Sports Medicine (ACSM), in its position statement on "The Recommended Quantity and Quality of Exercise for Developing and Maintaining Fitness in Healthy Adults," emphasizes that the total energy cost of activities or total amount of work done within the training session is what determines improvement in fitness.

3. A *maintenance phase*, in which you strive to retain the benefits of training. According to the ACSM, a significant reduction in working capacity (training effect) occurs after two weeks of detraining (cessation). After about 10 weeks to 8 months of detraining, you may expect to return to your pretraining level of fitness. After about 4 to 12 weeks of detraining you will lose approximately 50 percent of your improvement in cardiorespiratory fitness. To maintain cardiorespiratory fitness and muscular strength gains achieved through training, you should train 3 to 5 days per week at 50 percent to 85 percent of maximum oxygen uptake.

WARMUP

The organs and systems of your body must be alerted to their forthcoming responsibility. Cardiorespiratorially, muscularly, biochemically, and metabolically, you must crank up and get ready.

Without careful preparation, the likelihood of injury is increased. Regardless of the level of your motivation, clarity of goals, and quality of planned fitness program, if you are frequently injured or if you are organically incapable of dealing with the stresses accompanying vigorous exercise (minor though they may initially be), then you can't very well train effectively. Unless you are in very good physical condition, it is very important that you warm up.

The nature of warmup activity varies in accordance with the type of exercise you do during the conditioning part of your session. Stretching, calisthenics, light jogging, manipulation of equipment, mental imaging, and limited physical performance of selected skilled movements are all examples of warmup activities.

Stretching.   Stretching is an important aspect of warmup activities. Figures 3.1 to 3.10 demonstrate the correct way(s) to perform some stretching exercises. (Others that are specific to running and jogging are included in Chapter 14.)

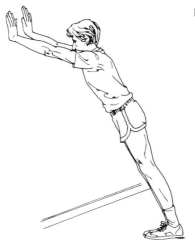

FIGURE 3.1   Achilles tendon

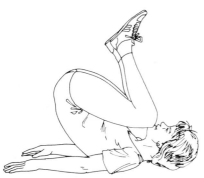

FIGURE 3.2   Back stretch

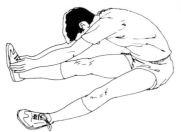

FIGURE 3.3   Hamstring stretch

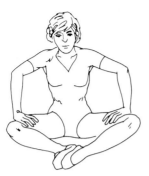

FIGURE 3.4   Groin stretch

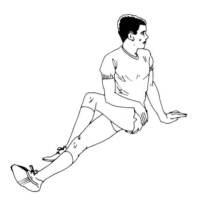

FIGURE 3.5   Spine and waist stretch

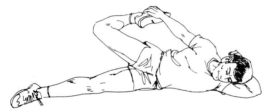

FIGURE 3.6   Quadriceps stretch

FIGURE 3.7   Shoulder and chest stretch

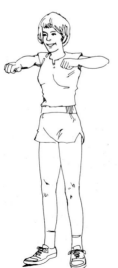

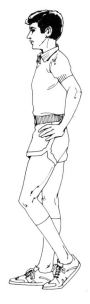

FIGURE 3.8   Ankle stretch

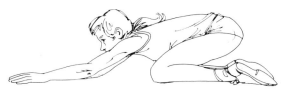

FIGURE 3.9   Abdominal stretch

FIGURE 3.10   Hip stretch

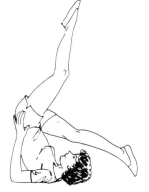

Let's review a few things that happen when you stretch before exercising. Many gross movements in physical exercise tend to tighten muscles. For example, tennis players spend a lot of time on their toes, which causes contraction of the calf muscles. Then suddenly, they must get off the balls of their feet to move sideways or to the rear. This dramatic shift in demand on the muscle from contraction to elongation can be troublesome. Therefore, training must also emphasize movements that stretch and relax muscles.

Stretching not only loosens muscles in preparation for vigorous contraction, it "trains" them to be loose during exercise. And while stretching, large skeletal muscles and surrounding connective tissue are strengthened. This is important, because many sport and physical activity injuries involve connective tissue rather than muscle itself.

Stretching exercises increase body as well as muscle temperature and thereby tend to protect muscle from tearing or injury during exercise. A so-called cold muscle is vulnerable to injury, particularly when the exercise is vigorous. In fact, it is recommended that you even walk and move your limbs for a few minutes before stretching to prepare for stretching.

Stretching also increases the amount of blood and oxygen reaching the muscles. All in all, skeletal muscle contracts more efficiently and more safely when it has been warmed up through stretching. It makes a lot of sense to stretch all major muscle groups in the body systematically and slowly before beginning the conditioning phase of training.

Other Warmup Activities.   If your physical activity includes use of special equipment (tennis racket, baseball bat), then it's a good idea to manipulate, handle, or get the feel of the instrument during warmup. Going through the basic movement patterns with the equipment will help prepare muscles for the much more vigorous movements they will make during the conditioning phase. It will also activate neuromuscular and hand-eye coordination mechanisms. If you are training on new or different facilities, get the feel of the floor, turf, court, or exercise environment during warmup. Don't rush. Bring body, equipment, and environment into an easy relationship.

If the conditioning period entails a new or particularly difficult movement or movement pattern, try to conceptualize or imagine it in your mind before actually doing it. Experience it mentally during warmup.

Perhaps calisthenics or a little light jogging (slow speed, short distance) are good warmup activities for *you* and *your* specific program of physical activity. Take some time now to think about *your* exercise activity. Will you be using equipment, balls, or special facilities? Will complex motor skills be involved? Identify some appropriate warmup experiences. Give careful consideration to including some kinds of stretching movements.

TRAINING

Training means preparing for something: an event, a season or athletic competition, a nursing career, an operatic performance, or military combat. Much growth and change occur during training. It usually involves learning or polishing skills, changing attitudes, and developing and strengthening organs and their functions. When you train, you have something in mind: a goal, a level of competence, a performance of some kind. An aspiration is established in your mind which you systematically pursue. You're preparing to meet increased demands of some kind on your current mental and physical resources. You seek in some way to change and better your present status, to improve on your previous level of performance.

Training involves periodic assessment of your status and progress. You have to know pretty much where you *are* in relation to the behavior, attitude, or skill for which you seek change. You also need to develop a clear vision of where you want to *be* when you embark upon a training program.

Training usually requires regular increase in the difficulty of task performance. When the essence of the training program is physical, adjustment of resistance, load, or level of skill difficulty is typically incorporated. If you are preparing for a race, you must increase the speed or distance over which you run, swim, cycle, ski, or row. Sometimes the terrain over which these activities are performed can be periodically made more difficult or challenging. You may swim in a specially constructed suit that creates drag in the water. You may run up hills or stairs, or cycle with weights on your legs or back. Training suggest some form of gradual increase in your performance output over an extended period of time. Most kinds of training entail regularly repeated and correct, trial-by-trial repetition of the same or similar movements. And invariably, training implies hard work.

Principles of Training

When you decide to train, you should understand the nature of your commitment—what you're getting yourself into. Here are some of the important features of most training regimens:

1. Training is done over an extended period of time. Sometimes it takes months or years to achieve training goals.
2. Training should be done 3 to 5 times a week (preferably every other day) at your target heart rate for about 30 minutes per session.
3. Training may mean alteration of aspects of your life that are not basically physical, such as attitudes, schedule of daily activities, eating and resting habits, as well as social relations.
4. Training may affect your psychological and emotional as well as your physical status. It is usually intended to produce positive or desirable change.
5. Training should result in a level of personal fitness associated with good health.
6. Training sessions should be preceded by warming up and followed by cooling down.
7. Training programs should incorporate the principle of overload.
8. Training increases the size of the heart and the efficacy of nerve impulse transmission.
9. Training results in increased ability of the cardiorespiratory system to distribute oxygen throughout the body.
10. Training results in muscle fiber thickening.
11. Training may have an impact on your sexuality, since it can result in change in the way you look and feel about yourself.

Frequency.   To obtain a training effect, you need to exercise at least 3 to 5 days a week (preferably every other day) at the levels of intensity and duration described shortly. You can *objectively* determine whether you are obtaining a training effect by determining your resting pulse rate. If it is lower than before you began your training program, you are probably exercising in a manner that is beneficial to your heart and circulatory system. You should also be able to detect the benefits of your program *subjectively*. You should feel you have more energy, are more alert, less fatigued at day's end, and more confident in your ability to take control of your health.

Intensity.   To obtain the optimal effects of exercise, you should train at a level of intensity vigorous enough to raise your heart rate. The increased heart rate indicates the body needs oxygen in greater amounts than at rest, and this need in turn leads to development of the body's oxygen transport system (heart, lungs, and blood vessels). The question you may now be asking is: "How fast does my heart have to beat to get this training effect?" The answer is that it should beat at your *target heart rate* and that varies depending on your age and initial physical condition. We will show you how to determine *your* target heart rate in Chapter 4.

Obviously, you need to take your pulse during exercise to determine if the intensity of your workout is too light, too heavy, or just right. Take your pulse in the middle of exercising, if possible. A 10-second pulse count multiplied by 6, to arrive at your heart rate per minute, is recommended. However, if it is not possible or is inconvenient to take your pulse while exercising, do it immediately upon the completion of exercising.

Duration.   If you follow these recommendations (3 or 5 days of exercise at your target heart rate), you will need to exercise for only about 30 minutes per session to obtain a training effect, although you should work up to that amount of exercising over a period of time. A range of 15 to 60 minutes probably accomodates the capabilities of most participants. Eventually, 1-1/2 to 2 hours of exercise each week will be enough to obtain improvement in your level of physical fitness. Of course, you can obtain even greater improvement by spending more time exercising. Preferred activities are those that use large muscle groups, are sustained and rhythmical.

Warmup and Cooldown.   When we get more specific about how you should plan your training program (Chapter 6), we will describe how to warm up and cool down during exercise. Suffice it to say here that concentrating on warming up *before* training is the wrong idea. You should warm up as *part* of training. You prevent injury and prepare the body for the demands of the activity to follow by warming up. Similarly, you cool down to help the body recover from the physical demands it has just encountered.

The Overload Principle.   To improve any component of physical fitness, you need to stress that component more than normally. This is called the *overload principle*. For example, if you want to improve your muscular strength, you need gradually to lift more and more weights. If you want to run faster, you need to increase the speed and/or distance at which you run at that speed. If you want to improve your cardiorespiratory endurance, you need to add distance to your training runs. The only way to improve your fitness is to apply the overload principle.

How to Train

A close look at any effective training program reveals that in one way or another the principles we've just reviewed are included. Programs may differ in *how* they incorporate overload, but it's got to be there in some way if the program is intended to increase muscular strength. Since your muscles are incapable of distinguishing among various *kinds* of resistance, it makes little or no difference whether they contract against loads created by metal weights, sand bags, rubber bands, springs, or cables. Some strength training equipment uses hydraulic (liquid) or pneumatic (air) pressure to create resistance. Even your own body weight can be used (pullups, bar dips). Factors such as portability, expense, and comfort will help you determine which are appropriate for your use. But as far as your muscles are concerned, resistance is resistance and overload is overload.

Certain kinds of programs emphasize muscular endurance (repetition of contractions); others, muscular strength. Some are more effective in preparing you for events that require considerable cardiorespiratory efficiency, such as the marathon. Other programs are geared toward activities that demand a lot of short bursts of sprinting, such as in soccer or tennis.

The ways in which you schedule your program's rest intervals between bouts of exercise (sets) will have an impact on the development of your body's energy systems and the movement patterns required in various sports and physical activities. Therefore, the program you select and the way you train can make an important difference in your fitness development.

A number of training methods have been developed by physical educators and track coaches throughout the world. By and large, they are intended to increase sprinting or endurance capacities. Although directed primarily at track and field events, their effects are applicable to a wide assortment of physical activities if movements peculiar to a particular sport are used. The following are five widely used training methods:

1. *Sprint training*, which emphasizes running at maximum or near-maximum speed for short distances.
2. *Fartlek or speed play*, in which fast and slow running is alternated, with no intervals of rest.
3. *Interval training*, in which bouts of hard running or work are separated by periods of light exercise, with no pause for rest.
4. *Continuous training*, in which exercise is maintained at a constant level of intensity for a fairly long and uninterrupted period.
5. *Circuit training*, in which a participant is expected to complete a round or circuit of certain exercises or movements at less than maximum

repetitive capacities within a specified period of time. Sometimes more than one round may be used.

We will devote special attention to three of these training methods: interval, continuous, and circuit training. Most programs are modifications of these.

Interval Training.   As the name implies, interval training involves intervals of intense exercise interspersed with intervals of relatively light exercise. To improve cardiorespiratory functioning, the strenuous intervals should be done at near-maximum heart rate intensity. This form of training usually results in a greater buildup of lactate, accompanied by greater pain and discomfort. However, since the overload principle is applied—that is, the length or intensity of the intervals can be increased—great improvement in fitness can occur in a short period of time.

If you were applying this kind of training approach to running, your regimen might look like this: Run 100 yards at half speed, slowly jog 200 yards, run 100 yards at half speed, slowly jog 100 yards; repeat for approximately 1 to 2 miles. Your present level of conditioning will determine how long you repeat this cycle of alternate running and jogging. The speed with which you run and the distance you run and jog are also related to your present level of fitness. You may eventually define work and rest intervals in terms of number of minutes or seconds instead of distance.

Continuous Training.   Continuous training involves engaging in an activity at about the same level of intensity throughout the exercise session. When applied to continuous training, the overload principle may result in an increase in the *length of the session* while maintaining the level of intensity, or an increase in the *level of intensity* while keeping the duration of the exercise the same.

In Chapter 2 we discussed the difference between slow- and fast-twitch muscle fibers. Continuous training seems to work to improve the functioning of slow-twitch muscle fibers, whereas interval training seems to improve both fast- and slow-twitch functioning. If you are training for an activity that uses predominately slow-twitch muscle fibers (for example, jogging), then continuous training is fine. However, if you are training for activities requiring bursts of fast movement (for example, tennis or racketball), you would be wise to include some interval training.

Using running as an activity, a continuous training workout would typically involve 2 or 3 miles of slow-speed, uninterrupted running. The speed at which you would run and the number of times per week you would train would depend upon your goals (do you wish to compete?) and present level of fitness.

Circuit Training.   A training program that moves you from one exercise station to another—that is, takes you through a *circuit*—is called circuit training. Some of you may have Par Courses in your neighborhood. Signs

A CIRCUIT TRAINING PROGRAM

Station Number	Activity
1	440-yard run or jog
2	Situps
3	Bench press
4	Hamstring stretch
5	Pullups (wide grip, knuckles toward you)
6	Rope skipping
7	Arm curl
8	Standing (overhead press)
9	Leg raising
10	Upright rowing
11	440-yard run

at various places along the Par Course instruct you to do a particular physical activity at each location. You may be asked to do pullups at a bar, or situps on the ground, or any other physical fitness activity. Once you've completed that activity, you jog to the next station on the course. Since many different exercises can be used within any one circuit, circuit training is an excellent way to train on all components of physical fitness.

In this method of training, the overload derives from any of three program adjustments: (1) increasing the number of repetitions at each station; (2) increasing the resistance against which the muscles contract at each station (for example, adding more weights to barbells); or (3) requiring that the entire circuit be completed in less time.

If strength is an important training objective, then weight resistance exercises for specific muscle groups should be emphasized in the circuit. Running, swimming, or cycling should be included if your objective is cardiorespiratory endurance.

To determine the number of repetitions you should do at each station, you need to test yourself on each exercise. In the beginning, your work prescription for each exercise (at each station) should be one-half your maximum number, as determined by the test. For example, if you include pullups as an activity, and you determine that you can do 6, then prescribe 3 repetitions for that station. Be sure that you are well rested between each test to determine your true maximum.

As your fitness improves and your time for the entire circuit has been decreased a few times, you might add a second or third circuit. Circuits should contain between 6 and 15 stations and should take about 10 to 20 minutes to complete. The box shows a circuit training program that includes muscular strength and endurance as well as cardiorespiratory activities.

PHYSIOLOGICAL RESPONSES

Neuromuscular Changes

Training has a positive effect on the functional capacities of the synapse as well as the myoneural junction (see Figures 2.6, 2.7). Apparently, transmission of the nerve impulse occurs more efficiently in the trained than in the untrained individual. Although this can be demonstrated in the laboratory, it has not yet been determined whether this result has any real application to performance on the athletic field or other kinds of physical activity. It may be that this will never be definitively shown, because of the complex nature of many of our motor and athletic skills. The skills we use on the sport field, for example, involve so many different kinds of coordinated movements that the contribution of improved nervous impulse to an actual performance in an applied situation is difficult to assess. However, it seems logical to assume that if the transmission is occurring with improved efficiency, then the quality of the overall performance will be improved.

The most dramatic changes in muscle tissue due to training occur in skeletal muscle. Smooth muscle changes undoubtedly also occur, but they are more difficult to observe. Their responses to training are of necessity monitored indirectly. That is, we make the assumption that the smooth muscle lining the intestines, coronary (heart) arteries, and blood vessels is strengthened as a result of training, since the functions of these organs are improved. To an extent, this is also true of cardiac muscle.

Effects of training on muscle tissue are also specifically related to the type of training used. Endurance training (for example, distance running and cycling), which emphasizes ST fibers, will yield different effects than sprint-type (FT) training.

Training causes the following overall improvements in muscle function:

1. The efficiency of the nervous stimulation of the muscle is improved.
2. More fuel for muscular contraction is available, and the distribution of fuel is more efficient.
3. Less metabolic waste is produced in the muscles, and fatigue is therefore delayed.

Endurance Training Effects.   Muscle cells require oxygen to sustain their metabolic activity. *Myoglobin* is the chemical compound in muscle in which oxygen is stored. Obviously, its function is critical in skeletal muscle contraction. Endurance exercise training has been shown to increase skeletal muscle myoglobin content significantly. The muscle's ability to utilize fuel for contraction is also improved as a result of training. This is believed to be due to an increase in the activity of certain chemicals called *enzymes*, which occur in muscle cell parts called *mitochondria*. In fact, endurance training causes an increase in the number of mitochondria.

Also, the fuel supplies in the muscle itself (*glycogen, triglyceride,* and *phosphagen*), which are necessary for metabolism, are increased as a result of exercise. And as you might expect, endurance training results in an increase (or *hypertrophy*) in the size of ST fibers.

Sprint Training Effects.   Biochemically and histologically (with reference to tissues), the responses of skeletal muscle to sprint training or exercise routines that emphasize short bursts of fast running or other such movement are not nearly as dramatic as the response to endurance training. It appears that skeletal muscle does not have to adapt very much to the demands of sprint activities—or at least, not as much as is necessary in endurance activities. Nonetheless, some responses to sprint training contribute to substantially improved physical performance: (1) an increase in certain enzymes important in muscle metabolism, (2) an increase in muscle storage of certain kinds of fuel needed for contraction (for example, *glycogen*), and (3) an increase in the amount of oxygen received by muscle tissue. Training results in an increased capacity to bring more oxygen to the body through the lungs.

Cardiorespiratory Changes

The common expression "the heart of the matter" indicates the importance attributed to cardiac function. Changes in cardiac function vitally influence a wide range of physical performance capacities. First, and perhaps foremost, the heart pumps blood to the muscles and thereby nourishes them. Second, it carries away the waste products of muscular contraction. But remember, when you embark on a training program with the intention of improving muscular strength and endurance, your heart is required to cope with additional loads and responsibilities. This is why it is wise to establish cardiac readiness for stress through a thorough medical exam (see Chapter 4).

What are the effects of training on the heart muscle itself? Some changes are evident even when you are at rest, and others are measurable only during exercise. As a rule, the longer the period during which training occurs (weeks, months, years), the greater the frequency of training, and the greater the intensity, the more marked will be the beneficial outcomes.

Training Effects at Rest.   Pulse is typically lower in the trained than in the untrained individual. The heart beats (pulses) fewer times per minute and pumps out a greater volume of blood (stroke volume) as a consequence of training (particularly training of the endurance kind). As a result, the heart muscle uses the energy necessary for its contraction more efficiently.

The size of the heart increases as a result of training (hypertrophy). Those participating in endurance-type training experience an increase in size, particularly in the left ventricle, the largest and most muscular of the heart's four chambers. In persons whose training emphasizes relatively short periods of heightened effort (wrestlers, track and field weight throwers, weight lifters), the walls of the left ventricle thicken, but there is no increase in size.

Training has also been shown to increase the volume of blood as well as its content of *hemoglobin*, the blood's oxygen-carrying element. Blood pressure is usually observed to be lowered in training for middle-aged or older persons whose beginning fitness levels are low. Younger persons of reasonably decent fitness levels typically experience no change in blood pressure as a result of training.

Training Effects During Exercise.   In the trained individual, less of the stored fuel for muscular contraction is used, and in the performance of moderate exercise, less waste materials (for example lactic acid) resulting from muscle tissue metabolism are produced. The pulse rate is lower, which means that the heart is working with less effort. Blood pressure is also lowered as a result of training.

As Table 3.1 suggests, the overall effect of training on the cardiovascular system is clearly positive. Training enables the heart to perform work more efficiently, which means its effort is decreased and its output is increased.

In well-trained individuals, the ability to distribute oxygen throughout the body is substantially higher than in untrained persons. Remember, when you exercise, your body organs require greater amounts of nutrient for cellular metabolism, as well as increased amounts of oxygen. If the delivery of oxygen by the blood is improved, more efficient organic function is to be expected. *Respiration* refers not only to the breathing in of air from the external environment, but also to the distribution of oxygen derived from environmental air throughout the body. As we have noted, stroke volume and heart rate are the cardiac factors that account for the amount of oxygen delivered to body parts. Training enhances the efficiency of these functions.

Table 3.1
Cardiovascular Changes as a Result of Training

Variable	Endurance-Type Training	Sprint-Type Training	Observable During Rest	Observable During Exercise
Pulse	Decreased	Decreased	Yes	Yes
Stroke volume	Increased	Increased (but not as much as in endurance-trained persons)	Yes	Yes
Hypertrophy	Left ventricular increase in size	Left ventricular increase in thickness of wall	?	?
Blood volume	Increase	Increase	Yes	?
Blood pressure	Lowered in middle-aged and older participants	Lowered in middle-aged and older participants	Yes	Yes

One very interesting observation some researchers have reported is that in trained individuals, blood flow to the working muscles is lowered during exercise. Evidently, well-conditioned muscles are better able to extract oxygen from the blood and thus require a relatively smaller amount of blood.

Metabolic Adjustments

Training influences metabolic processes in many different ways, but all its effects are positive. Muscle metabolism, in particular, is significantly affected by training. For example, the capacity of skeletal muscle to utilize oxygen and fuel is improved by training. Enzyme activity is increased, and so is the muscle's capacity to store fuel. Although training may not result in the generation of new muscle fibers, it does cause increased fiber size. Less lactic acid is produced by trained muscles when they are experiencing moderate exercise. (Few of us engage in maximal physical effort every time we exercise, so much of our exercise may be classified as moderate.)

One of the important fuels for muscular contraction, glycogen, is used in lesser amounts to satisfy the metabolic needs of skeletal muscle. Lactic acid derives from glycogen and its accumulation in the muscles is believed to be related to physical fatigue. Since less glycogen is used in contraction, less lactic acid is produced, and fatigue is delayed.

Body Composition Changes

Rigorous training, particularly when done against heavy resistance (weights), usually results in muscle fiber thickening. There is also an increase in the number of capillaries surrounding and nourishing the muscle, and a thickening of connective tissue surrounding the muscle (tendons that connect muscle to muscle and ligaments that connect muscle to bone). These kinds of changes are likely to result in a gain in body weight. However, for this to occur, exercise must be done regularly, over a fairly long period of time, and at significant levels of intensity. As you will discover in Chapter 11, such increased function will in all probability also cause the metabolism of significant amounts of stored body fat. Therefore, as a consequence of training, a net loss of body weight typically occurs, since more fat is usually lost than muscle and connective tissue (which are known as *lean body mass*).

These effects, however, vary according to (1) *sex* (females generally store more body fat and have less muscle tissue than males), (2) *age* (middle-aged and older people tend to be more fatty than young adults and teenagers), (3) *duration and intensity of training*, and (4) *heredity* (which influences the deposition of fat tissue and the amount of muscle tissue in the body).

Before you go on to read about psychological responses to training, see if you can recall the important physiological responses just reviewed. Write these responses in Figure 3.11 on the body location where they occur. Include in your summary the following aspects of our discussion: (1) neuromuscular, (2) cardiovascular, (3) respiratory, (4) metabolic, and (5) body composition.

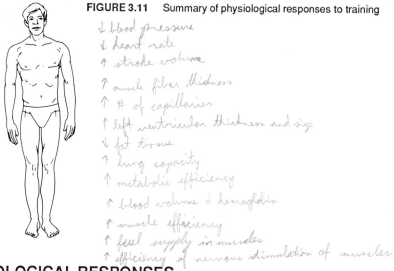

FIGURE 3.11   Summary of physiological responses to training

↓ blood pressure
↓ heart rate
↑ stroke volume
↑ muscle fiber thickness
↑ # of capillaries
↑ left ventricular thickness and size
↓ fat tissue
↑ lung capacity
↑ metabolic efficiency
↑ blood volume + hemoglobin
↑ muscle efficiency
↑ fuel supply in muscles
↑ efficiency of nervous stimulation of muscles

PSYCHOLOGICAL RESPONSES

Let us now consider specific psychological responses to training. Note that some of these responses are exaggerations or extensions of those we examined in Chapter 2. However, in the case of training, they are more pronounced, longer lasting, or both.

In general, the positive results of exercise are available to you in proportion to the duration of the program in which they are set. The more extended your program, the more dramatic will be your benefits. And with regard to psychological responses, the more enthusiasm, the more inspiration, the more verve and dedication you invest in your training program, the more profitable your reactions will be.

Once again we see evidence of the relationship between psychology and physiology, the mind and the body. When training results in specific biochemical alterations, changes in moods and feelings (known in psychological terms as *affect*) may occur. And these kinds of alterations may very well influence behavior. A cyclic model summarizing the interrelationships among physiological, affective and behavioral factors is presented in Figure 3.12.

Lowered Anxiety Levels

It is customary to distinguish between *state* and *trait* anxiety, so before we proceed, we consider the difference between these two forms. *State* anxiety is specific to a particular experience or set of circumstances (temporary); *trait* anxiety is the anxious feeling that persists across situations (it exists much of the time irrespective of environment or circumstances). Some of us tend to run high in trait anxiety and will therefore respond anxiously to many stimuli that would probably not evoke such emotion in those with low trait anxiety.

Many studies reveal that exercise-trained individuals tend to undergo stress-related physiological changes in comparatively less harmful ways than persons who are untrained. In other words, the altered physiology associated

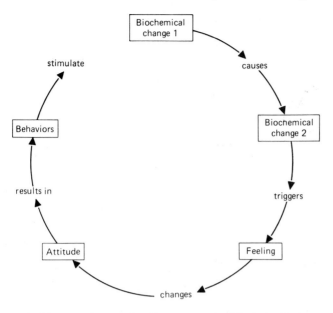

FIGURE 3.12   Interrelationships among physiological, affective and behavioral factors

with anxiety appears to be minimized by training. Certain of these biochemical changes may also cause behavioral and psychological changes, since some behaviors are believed to have chemical bases. For example, norepinephrine, or noradrenalin, when injected into an experimental subject, will cause arousal and increased metabolism. Norepinephrine levels in trained persons are lower than are those in the untrained. Highly-anxious individuals typically have higher levels of norepinephrine than do less anxious persons. Research studies also tell us that typical anxiety levels are lower in trained as compared to untrained subjects (for example, Cureton, 1963).

As fitness improves, anxiety scores decrease. More active groups of subjects usually demonstrate lower levels of anxiety and depression. Reasons offered for these observations include (1) reduction in muscular tension, which is often associated with anxiety; (2) physiological changes brought about by the alteration of brain chemistry; and (3) increase in stroke volume of the heart, which results in smaller quantities of the hormones related to anxiety (Mikevic, 1982; Morgan, 1979).

Better Stress Management

When events or stimuli are perceived to be stressful, levels of *cortisol* (a hormone secreted by the adrenal glands) rise in the blood. Training appears to result in reduced cortisol production. Also, some physiological parameters associated with stress reactions, such as heart rate, blood pressure, and muscular tension (known as *bracing*) are reduced as a result of regular participation in exercise (Balog, 1983).

TWENTY-FIVE YARDS TO CONFIDENCE

Derick stood about 6'5" tall and weighed well over 200 pounds. He was plump, rather shy, and absolutely petrified of any volume of water other than that found in a drinking cup.

He was in his senior year of engineering studies, but had been repeatedly unable to satisfy the college's swimming requirements. To graduate, a student had to traverse, unaided, one length of the pool (25 yards). His degree was in obvious jeopardy. The Department of Health and Physical Education extended to him an unprecedented opportunity: to enroll in a swimming section comprised of one student. On the very first day of the spring semester, I was given the job of teaching him to swim.

During the course of approximately 3 1/2 months, Derick came to class regularly—never an absence. Twice a week, always on time, a frightened and visibly trembling Derick would appear on the deck of the pool. We would work together for 40 minutes each time. As the weeks rolled by, we came to know one another in different ways. Derick began sharing personal experiences, aspirations, and troublesome aspects of his world. It appeared that he had a full measure of interpersonal difficulties which he was trying to resolve at the time.

In the beginning, Derick had little belief in his ability to succeed in endeavors outside the engineering classroom. In matters of physical performance, his confidence approximated zero. His unusual height compounded his problems, in that he was never able to fulfill the expectations often held by others for such a large and tall man.

Derick trained and trained and trained. He did exercises with weighted pulleys to strengthen his muscles. He did situps; he stretched. In short, he did whatever was asked of him. Little by little, subtle changes in his behavior and general outlook became noticeable. On a few occasions he expressed interest in his appearance and talked to me about a new sport coat he intended to buy. He began to talk about himself in different ways. He began to believe that he might be able, sometime in the future, to swim 25 yards and graduate.

After a while, we abandoned all attempts to get Derick to swim on his belly side and worked exclusively on getting him to make his way down the pool on his back. During the last class meeting of the semester, in the presence of the department's associate chairman, various colleagues and students in the department, and one very, very, proud swimming instructor, Derick jumped into the pool at its deep end, surfaced, leveled off onto his back and with an admittedly feeble flutter kick and nondescript flapping motion of his wrists, smilingly, happily, and proudly propelled himself ever so slowly and cautiously the full 25 yards to the other side of the pool. Never in the history of swimming had anyone applied a more literal interpretation of the term "free-style."

But Derick passed the course, graduated, and became an engineer. Later he stopped by to visit and share his reactions to the entire experience. Time and time again, when he spoke of his months of conditioning, anxiety, and almost phobic reaction to the water, Derick used the word "confidence." He learned important lessons about his physical capabilities, his courage, and about faith in another person. We talked at length about the importance of confidence in the physical part of self and its transferability to other dimensions of life. It is likely that Derick's wellness was expanded through his strengthened confidence, and that this effect will last. I believe he will always remember his swimming class. I know I will.

But training itself can be stressful for many persons. Training implies regular participation and an increase in the difficulty of movement, resistance, or speed. For some, this is interpreted as a commitment to exercise "without fail"; it means that you may feel obliged to jog or run, rain or shine, that you skip rope or swim every morning "no matter what." This sort of imposed regularity may become a stressor. Guilt may arise when you don't or can't exercise. In some cases, an addiction to regular exercise may develop.

In this sense, the self-imposed commitment to train may cause you stress, particularly if you have made the commitment irresponsibly. (By "irresponsibly," we mean without adequate thought being given to time management, degree of exercise difficulty, and extent of motivation to pursue the results of training.) When training is, or becomes, an agent of stress, you would do well to consider modifying your program or even withdrawing temporarily. (Signs of stress are described in Chapter 12.)

But for the most part, training apparently enhances stress-coping defenses. Participants in training programs report lower incidents of stress reaction. In fact, some individuals appear to do very well—or, indeed, thrive on certain degrees of stress. Habitual exercisers deprived of the opportunity to work out report experiencing stress. In fact, sometimes researchers find it very difficult to recruit habitual exercisers for experiments in which they have to agree to *not* exercise (Blakeland, 1970). Apparently, we seek a level of arousal that yields, for each of us, the best performance results throughout the day. In addition, physiologists who study mechanisms underlying reaction to stress have speculated that long-term training may cause an adaptation to the stimulating effects of certain chemically produced reactions to stress. In other words, after a while, if the daily run or swim is not made longer or more difficult, it loses it potential as a stressor.

Depression Reduction

Training does seem to cause depression to decrease, although some researchers (in particular, Griest et al., 1979) suggest that this effect may be observed only with moderately depressed subjects. It's important to note, too, that activities such as cycling, jogging, swimming, and cross-country skiing, rather than competitive sports such as softball, seem the most conducive to reducing depression. As fitness levels increase, depression seems to decrease.

The reasons for these antidepressant effects of training are speculative and include the following: (1) *Biochemical increase in neurotransmitter concentration,* which provides for improved impulse transmissions at synapses (Ransford, 1982); depression is believed to involve impaired nervous impulse transmission; also glucose, cholesterol, and androgen serum concentration are affected by training, and these are believed to be affiliated with depression; (2) *time-out,* changing the environment or doing something different; and (3) *social interaction,* opportunities for relating to others while exercising.

Increased Self-esteem

Mastery, or a sense of control over your day and where you are headed in life, may improve as a consequence of training. These positive feelings about yourself derive from the realization that you are fit and in shape. They may lead

Table 3.2
Exercise Checklist

Location	Environment— Social	Environment— Physical	Exercise Intensity	
Indoor ✓	Alone ✓	Pleasant ✓	Sustained maximum effort required	___
Outdoor ___	With others ✓	Unpleasant ___	Maximum effort required for brief periods	✓
			Sustained submaximum effort required	✓
			Submaximum effort required for brief periods of time	___

to heightened self-image and self-confidence, which may very well have a bearing on your attitudes and behaviors in other areas. Our physical appearance and the extent to which we succeed in physical endeavors correlate highly with our self-esteem.

Feeling good is a very important aspect of wellness and is a common outgrowth of training. When you feel good, you *are* good. Self-esteem is a measure of the regard you have for yourself. It influences your interactions with others, your personal decisions, your judgments, your moods and attitudes. Your fitness has a serious impact on it. And, of course, training directly influences fitness.

Enjoyment

If you presently exercise on a regular basis, pause for a minute or two and think about the following questions: (1) Do you enjoy your training sessions? (2) Are you disappointed when you miss a session?

When you select a training program with careful attention to safety factors and personal needs and interests, it should provide opportunity for joyful participation. The experience should be something to which you look forward. If you've responded negatively to the two foregoing questions, then it's probably time to take a close look at your training program. Perhaps you haven't taken the time to do this recently, or maybe you've really never analyzed aspects of your program that contribute to enjoyable participation.

Use the checklist in Table 3.2 to examine your training program. Analyze its elements and try to find weak spots. Perhaps you can manipulate some of these factors without much trouble, and thereby improve the enjoyment level of your training. The greater the degree of enjoyment, the greater the likelihood that high-quality participation will be sustained. The more regularly you participate in training and the longer the period of time in which you train (weeks, months, years), the higher will be your level of fitness. And as

Exercise Duration	Time of Day	Number of Days per Week	Nature of Exercise	
Less than 15 min ___	Morning ___	1 ___	Sportlike	___
	Afternoon ___	2 ✓	Calisthenics	___
From 15–30 min ___	Evening ✓	3 ✓	Aerobic	✓
From 30–45 min ✓		4 ___	Anaerobic	✓
		5 ___	Direct competition	___
From 45 min–1 hr ✓		6 ___		
		7 ___		
More than 1 hr ___				

we've been emphasizing all along, the higher your level of fitness, the more established and secure will be your wellness.

Researchers are fairly consistent in reporting that exercisers *feel better* after a workout. Participants themselves report being refreshed and rejuvenated after exercise. Long-term participation, which leads to higher levels of fitness, enables this pleasurable sensation to be sustained. As we've noted previously, when researchers try experimentally to deprive regular exercisers of participation in their training regimens, they are at a loss to find willing subjects. Exercise can add pleasure to your day.

Friendship

How did you respond to the environment—social section of Table 3.2? Do you train alone or with others? Training provides the opportunity to interact with others who are engaged in like activities. The fact that you and others have chosen to be at the same place at the same time while participating in a similar experience suggests that there is at least some sharing of personal interests. This overlap may spark new relationships. Exercising together and providing and receiving encouragement, motivation, and assistance (timing, counting repetitions, spotting, handling a weight) can enhance old relationships.

Frequency of contact is by no means a guaranteed solidifier of relationships. However, repeated interaction with others does afford the chance to observe aspects of personality that might otherwise go unappreciated. After all, how many times per week might you see some of your friends with whom you are supposedly close? Once or twice a week? You might easily spend time with an exercise partner (as much as three, four, or five times per week) that far exceeds time spent with a so-called close friend.

If your preferred exercise format requires friendship (for example, tennis), you are certainly obliged to seek out someone. In so doing, you telephone another to make arrangements; you talk; you call "out" or "fault" during the match. After, you share a drink; you discuss and evaluate together; you offer criticism and reinforcement and receive the same. In short, *you interact.* You have the opportunity to offer and accept friendship through exercise.

Sexuality

Regular participation in exercise usually results in marked physical changes. As your muscles become more firm and excess stored body fat is reduced, your body shape may assume new and desirable proportions (as defined by our society's view of desirable). Not only may this generate revision in your body and self-concept, but it may also alter the view others have of you. You may appear to be more physically attractive to others, more sexy. And according to a study by James White of the University of California at San Diego, regular runners *are* sexier.[1] They experience more sexual desire, arousal, and orgasms than nonrunners. Although White's data do not shed light on the causes of these sexual changes (are they biochemical or due to improvements in self-esteem?), they suggest that exercise plays an important role in the participants' sexuality.

Feeling of Health and Fitness

No remedy is yet available for restoring lost youth. But some physiological effects of aging can be postponed and some of the impairments associated with aging may be minimized through regular exercise. We'll have considerably more to say about age and physical fitness in Chapter 7, but we make this observation here because researchers tell us that physical inactivity causes the same physical and mental impairments that have been attributed to aging in people of all ages. Young people who are inactive show symptoms characteristic of aging. But training seems to reverse many of these impairments.

Exercise done regularly can result in a level of personal fitness associated with good health. And as we've repeatedly emphasized in this chapter, an impressive array of physiological and psychological responses to training affect your health in positive ways. In a nutshell, when you're in good shape, you feel good and you look good.

Cooldown

The cooldown period that follows the conditioning phase of the training session should be approximately the same length as the warmup routine. In this way you adjust to reduced physiological demands less abruptly. You also encourage the rapid dissipation of waste products of muscular contraction in the blood. You'll feel better. The key element here is continuation of exercise at a reduced level of intensity. If you've emphasized stretching in your warmup (and you should), then do the same movements while cooling down. If you've

---

[1]James White, personal communication, October 12, 1983.

included calisthenics, then do them in the cooldown period. Stretching should precede calisthenics in the warmup and follow calisthenics in cooldown, since stretching is less arousing physiologically than are calisthenics.

During exercise your heart should be working at approximately 75 percent of its workload. Try to reduce your heart rate to less than 100 beats per minute during the cooldown period. Slow jogging or walking for about 5 to 10 minutes after a training run is a sensible cooldown activity.

CONCLUSION

In this chapter we have defined training and discussed ways in which your body responds to this experience. You learned that there are various methods of training available. Some use different approaches, but all should have a few basic characteristics if they are to be effective in producing desired physiological and psychological results.

Every training session, regardless of method used, should have warmup, conditioning, and cooldown sections. All properly administered training programs should provide positive neuromuscular, cardiovascular, respiratory, and body composition changes. Training should also make you feel good.

SUMMARY

1. The principal components of a training regimen are the warmup, the conditioning period, and the cooldown.
2. A good training regimen emphasizes participation three or more times per week. The target heart rate should be maintained for a total of 30 minutes during the workout.
3. Training may involve changes that are not basically physical. Attitudes, schedule of daily activities, eating and resting habits, as well as type and frequency of social interactions may be revised.
4. Training may affect your psychological as well as your physical status. Such change is intended to produce positive or desirable change.
5. Training should result in a level of personal fitness that is associated with good health.
6. Training increases the size of the heart and the efficiency of nerve impulse transmission.
7. Training results in increased ability of the cardiorespiratory system to distribute oxygen throughout the body.

REFERENCES

AMERICAN COLLEGE OF SPORTS MEDICINE. "The Recommended Quantity and Quality of Exercise for Developing and Maintaining Fitness in Healthy Adults." *Medicine and Science in Sports,* 10(3) (1978): 7-10.

BALOG, L.F. "The Effects of Exercise on Muscle Tension and Subsequent Muscle Relaxation Training." *Research Quarterly for Exercise and Sport* 54 (1983):119-25.

BLAKELAND, F. "Exercise Deprivation." *Archives of General Psychiatry* 22 (1970): 365–369.

CURETON, T.K. "Improvement of Psychological States by Means of Exercise-Fitness Programs." *Journal of the Association of Physical and Mental Rehabilitation* 17 (1963): 14–17.

GRIEST, J.H., M.H. KLEIN, R.R. EISCHENS, J. FARIS, A.S. GURMAN, AND W.P. MORGAN. "Running as Treatment for Depression." *Comparative Psychiatry* 20 (1979): 41–54.

MIKEVIC, P. "Anxiety, Depression and Exercise." *Quest* 33 (1982):140-53.

MORGAN, W.P. "Anxiety Reduction Following Acute Physical Activity." *Psychiatric Annals* 9 (1979).

RANSFORD, C. P. "A Role for Amines in the Antidepressant Effect of Exercise: A Review." *Medicine and Science in Sports and Exercise* 14 (1982): 1–10.

RORST, R. *Athletics and the Heart.* Chicago: Yearbook Medical Publishers, 1987.

4

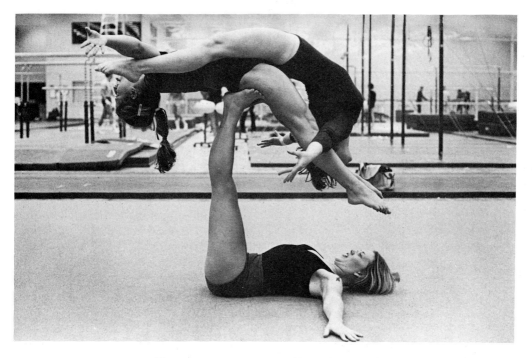

Assessment:
Medical Evaluation
and Fitness Appraisal

Some people are just plain lucky. The comedian George Burns is certainly one of these. In his nineties, George Burns is well known for his perplexing lifestyle—that is, perplexing to everyone but him. His dates with women in their twenties and thirties are notorious; they alone would be enough to tax the health of a man in his sixties. When asked about his unusual appendage—his cigar—Mr. Burns admits to smoking 15 to 20 a day. That alone would have finished most of us off at a much younger age—say, in our seventies. Added to this brew, however, is George Burns's practice of drinking four or five martinis each day. Certainly we would have great difficulty living into our eighth decade under these circumstances. Not surprisingly, when asked what his doctor says about his health-related behavior, George Burns replied: "My doctor's dead."

Stories such as this one often fuel the rationalizations used by some of us to explain our health risk behavior. Yes, some people are just plain lucky. You may be one of them—or you may not be. If you don't want to take the chance of finding out eventually, you'll do something to reduce your health risks now. In this chapter we discuss activities that will provide you with the baseline information you need to begin planning your fitness program. In a subsequent chapter, you will actually use this information to develop your own individualized program. We begin with the need for a medical evaluation.

THE MEDICAL EVALUATION

There is an abundance of literature regarding the need for a medical examination prior to beginning a program of regular exercise. However, not all experts agree on what the medical evaluation should entail, who should be sure to have a medical examination, and whether the examination is necessary at all. We will do our best to present these viewpoints as objectively as possible so you can decide whether a medical evaluation is wise for you.

The Controversy: Is It Needed?

Most physicians state that all those over 40 years of age or those who have previously been sedentary should have an exam. Some disagree (as we shall soon see). Some believe the exam should be comprehensive; others believe it should be more of a screening procedure. We have chosen to ignore individual recommendations for two reasons: first, they are so varied that it would be difficult to make sense of them; and second, because we agree with Dr. Steven Havas, a physician previously with the National Heart, Lung and Blood Institute and now chief of the Bureau of Health Promotion and Disease Prevention of the Connecticut Health Department, when he states: "The fact is that most doctors don't know much about exercise. Medical schools don't teach it" (Ryan, 1981, p. 5). Instead, we will concentrate on the recommendations of authoritative organizational sources.

The American College of Sports Medicine's recommendations are related to the health, status, and age of the participant. They separate individuals who may undergo exercise testing into three categories (American College of Sports Medicine, 1986, p. 2):

1. *Apparently healthy*—those who are apparently healthy and have no major coronary risk factors.
2. *Individuals at higher risk*—those who have symptoms suggestive of possible coronary disease and/or at least one major coronary risk factor.
3. *Individuals with disease*—those with known cardiac, pulmonary, or metabolic disease.

Based upon this classification, the American College of Sports Medicine recommendations appear in Table 4.1.

On the other hand, the National Heart, Lung and Blood Institute advises that most people up to 60 years of age do not need a medical examination prior to beginning a gradual and sensible exercise program (National Heart, Lung, and Blood Institute, 1981). The rationale behind this recommendation is the realization that not exercising regularly is far more dangerous than exercising without a physician's approval and that many people will not seek their physician's approval to exercise and therefore will not exercise regularly if such a recommendation is made.

The commonsense approach is perhaps best summed up as follows (Pollock et al., 1978, p. 76):

> If possible, it would be desirable for all persons to have a complete physical examination . . . prior to their physical fitness evaluation . . . the more information known about a participant before training, the safer and more accurate the exercise prescription.

At best, without a medical examination, certain categories of people are at minimal risk engaging in fitness programs, not at no risk. However, as with most things, only you can decide what is best for you.

Components of the Medical Evaluation

The medical evaluation should include a medical history that asks questions about your own and your family's history of coronary heart disease and as-

Table 4.1
Guidelines for Exercise Testing

	Apparently Healthy		Higher Risk			With Disease
	Below 45	45 and above	Below 35 and no symptoms	35+ no symptoms	Symptoms	Any age
Maximal exercise test recommended prior to an exercise program	No	Yes	No	Yes	Yes	Yes
Physician attendance recommended for maximal testing	No (under 35)	Yes	No	Yes	Yes	Yes
Physician attendance recommended for submaximal testing	No	No	No	Yes	Yes	Yes

Source: American College of Sports Medicine, *Guidelines for Exercise Testing and Prescription* (Philadelphia: Lea and Febiger, 1986), p. 7.

sociated risk factors (for example, hypertension), present illnesses and medications being taken, eating habits, smoking history, current physical activity level, and physical disabilities. The physical examination should include a measurement of blood pressure, listening to the heart's sounds, determining pulse rate, listening to the lungs, and a chest X ray, blood tests for blood fats and for the ratio between high- and low-density lipoproteins, a resting electrocardiogram (ECG), and a graded exercise test (stress test).

The results of the medical evaluation should be discussed with the patient and any restrictions on physical activity or fitness testing identified. Remember: The fact that your physical activity may have limits does not mean it need be eliminated. Try to find regular exercise that meets your fitness needs and that does not otherwise threaten health.

THE FITNESS APPRAISAL

After the medical evaluation, you need an appraisal of your present level of physical fitness. Here is where you need to participate. You will be asked to put this book down and actually assess components of your physical fitness. We will use these assessments—rather *you* will use these assessments—when we come to developing an individualized fitness prescription.

Caution: If you begin to feel chest pains, feel faint or dizzy, develop an excruciating headache, or you can't seem to get enough air, cease the activity immediately. If you experience any other disturbing sensations, also stop right away. If these signs or symptoms appear, you should consider consulting a physician to determine their causes. It may be that you were just so out of shape your body couldn't stand strenuous activity, or there may be something more seriously medically. Rather than worry, check it out and find out for sure.

Cardiorespiratory Assessment

Many exercise programs focus on cardiorespiratory endurance. The publicity surrounding the benefits of exercise for the nation's leading killer (heart disease), whether justified or not, is probably responsible for the emphasis on improving the functioning of the heart, circulatory system, and lungs. If you were to concentrate on only one component of fitness, this is the best one to choose. Exercises that overload the oxygen-transport system (aerobic exercise) lead to an increase in cardiorespiratory endurance and often an increase in strength for selected large muscle groups.

The 1.5-Mile Test.   To assess your cardiorespiratory endurance, you can get out and run or stay indoors. If you can get out, measure a 1.5 mile level route or go to a track where you can run or walk 1.5 miles. Complete that distance as quickly as possible. You can run the whole time or walk some, but in any case, to get an accurate assessment you must attempt to complete that distance as fast as you can. Consult Table 4.2 to determine the cardiorespiratory fitness level at which you are functioning. Remember to determine the desirability of a medical evaluation before this test.

The Harvard Step Test.   An alternate assessment is an old procedure which is as good and as feasible as any developed since. It is called the Harvard Step Test (Brouha, 1943), since it involves stepping up and down. All you need is an 18-inch bench or stool (or something sturdy and close to that height), and a wristwatch with a second hand. Here is the procedure:

1. Step on the bench with one foot and then the other until you are standing erect, and then down with one foot and then the other.
2. Step at a cadence that will result in 30 such repetitions each minute for 4 minutes for females and 5 minutes for males.
3. When the stepping is completed (being sure to straighten the knees), be seated.
4. After one minute of sitting, take your pulse for 30 seconds (if you can get a partner to do this test with you, have your partner take your pulse), and record that number.
5. Wait 30 seconds more, and then take your pulse for the next 30 seconds and record that number.

Table 4.2
1.5-Mile Run Test (Time in minutes)

Fitness Category		13-19	20-29	30-39	40-49	50-59	60+
				Age (years)			
I. Very poor	(men)	>15:31*	>16:01	>16:31	>17:31	>19:01	>20:01
	(women)	>18:31	>19:01	>19:31	>20:01	>20:31	>21:01
II. Poor	(men)	12:11–15:30	14:01–16:00	14:44–16:30	15:36–17:30	17:01–19:00	19:01–20:00
	(women)	16:55–18:30	18:31–19:00	19:01–19:30	19:31–20:00	20:01–20:30	21:00–21:31
III. Fair	(men)	10:49–12:10	12:01–14:00	12:31–14:45	13:01–15:35	14:31–17:00	16:16–19:00
	(women)	14:31–16:54	15:55–18:30	16:31–19:00	17:31–19:30	19:01–20:00	19:31–20:30
IV. Good	(men)	9:41–10:48	10:46–12:00	11:01–12:30	11:31–13:00	12:31–14:30	14:00–16:15
	(women)	12:30–14:30	13:31–15:54	14:31–16:30	15:56–17:30	16:31–19:00	17:31–19:30
V. Excellent	(men)	8:37–9:40	9:45–10:45	10:00–11:00	10:30–11:30	11:00–12:30	11:15–13:59
	(women)	11:50–12:29	12:30–13:30	13:00–14:30	-13:45–15:55	14:30–16:30	16:30–17:30
VI. Superior	(men)	<8:37	<9:45	<10:00	<10:30	<11:00	<11:15
	(women)	<11:50	<12:30	<13:00	<13:45	<14:30	<16:30

* < means "less than"; > means "more than."

Source: From *The Aerobics Program for Total Well-being* by Kenneth H. Cooper, M.D., M.P.H. Copyright © 1982 by Kenneth H. Cooper. Reprinted by permission of Bantam Books. All rights reserved.

6. Last, wait 30 more seconds and then take your pulse for the next 30 seconds and record that number. In other words, you will have taken your pulse between 1 and 1-1/2 minutes after stepping, 2 and 2-1/2 minutes after stepping, and 3 and 3-1/2 minutes after stepping.
7. Using the three pulse counts, compute the following formula:

$$\text{index} = \frac{\text{duration of exercise in seconds x 100}}{\text{2 x sum of the 3 pulse counts in recovery}}$$

Your cardiorespiratory fitness can then be judged using this scale:

Below 55   Poor
55–64   Low average
65–79   Average
80–89   Good
90 and above   Excellent

Now put this book down, assess this component of fitness, and record your appraisal in the Fitness Profile at the end of this chapter.

Muscular Strength Assessment

In the laboratory, muscular strength—or the absolute maximum force that a muscle can generate—can be measured using elaborate and expensive equipment. Dynamometers, cable tensiometers, and force transducers and recorders have all been used this way. For our purposes, we will use a more practical, and yet valid, assessment. One problem with such practical methods, however, is that we need to test numerous muscle groups to obtain an accurate measure of muscular strength. Feasibility dictates testing only several limited muscles: in the legs, the abdomen, and the arms. These muscles cover such diverse body parts that we can safely assume their levels of muscular strength are representative of the total body's strength.

To begin, you need weight-training equipment: a bar and weights that can be attached to it. Start with a level of weight you can comfortably lift and proceed to increase the weight until you have reached the maximum you can lift in one repetition. This one-repetition maximum test should be done for each of the four exercises that follow.

Bench Press.   This exercise measures the strength in the chest, anterior shoulder, and posterior arm muscles. As can be seen in Figure 4.1, you lie on your back on a bench that is approximately 10 to 14 inches wide. Have partners help lower the weight slowly to your chest and then attempt to raise the weight until your arms are straight. The maximum weight you can raise once is your strength score. Record this score on the Fitness Profile at the end of this chapter.

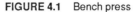

FIGURE 4.1   Bench press

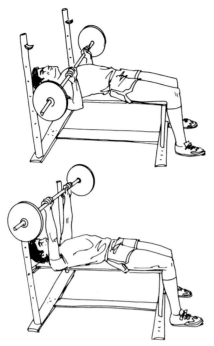

Standing Press.   To test the strength of the muscles of the shoulders and upper arms, stand with the feet shoulder-width apart, with the bar evenly supported up both arms and chest high (see Figure 4.2). Make sure you use an overhand grip, and keep your back straight as you press the weight straight up until your elbows are locked. Record your score on the Fitness Profile.

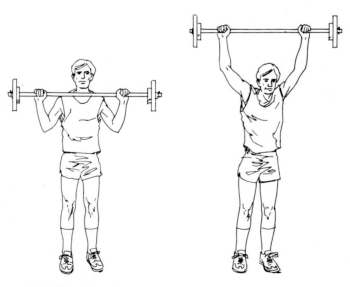

FIGURE 4.2   Standing press

Curl.   To test the anterior arm muscles, stand with your feet shoulder-width apart and the weight held with an underhand grip, at your thigh. Now bring the weight up to your chest by bending your arms (see Figure 4.3), and then lower it again to your thigh. The greatest amount of weight you can curl once should be recorded on the Fitness Profile.

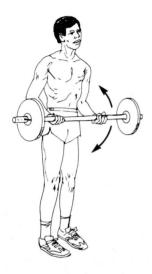

FIGURE 4.3   Curl

Leg Press.   Using a mat to lie on and holding onto the equipment with your hands, press up on the weight with your feet until your legs are straight (see Figure 4.4). Those with back problems should skip this exercise. Record your leg press score on the Fitness Profile. This test measures the strength of the muscles on the front of your upper legs.

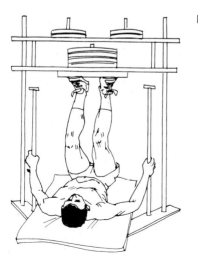

FIGURE 4.4   Leg press

AN ASSESSMENT EXAMPLE: 42-YEAR-OLD BILL

Bill has been sedentary for most of his adult life. Now, approaching the coronary-prone years, he has decided that an ounce of prevention is worth a pound of cure. Consequently, Bill spoke with his physician about beginning a regular program of exercise. His physician classified Bill in the C category of the American College of Sports Medicine's guidelines for exercise testing because Bill was over 35 years old, and physically inactive, and was without coronary heart disease or its risk factors. As a result, Bill needed a complete medical exam prior to organizing for exercise. Bill related his medical history as part of this examination: There was little CHD in his family; there were a few cases of hypertension, but most family members had lived well into their eighties. He was not currently ill or taking any medication, did not smoke, and had no physical disabilities of which he was aware. His physician tested Bill's blood pressure (135/85), took his pulse (80), listened to his lungs and heart, took a chest X ray, tested his blood for blood fats and for the ratio of high- and low-density lipoproteins, and administered a resting electrocardiogram, and a stress test. All these procedures determined Bill to be within normal limits and fit for exercise.

Bill's physician then recommended he consult with a fitness expert and gave him the telephone number of the local university physical education department. When he called, Bill was referred to the fitness program conducted at the university, and an appointment was made for him to be screened.

The screening consisted of Bill's completing a 1.5-mile run/walk on the track to determine his cardiorespiratory endurance; several weight-lifting one-repetition maximum tests to determine his muscular strength; situps and pullups to determine his muscular endurance; shoulder reach, trunk flexion, and trunk extension tests to determine his degree of flexibility; skinfold tests to determine his degree of body fat; and the Illinois agility run to determine how much agility he possessed. The results of these tests were as follows:

1. Run/walk: 14 minutes, 10 seconds (fair)
2. 1-RM tests
   Bench press: 130 pounds (below average)
   Standing press: 90 pounds (below average)
   Curl: 65 pounds (below average)
   Leg press: 325 pounds (average)
3. Situps: 30 (below average)
4. Pullups: 2 (below average)
5. Shoulder reach: 2/0 inches (below average)
6. Trunk flexion: 5 inches (below average)
7. Trunk extension: 6 inches (below average)
8. Skinfold: 18% (average body fat)
9. Agility: 19.5 seconds (average)

Based upon these results, Bill's exercise program emphasized cardiorespiratory endurance (by beginning a walking program, progressing to run/walks, and leading up to jogging), development of greater upper body strength (with bench press, standing press, and curl exercises with low weights progressing to greater weights), muscular endurance (situps beginning with just the head and shoulders lifting off the ground and progressing to the whole upper body lifting, with increasing repetitions, and pullups beginning with flexed-arm hangs), and flexibility (with hamstring, shoulder and chest, and spine and waist stretches).

Because Bill seemed to be a gregarious person, it was recommended he join an ongoing group of exercisers who met at a predetermined time 4 days a week. In that way he would be more apt to maintain his exercise regimen and would also be improving his social health.

Bill was enrolled in this physical fitness program with the confidence of knowing the program was individualized to his capabilities and to his needs. Periodic reassessments would continue to ensure this degree of individualization and Bill's further participation in regular exercise.

Half-Squat.   For those with back problems, an alternative to the leg press is the half-squat. As shown in Figure 4.5, the bar is placed on the shoulders by partners. Your feet should be shoulder-width apart, with toes pointed slightly outward. The head should be kept up and the shoulders unrounded to prevent undue strain on the lower back. Next, lower your body by bending your knees until your buttocks are about the height of the seat of a chair. If you go down lower than that and do a full squat, you could damage your knees. Your score should be recorded on the Fitness Profile.

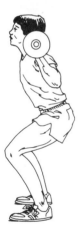

FIGURE 4.5   Half-squats

Muscular Endurance Assessment

There is a big difference between muscular endurance and muscular strength: strength is the maximum that can be done, and endurance is the ability to do continuous muscular work (Berger, 1982, p. 240). We will use three tests of muscular endurance: the situp, the pullup, and the flexed-arm hang.

Situp.   This test measures the endurance of the abdominal muscles and needs a partner to hold your feet. Lying on your back with your feet drawn back to your buttocks until they are flat on the floor and your hands folded across your chest (see Figure 4.6), sit up until your lower back is perpendicular to the floor. Then gently return to the starting position. Your partner should

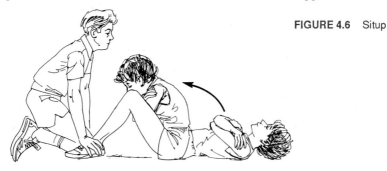

FIGURE 4.6   Situp

keep count of how many situps you can do in 2 minutes, and that number should be recorded in the Fitness Profile.

Pullup.   If you are a man, to measure the muscular endurance of the muscles in the arms, shoulders, and upper back, a bar approximately 1.5 inches in diameter is placed high enough for you to hang from with the arms fully extended and your feet not touching the ground. Grasp the bar with the overhand grip (palms facing away), and hang with the arms and legs fully extended (see Figure 4.7). Next, raise your body until your chin is above the bar and then lower yourself so that your arms are once again fully extended. Record the maximum number of pullups you can do on the Fitness Profile.

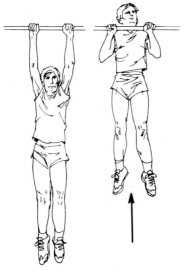

FIGURE 4.7   Pullup

Flexed-Arm Hang.   Some studies have found the pullup to be a poor measure of muscular endurance in women. Consequently, the flexed-arm hang is used to measure the endurance of the arms, shoulders, and upper back muscles in women. A bar similar to that used for the pullup, and at the same height, is grasped with the overhand grip. In this case, however, your body is initially positioned so that it is stationary, with the chin just above the bar (see Figure 4.8). Your score, which should be recorded on the Fitness Profile, is the amount of time (in seconds) you can remain in this position.

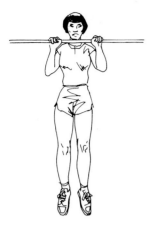

FIGURE 4.8   Flexed-arm hang

Flexibility Assessment

A doctoral student once submitted a draft of her dissertation that was replete with spelling errors. Becoming upset and embarrassed about all the corrections, she shouted: "It's a small mind that can spell a word only one way!" Well, the story may be *stretching* the point (pun intended), but flexibility is an important part of our needs—and certainly of our fitness needs. *Flexibility* is the ability to move the body throughout a range of motion and concerns the stretching of the muscles and tissues around skeletal joints (Berger, 1982, p. 240). We will measure flexibility with three tests: shoulder reach, trunk flexion, and trunk extension.

Shoulder Reach.   Standing against a pole or a projecting corner, raise the right arm and reach down behind your back as far as you can. At the same time, reach up from behind with the left hand and try to overlap the palm of the right hand (see Figure 4.9). Have a partner measure the overlap, or by how much you miss overlapping, to the nearest half-inch. If you overlap, place

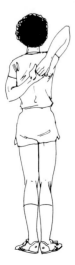

FIGURE 4.9   Shoulder reach

a plus sign in front of the amount of overlap; if you are short of touching fingers, place a minus sign in front of the amount of the gap between the fingers of one hand and those of the other. If the fingers of one hand just barely touch those of the other, score that a zero. Repeat this test with the arms reversed; that is, the one that reached down over the shoulder now reaches up from behind the back. Enter both scores on the Fitness Profile at the end of the chapter.

Trunk Flexion.   To measure the ability to flex the trunk and to stretch the back and the backs of the thigh muscles, sit with your legs straight and your feet flat against a box set against a wall. Place a ruler on top of the box and then stretch over the box (and the ruler) as far as you can (see Figure 4.10). Your score is the number of inches beyond the edge of the box you can stretch (a plus sign in front of that value) or the number of inches short of the edge of the box you can reach (a minus sign in front of that value). Just to the edge of the box is a zero score. You must, however, maintain the stretched position for 3 seconds. Enter your score on the Fitness Profile.

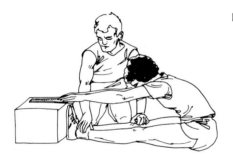

FIGURE 4.10   Trunk flexion

Trunk Extension.   To determine the flexibility of your back, lie on the floor face down with a partner holding your legs and buttocks down (see Figure 4.11). Claps your hands behind your neck and raise your head and chest off the ground (for 3 seconds) as high as you can. Have another partner measure the distance (to the nearest inch) between your chin and the floor. Enter that value on the Fitness Profile.

FIGURE 4.11   Trunk extension

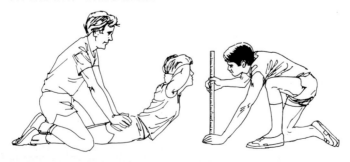

Body Composition Assessment

One of our friends and colleagues, Dr. Jack Osman, goes around the country delivering a lecture called "Fat Is Where It's At." A good speaker, and well informed, Jack is always looking for new ways to help his audience appreciate that the charts listing how much you should weigh for your sex and height (and sometimes body build) are invalid. We were sitting in my office one day when Jack described his latest motivational device.

"I'm going to purchase old bathroom scales from junkyards. They'll probably cost a dollar a piece. Then I'll get a sledgehammer. The first thing I'm going to do after I'm introduced to the audience is use that sledgehammer to whack the hell out of a scale. I'll hit that sucker until it begs for mercy." Jack cares about those he educates. He wants them to know that weight charts do not consider body fat, but rather total weight. A well-developed weightlifter, for instance, may weigh more than the weight chart advised but not be "overfat."

To assess your body composition, you will need to estimate your body's proportion of fat. We will do this using skinfold calipers that you will make following the instructions in Figure 4.12.

FIGURE 4.12   Skinfold measurement

Source: George B. Dintiman and Jerrold S. Greenberg, *Health Through Discovery* (Reading, MA: Addison-Wesley, 1983), p. 188.

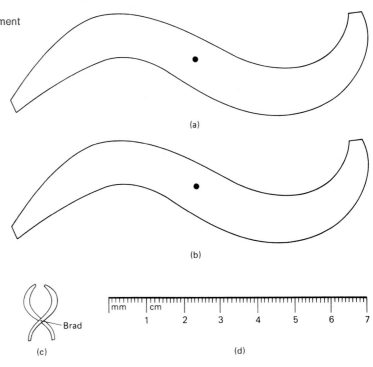

(a)

(b)

Brad

(c)

(d)

Procedures

1. Trace the skinfold calipers (*a*) and (*b*) on a piece of paper.
2. Cut out the traced calipers and paste onto a very stiff piece of cardboard or 1/16 in. plywood backing.
3. Place a brad through the dot in each section of the skinfold calipers as shown in (*c*).
4. After measuring a skinfold, place the calipers on the millimeter scale (*d*).
5. Use the calipers to measure the fat on the body parts listed below. Record the average of three measures on each site.

Men:	Back of the arm (tricep)	_____ mm
	Abdominal	_____ mm
	Chest	_____ mm
Women:	Back of the arm (tricep)	_____ mm
	Iliac crest	_____ mm

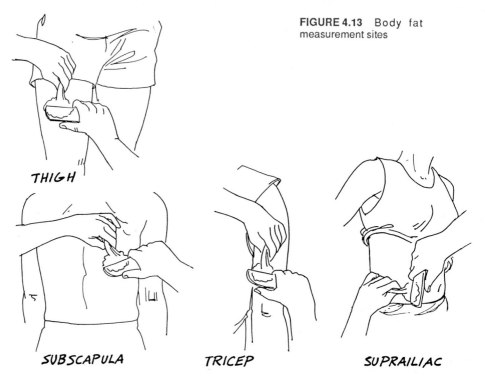

FIGURE 4.13 Body fat measurement sites

THIGH

SUBSCAPULA   TRICEP   SUPRAILIAC

With a partner, if you are a man, measure the body fat on the bottom part of the shoulder blade (subscapula) and the thigh. If you are a woman, measure the body fat at the back of the upper arm (tricep) and the side of the waist (suprailiac) (see Figure 4.13). Be sure to pinch the skin vertically for all measures except at the suprailiac.

The results you get are *estimates* of body fat. To get a more accurate body fat measure, you would need to be weighed while supported underwater (hydrostatic weighing). Since underwater weighing facilities are often unavailable and/or expensive, we have chosen the skinfold measurement as an estimate of body fat.

Motor Skill Assessment

Your *motor skill* refers to your ability in various physical activities. Included in this category are speed, power, balance, agility, reaction time, and coordination (Getchell, 1983, p. 63). Given our interests and limitations, we will measure only agility, since that trait seems a vital one for motor proficiency. To begin, mark off a course, as shown in Figure 4.14.

Use chairs or cones where the four squares are marked (10 feet apart from each other). Start lying on the floor on your stomach, with your hands placed on the floor just under your shoulders. At the signal, jump to your feet and follow the course, completing it as quickly as possible. Your score is the time it takes to complete the course (to the nearest tenth of a second). Record that value on the Fitness Profile. Make sure not to touch the chairs as you go around them.

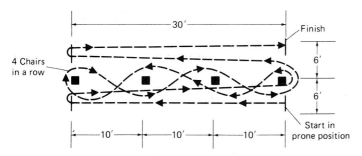

FIGURE 4.14   Illinois agility run

Source: T.K. Cureton, *Physical Fitness Workbook* (Urbana, IL: Stipes Publishing Co., 1944) p. 24.

AN ASSESSMENT EXAMPLE: 66-YEAR-OLD JOAN

Joan was older than Bill, and her fitness profile differed in some respects. Her physician classified Joan in the D category of the American College of Sports Medicine's guidelines for exercise testing because she was asymptomatic, physically inactive, had no coronary diseases, but did have a high cholesterol level and elevated blood pressure readings. Joan's medical history was without incident except for her 20-year-old cigarette smoking habit, and her screenings revealed only the concern for her hypercholesteremia and hypertension.

She too was put in touch with the local university's physical fitness program. When tested, her results were

1. Run/walk: 21 minutes (poor)
2. Situps: 31 (below average)
3. Shoulder reach: 3 inches (average)
4. Trunk flexion: 8 inches (average)
5. Trunk extension: 16 inches (average)
6. Skinfold: 32% (above-average fat)

It was determined to withhold the muscular strength and agility testing at this time, since the concern was to devise a program to respond to the hypercholesteremia and the hypertension. Consequently, an aerobic exercise program would be needed, and to develop one required a determination of Joan's present endurance fitness. It was decided to test flexibility as well, since the program the fitness experts had in mind had a tendency to result in less flexibility and thus possible injury.

The analysis of Joan's fitness testing concluded she needed to develop cardiovascular and muscular endurance and to decrease her body fat. Her flexibility was just fine.

Based upon these findings, a program was developed to get Joan jogging. Jogging has a tendency to burn up calories, strengthen muscles, improve the ratio of high- and low-density lipoproteins, and decrease blood pressure. To begin, however, and because Joan's run/walk test placed her in the poor category, she was instructed to walk 4 days a week for a distance that did not exhaust her (perhaps 1.5 miles initially) and gradually work up to a slow jog after several weeks or months. When she could begin jogging would be determined by how Joan felt walking and by her target heart rate.

Prior to jogging, however, Joan was instructed to walk some and jog some of her route. The program, then, progressed gradually from walking, to walking some and jogging some, to jogging. Joan was told though that even if she stayed at the walking stage and could do that while maintaining her target heart rate, she would be benefiting physically.

In addition to the walk/run program, Joan was instructed on which stretches to do before and after each exercise session. In that way she could maintain a satisfactory level of flexibility.

Since it has been found that regular exercisers tend not to smoke cigarettes, it was hoped that Joan would give up her habit. In particular, aerobic exercise is incompatible with cigarette smoking. However, to be assured to responding to Joan's high cholesterol and blood pressure, her physician recommended she enroll in a stop-smoking program and also put her in touch with a registered dietitian who would develop a diet for her.

All things considered, Joan was well on her way to taking greater control of her health. With the support of loved ones, the fitness program personnel, the dietitian, the stop-smoking staff, and her physician, we can expect that Joan's health will soon improve—especially if *she* is committed to that goal.

YOUR FITNESS PROFILE: A STEP TOWARD WELLNESS

At this point, your Fitness Profile should have recorded on it your cardiorespiratory, muscular strength, muscular endurance, flexibility, body composition, and motor skills scores. Now, let's interpret these scores. Consult Table 4.2 and the ratings presented earlier for the Harvard Step Test index and place a check mark on the Fitness Profile that rates these scores as poor, average, or above average.

Next, consult Table 4.3 to interpret your muscular strength scores. If you lifted more than 10 pounds over the optimal strength values for your body

Table 4.3

Optimal Strength Values for Various Body Weights (based on the 1-RM test)[*],[†]

Body Weight	Bench Press		Standing Press		Curl		Leg Press	
(lb)	Male	Female	Male	Female	Male	Female	Male	Female
80	80	56	53	37	40	28	160	112
100	100	70	67	47	50	35	200	140
120	120	84	80	56	60	42	240	168
140	140	98	93	65	70	49	280	196
160	160	112	107	75	80	56	320	224
180	180	126	120	84	90	63	360	252
200	200	140	133	93	100	70	400	280
220	220	154	147	103	110	77	440	308
240	240	168	160	112	120	84	480	336

[*] *Note:* Data collected on Universal Gym apparatus. Information collected on other apparatus could modify results.

[†] Data expressed in pounds.

Source: Michael L. Pollock, Jack H. Wilmore, and Samuel M. Fox, *Health and Fitness Through Physical Activity* (New York: John Wiley, 1978), p. 106.

weight, check "Above average"; if 10 pounds were under the optimal strength values, check "Below average"; and if within 10 pounds, check "Average". For those who did the half-squat instead of the leg press, if you lifted more than 10 pounds over two-thirds of your body weight, score that above average; less than 10 pounds of two-thirds your body weight, below average; and within 10 pounds, average. For your muscular endurance ratings, see Table 4.4. For your flexibility ratings, see Table 4.5.

Table 4.4
Muscular Endurance Interpretations

	Situps (No.) Men/Women	Pullups (No.)	Flexed-Arm Hang (sec.)
Above average	69+/58+	9+	27+
Average	44–68/40–57	3–8	15–26
Below average	0–44/0–40	0–2	0–14

Table 4.5
Flexibility Interpretations

	Shoulder Reach (Rup/Lup)	Trunk Flexion	Trunk Extension
For Men			
Above average	6+/3+	11+	15+
Average	4–5/0–2	7–10	8–14
Below average	Below 4/below 0	Below 7	Below 8
For Women			
Above average	7+/6+	12+	23+
Average	5–6/0–5	7–11	15–22
Below average	Below 5/below 0	Below 7	Below 15

To interpret your body composition scores, use Figure 4.15 if you are a woman or Figure 4.16 if you are a man, and place a mark on the two sidebars to indicate your skinfold measures for those sites. Then draw a straight line connecting these two measures, and you will have your body density (body weight divided by body volume) and your percentage of body fat. Once you obtain your percentage of body fat, consult Table 4.6 to interpret that score.

To interpret your motor skill (agility) score, use the following classifications:

1. Above-average agility   17.0 seconds or less
2. Average agility   17.5–21.5 seconds
3. Below-average agility   More than 22 seconds

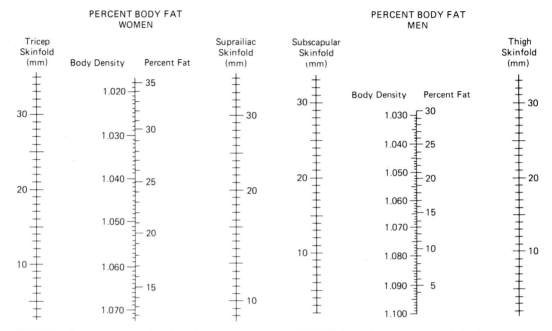

FIGURE 4.15   Percentage of body fat for women   **FIGURE 4.16**   Percentage of body fat for men

Sources: For body density, A.W. Sloan et al., *Journal of Applied Physiology* 17 (1962):967. For percent body fat, J.F. Brozek et al., *Annals of the New York Academy of Science* 101 (1963):113.

Table 4.6
Body Composition Interpretation

	Women (%)	Men (%)
Above-average fat	27+	20+
Average fat	20–26	13–19
Below-average fat	Below 20	Below 13

CONCLUSION

Now your Fitness Profile is complete. You can evaluate your physical fitness in absolute terms (are you satisfied with your levels of each component?) or in relative terms (are you happy with how you compare with others?). Wellness requires information. Where are you now? Where do you want to be? How can you get there? Now that you have your current fitness level, you can decide on what goals you will set for yourself. For example, if you are not satisfied with your cardiorespiratory fitness, read the remainder of this book with a view toward improving that component. Or for muscular strength and endurance, flexibility, body composition, or motor skill. We have included means for you to be successful at enhancing your level of physical fitness. All you need do is apply them. But remember that improving one aspect of your health (or fitness) should not mean a diminishing of another component. Keep that ride smooth; keep that tire round. Then you will have improved your physical fitness with a wellness approach.

YOUR PHYSICAL FITNESS PROFILE

Directions: As you complete each test, place your score where requested. After all tests are completed, consult the latter part of this chapter for the means of determining the ratings for your scores.

I. Cardiorespiratory Fitness
A. 1.5-Mile Test
Score _____

Rating (check one):
_____ Very poor
_____ Poor
_____ Fair
_____ Good
_____ Excellent
_____ Superior

B. Harvard Step Test
Index _____

Rating (check one):
_____ Poor
_____ Low average
_____ Average
_____ Good
_____ Excellent

II. Muscular Strength
A. Bench Press
Amount lifted _____

Rating (check one):
_____ Below average
_____ Average
_____ Above average

B. Standing Press
Amount lifted _____

Rating (check one):
_____ Below average
_____ Average
_____ Above average

C. Curl
Amount lifted _____

Rating (check one):
_____ Below average
_____ Average
_____ Above average

D. Leg Press
Amount lifted _____

Rating (check one):
_____ Below average
_____ Average
_____ Above average

E. Half-Squat
Amount lifted _____

Rating (check one):
_____ Below average
_____ Average
_____ Above average

III. Muscular Endurance
A. Situps
Number done _____

Rating (check one):
_____ Below average
_____ Average
_____ Above average

B. Pullups (Men)
Number done _____

Rating (check one):
_____ Below average
_____ Average
_____ Above average

C. Flexed-Arm Hang (Women)
Seconds hung _____

Rating (check one):
_____ Below average
_____ Average
_____ Above average

IV. Flexibility
A. Shoulder reach
Score _____

Rating (check one):
_____ Below average
_____ Average
_____ Above average

B. Trunk Flexion
Score _____

Rating (check one):
_____ Below average
_____ Average
_____ Above average

C. Trunk Extension
Score _____

Rating (check one):
_____ Below average
_____ Average
_____ Above average

V. Body Composition
Percent Body Fat _____

Rate (check one):
_____ Above-average fat
_____ Average fat
_____ Below-average fat

VI. Motor Skill (Agility)
Time _____

Rating (check one):
_____ Below-average agility
_____ Average agility
_____ Above-average agility

VII. Summary
   A. List those components of physical fitness for which you rated:
      1. Above Average

           _____

           _____

           _____

      2. Average

           _____

           _____

           _____

      3. Below Average

           _____

           _____

           _____

SUMMARY

1. Not all experts agree whether everyone starting an exercise program should obtain a medical examination.
2. Even when there is agreement regarding the need to have a medical examination before starting an exercise program, there may be disagreement among the experts as to what that examination should entail.
3. Possible components of the medical examination include taking a medical history, measurement of blood pressure, listening to the heart's sounds, determining the pulse rate, listening to the lungs, taking a chest X ray, administering a resting electrocardiogram and a graded exercise test (stress test), and administering blood tests for blood fats and for the ratio between high- and low-density lipoproteins.
4. The physical fitness appraisal includes measures of cardiorespiratory endurance, muscular strength and endurance, flexibility, body composition, and motor skill.
5. Cardiorespiratory endurance can be measured by a 1.5-mile test or the Harvard Step Test.
6. Muscular strength can be determined by the bench press, standing press, curl, leg press, and half squat.
7. Muscular endurance can be determined by the situp, pullup, and the flexed-arm hang.
8. Flexibility can be determined by the shoulder reach, trunk flexion, and trunk extension.
9. Body composition can be estimated by use of underwater weighing (hydrostatic weighing) or by taking skinfold measures at various body locations.

10. Motor skills (speed, power, balance, agility, reaction time, and coordination) can be estimated by measuring agility (a trait that seems a vital one for motor efficiency). Agility can be determined by administering the Illinois Agility Run.

REFERENCES

AMERICAN COLLEGE OF SPORTS MEDICINE. *Guidelines for Exercise Testing and Prescription.* Philadelphia: Lea and Febiger, 1986.

BERGER, RICHARD A. *Applied Exercise Physiology.* Philadelphia: Lea and Febiger, 1982.

BROUHA, LUCIEN. "The Step Test: A Simple Method of Testing the Physical Fitness of Boys." *Research Quarterly* 14 (1943): 23.

GETCHELL, BUD. *Physical Fitness: A Way of Life.* New York: John Wiley, 1983.

NATIONAL HEART, LUNG AND BLOOD INSTITUTE. *Exercise and Your Heart.* Washington, DC; U.S. Public Health Service, 1981.

POLLOCK, MICHAEL L., JACK H. WILMORE, AND SAMUEL M. FOX. *Health and Fitness Through Physical Activity.* New York: John Wiley, 1978.

RYAN, BILL. "The Government's Surprising New Position: It May Be Okay to Start Exercising Without Seeing a Doctor First." *Parade*, November 15, 1981.

5

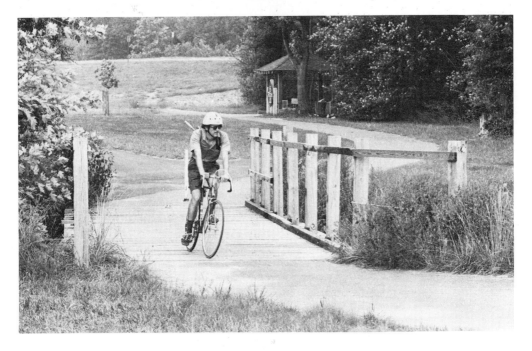

How to Get Where You Want to Be: Choices

1. To be able to identify the important criteria for choosing an appropriate activity.
2. To know how often and how long you should participate in physical activity.
3. To be able to discuss factors that limit participation in exercise.

Let's assume that you are a person in search of activity. You've never participated much in outdoor or indoor games, sport or exercise. And now you're ready for action. You've bought the argument that exercise will be good for you. Chapters 1 through 4 have convinced you of the benefits of physical activity.

What's your cup of tea? A little heavy body contact, as in wrestling, football or basketball? Or are the stimulating and risk-taking aspects of rock climbing, sky diving, or scuba diving your thing? Perhaps racket sports such as tennis, squash, or paddleball are for you. Do you enjoy the sensation of speed, or the wind whistling through your hair and assaulting your face? Then maybe you want cycling or downhill skiing. Perhaps activity that combines an esthetic dimension with solitude and vigorous movement is what you're looking for. If so, cross-country skiing or backpacking may be it.

MAKING A CHOICE OF ACTIVITY

What should you choose? Remember the sporting goods store in the neighborhood or the town where you grew up? Or the section of your local department or hardware store devoted to sporting goods? As a young child you may have absolutely reveled in the opportunity to browse in these places. Baseball gloves, dumbbells, roller skates, surfboards, bicycles, rowboats: equipment galore to delight the young and titillate the fantasies of the not so young. When we were kids, the sporting goods store and the bakery probably ranked highest of all on our list of favorite stores to visit. For many of us, this priority is still valid.

Now that you're ready for exercise, you're faced with some important decisions. Among the first is what activity to choose. But don't let this decision overwhelm you. Your choice doesn't have to be final or etched in stone. You can try on an activity for size and, if it doesn't work, try on another. Find someone who participates in an activity that interests you. Ask questions about it, observe this person engaging in the activity, borrow his or her equipment and try it out. The library is loaded with books on almost every sport, game, and physical activity you can imagine. If you can spell it, you can find it somewhere in the library or bookstore. Many of the books are of the "how to" variety and contain diagrams and photographs of basic techniques, movements, and skills. Your local recreation department probably offers a full range of activities with free or very modestly priced instructional fees, conducted during evening or after-school hours. So do the YMCA, Boys Clubs, and other similar service organizations.

Some Criteria

The really important thing is to make a selection and get started. Here are some criteria to consider when choosing an appropriate activity.

Enjoyment.   Select something that carries a high probability of being enjoyable. Think about past experiences that have been fun for you, and see if you can think of a sport or activity that is close. If you very much like to be with other people and to talk while you perform, don't select swimming or skydiving (you can't talk). If manipulating balls or objects, where accuracy and motor control are important, produces anxiety, stay away from basketball, juggling, or handball. There are plenty of other terrific activities.

Cost.   Check into necessary expenses for an activity before making a commitment. Remember, equipment purchasing or rental costs can be prohibitively high in some cases. Jogging and jumping rope are cheap; skiing is not. Tennis may involve some sort of club membership in some communities.

Previous Experiences.   You can often borrow or transfer skills learned in one area to another. Therefore, it is not necessary to enter an activity as a rank beginner even if it is new to you. If you've previously played squash, you might easily take to racketball or badminton. If you've played high school football, you might find that your college or community rugby club is worth looking into.

Social Aspects.   Give some thought to your interest in being with others when you exercise. Do you need and desire the company of others? Are you looking for new social contacts? Most activities provide opportunity for meeting new acquaintances and establishing friendships, but certain ones do this better than others. Backpacking is usually done alone or in groups. Sometimes someone will organize an expedition of people who know one another casually. Tennis usually requires preestablished relationships, but finding someone to chat with while you exercise at your YMCA or health club should be easy.

Level of Readiness.   How much preparation is necessary for you to be ready for participation? Are you able realistically to meet the physical and psychological demands of the beginning stages of activity *now*? Or is some degree of training necessary. If so, how much? Do you have time to get ready to enter the activity safely?

Participation Time.   Do you have blocks of time necessary to participate in the activity to the extent that tradition and rules dictate or playing partners expect? For example, golf is time consuming: 18 or even 9 holes require hours of play. Tennis also presents a time problem. It may be difficult to find a partner who is willing to play for 15 or 30 minutes (assuming that is what you want). Rock climbing, swimming, and scuba diving may involve transporting yourself to appropriate locations, which can be very time consuming. But you can jog, cycle, skip rope, or do calisthenics to your heart's content within a time frame that suits you.

EVELYN: BUILDING A PROGRAM AROUND A CAREER

Evelyn, who is in her late twenties, has intended to start a regular exercise program for some time.

Evelyn has recently been promoted to the vice presidency of a large company and earns a high salary. She is interested in establishing new social relationships with men and women of her own life-style and interests.

Evelyn is an avid skier. Among her important objectives is to prepare her large leg muscles and increase her cardiorespiratory efficiency for the forthcoming skiing season. Evelyn is looking for a training program whose workouts can be accomplished in short blocks of time. She is product oriented and seeks clearly definable results.

Evelyn's professional responsibilities often require that she remain in her office until 7 P.M. She is frequently at work on Saturdays. Few of her acquaintances have similar schedules, and it is therefore difficult for her to arrange sport or exercise dates. She has tried being part of volleyball and softball teams, but she was absent from too many practice sessions and games. Her professional responsibilities similarly interfere with tennis and racketball arrangements.

A private health club or community recreational center near her office would serve Evelyn's needs nicely. Such places are usually open late in the evening, and membership fees are not likely to be a deterrent for Evelyn.

Other exercisers with whom Evelyn might interact are likely to have daily professional schedules that are compatible with hers.

Circuit training makes sense for Evelyn. It would enable her to use a variety of movements and exercises that could be related to her fitness goals. Rapid movement from one station to another would place demands on her cardiorespiratory system. Progress would be easy to monitor by maintaining a record of her repetitions and the total amount of time necessary for their completion. Moreover, Evelyn would be able to predict reasonably accurately the amount of time necessary to complete her workout. She could begin her training any time she arrived at the exercise facility. Approximately 20 minutes of circuit training should provide a productive and challenging training session.

Health clubs and community recreation centers usually have weight-training facilities and various kinds of resistance-training equipment. Evelyn's circuit would include stations that emphasize development of leg strength and endurance (leg pressing, rope skipping, partial squats).

HOW OFTEN SHOULD YOU EXERCISE?

Obviously, some of the criteria used to select an appropriate type of activity are also applicable when thinking about how often you will exercise.

Time constraints, your ability to meet the financial demands of certain sports or activities, and your personal level of fitness or readiness to participate by and large determine the frequency with which you will exercise.

Imagine that you've just come off the tennis court on a beautiful Saturday morning. The weather is perfect. You've played very well, and you've enjoyed the company of your opponent. Her skill level was close to your own, and her congeniality made you feel comfortable. Not only was she fair and honest in calling "outs," "lets," "nets," and "faults," but she was supportive of your efforts. When you made a nice return, she said so; when you fired an ace into her service box she smiled in acknowledgment. She won, but the match was close. You really had a terrific morning and as you walk off the court you can't help but think how much you'd like to recreate the experience as soon as possible (next time you'll win).

If your interests are essentially social and recreational, by all means play again as soon as you can. If a hefty court fee is involved, temper your appetite for tennis in accordance with your purse. Or find an inexpensive backup court on which to play occasionally. Plan in advance to make necessary arrangements. The weather, court, and partner availability are probably important considerations that will influence frequency. But by all means, play again as soon as you can.

If your goals emphasize preparation for serious competition or tournament play, then participation assumes the proportions of training. Regularity and structure become overriding influences in your tennis activity. Here, the recreational component is subordinated to the hard work and dedication typically associated with training. Pleasure will be delayed until success in competition can be achieved. Your frequency of exercise or play depends on your goals. Are they purely social and recreational, or do they include a competitive component?

Bear in mind that competition can also be recreational. A good case in point is the very popular weekend road race frequently held in innumerable communities across the nation. Most participants run to best previous times, win a T-shirt, or perhaps beat a friend or two. Their primary motivation seems to be fun. A small hard core of runners actually aspire to win all the marbles.

These different goals reflect different preparatory experiences. If an age-group victory is your quest, then training is an essential prerequisite. Perhaps a 6- or 7-day per week training schedule with some twice-a-day workouts is indicated. The T-shirt runner, in comparison, may take to the roads three or four times a week and permit the physical beauty of the running trail or the clear, blue sky rather than the stopwatch to dominate the run.

As we noted in Chapter 3, training means a strong commitment to regular participation. Recreational exercise, with modest fitness goals, involves less stringent regularity in participation. Tournament tennis players probably need 6 or 7 days of play a week. Recreational players are bound only by the

KEN: TRAINING FOR TOURNAMENT PLAY

Ken works in a meatpacking plant. His passion is handball, which he plays in weekend tournaments. He is a skilled player; he executes a large repertoire of shots very well.

Ken is finished with his workday at approximately 3 P.M., when he likes to go to the courts for about an hour and a half before heading home. Ken's arms and upper body are well developed because of his handling large and heavy sides of beef. However, he realizes that to improve his performance on the handball court, he must strengthen his abilities to move quickly and to generate short bursts of speed on rapid demand.

Interval training would satisfy Ken's specific training needs. Fifty-yard sprints at approximately three-quarter to full speed would be alternated with jogging for about 100 yards. Three bouts of sprinting and jogging would comprise a set. Two such sets with a rest between (walking or stretching) three times a week would suffice. Ultimately, more sets could be added to the routine. A nearby running track, gymnasium, or flat, even surface such as a deserted road would be an adequate facility for Ken's training. In order to provide the opportunity to train in this manner a few days a week, Ken would relinquish some of his handball playing time. Since his athletic skills are highly developed, he would do well to cultivate speed and anaerobic fitness. In the long run, he is likely to be a more effective tournament competitor.

constraints of their personal schedules, availability of playing partners, costs associated with court rentals, and so on. But these factors are realistic deterrents to daily play. Fitness joggers probably need to get out three times a week for about 30 to 40 minutes to satisfy their goals (cardiovascular efficiency and body weight maintenance). Competitive runners, on the other hand, run 6 or 7 days a week on a planned schedule in which distance, intensity, and speed are emphasized.

So you see, before answering the question "How often should I exercise?" ask, "Why do I wish to participate in this activity?" If your answer is enjoyment, fun, or recreation, then the frequency of participation is likely to be less than if your answer indicates preparation for a particular event or competition. You'd probably be surprised to learn that fairly high degrees of fitness for health and wellness can be achieved by exercising for approximately a half-hour, three days a week.

Now let's put a few of the things we've just mentioned into a personal perspective. Answer the following questions to determine how often you should exercise.

1. What are your most important exercise goals?

   _____

   _____

   _____

2. What forms of exercise do you prefer?

_____

_____

_____

3. When was the last time you participated in regular exercise?

_____

_____

_____

4. How much time do you have during the day to devote to exercise?

_____

_____

_____

Answers to these questions should be helpful in leading you to an understanding of your individual exercise program's general shape and form.

HOW LONG SHOULD YOU EXERCISE?

Very young children usually do not need encouragement to play. They seem to find and even make opportunities for participation in games and playful activities. And by playing, kids exercise. No one has to tell a typical 6- to 10-year-old child to play (unless the child's presence is not desired and an effort is being made on behalf of adults to secure privacy). But adult intervention is often necessary in helping the child terminate the period of play or exercise. In a word, sometimes kids don't know when to stop. Older children, teenagers, and even adults occasionally need reminders about when to stop playing and exercising. Basically, an exerciser must *learn* about appropriate stopping points.

In previous chapters we've extolled the benefits of physical activity, and if its virtues are indeed defensible, then it's not difficult to understand how disengagement may be a problem at times. Exercise has the capacity for being an exciting and enjoyable experience, but most good things should come at least to a temporary end.

Fatigue

Perhaps the most influential factor limiting participation in exercise is *fatigue*. There are two kinds of fatigue: physiological and psychological. The former relates to internal chemical and metabolic changes that occur as a consequence of prolonged exercise (or many repetitions of a particular movement); and the latter, to perceptions and intellectual awareness of these changes. Training increases performance time before the onset of physiological fatigue. Although the effects on psychological fatigue are less well known, it is likely that it too is delayed by training.

The buildup of waste products due to muscular contraction and depletion of fuel supplies in the muscles needed for contraction causes inhibition of further muscular contraction. What this means is that when your skeletal muscles become biochemically *tired*, legs and arms feel heavy, and a sensation of weariness develops. It becomes increasingly difficult to continue your activity. The muscles function with less efficiency, and your control of them is diminished. This is why athletes are temporarily replaced during a game in team sports. Coaches "go to the bench" to provide reprieves for tired players. Tired players perform at less than optimal levels, and they are also vulnerable to injury.

But if no parent or coach is available to make decisions for you, then *you* must understand the telltale signs of fatigue; you must learn when it's time to stop.

It is important to understand your limitations and to anticipate your personal appropriate stopping time even before you feel the sensation of physiological fatigue. The idea is to avoid dramatic decreases in performance efficiency, accuracy, enjoyment, or safety as a result of fatigue. Fatigue is unavoidable, but if you can anticipate its arrival and stop or alter your performance in some sensible fashion, then you are in effect preventing its effects.

Fatigue is real, so be prepared to deal with it. Training and the confidence it generates can lengthen the distance between physiological and psychological fatigue. That is, as a result of training you may develop a sort of complacency or acceptance about early sensations of fatigue. You don't panic; your performance doesn't fall apart. You are familiar with what you are feeling. You recognize the symptoms of fatigue and act accordingly. Training helps you learn to spread out your energy during your exercise so that you have enough reserve to carry you through to completion.

Of course, the higher your level of readiness for physical activity (fitness), the longer you will be able to exercise. The longer you have been involved in training, the longer you will be able to perform before physical fatigue sets in. But unless you are preparing for an unusually demanding physical experience (such as Olympic trials or National Football League training camp) you probably need to exercise for a shorter duration than you believe to satisfy adequate fitness goals. If you wish to attain a fairly high degree of cardiovascular fitness, jogging for about 30 minutes a few days a week will do it. If muscular strength is your concern, approximately 10 repetitions of each of a few selected movements done three times (each group of 10 is a set) will be adequate.

In simple and direct terms: *You don't have to kill yourself to get into shape.* Regularity of exercise and tuning in to what your body is telling you about biochemical changes are, however, very important. If you haven't learned to identify and understand the signs of fatigue, you're headed for trouble.

Extending your exercise bouts beyond an optimal duration may encourage the onset of fatigue. The result is reduced enjoyment, lower motivation for exercise, and vulnerability to injury. (We will talk about injury prevention in considerable depth in Chapter 13.)

Prescriptions for precise lengths of exercise bouts for all individuals in all kinds of activities cannot be prudently made. In addition to some forms of exercise being more strenuous than others, some obviously require longer periods of time to complete. For example, if you are a cyclist, you can very well determine the distance or amount of time you will spend pedaling on a given day. But if you are a racketball player, you cannot accurately predict the amount of time necessary to finish a match. Unless you can convince a friend to play for a specified number of minutes, you are obliged to remain on the court until the match is over. Nonetheless, you must learn when you have overextended yourself, when you have reached your limit for safe, enjoyable competition. Even if this point is reached in the middle of a match, it may be best to withdraw.

Stress

As a rule of thumb, if your goals are recreational, social, and/or health-related, stop exercising when the activity ceases to be fun, invigorating, stimulating, or exciting. A bit of physical stress is typically a necessary accompaniment to exercise. So don't use awareness of stress per se as a criterion for withdrawing from activity. In fact, for many persons it is precisely their reaction to moderate physical stressors that make an activity fun and exciting. And if your exercise takes the form of athletic competition, you'll undoubtedly have to deal with a number of psychological stressors. But when your stress reactions become srong, bothersome, or overwhelming, it may be time to modify or stop the exercise. It's better to withdraw a little early than a little late.

Perceived Exertion

About 25 years ago, Swedish psychologist Gunnar Borg introduced the concept of perceived exertion. This notion suggests that you are capable of making subjective evaluations about the intensity of work (in this case, exercise). Therefore, use such evaluative approaches to help you determine your exercise effort. Your effort may be high without necessarily experiencing fatigue. In fact it may be arousing and invigorating. The point is that you should be able to judge your level of exercise intensity and use this information to evaluate your progress.

HOW MUCH EFFORT DO YOU EXPEND?

"When the going gets tough, the tough get going," "No pain, no gain," "Winning isn't everything, it's the only thing." The world of professional football is famous for its slogans and mottos, which are often flaunted as guiding principles in all kinds of sports and physical activities, at all levels of age and skill. Unfortunately, many of them are invalid or at least inappropriate for many exercise participants. As we have tried to point out, not all those who exercise are necessarily committed to serious training programs; moreover, not all who are so committed are preparing for professional or very high levels of competition.

Don't permit these mottos to become your modus operandi without a careful evaluation of your goals and aspirations. Many of us are not destined for careers as professional athletes, nor do all of us desire such a future. A great deal of skill improvement, insight into competitive sports strategy, comradeship, fun, and of course enhanced wellness can be derived through exercise without physical pain, mental anguish, or physiological exhaustion. In fact, you would do well to avoid these responses altogether. If your intensity of exercise does yield these reactions, chances are you are sacrificing many of the positive payoffs we have been continually emphasizing in this book. Pain, anguish, and exhaustion are probably not good supporters of wellness (although, admittedly, they are not necessarily always deterrents).

On the other hand, complete comfort and ease of movement will not always characterize your exercise performance. But as your skill and fitness levels improve, efficiency, grace, confidence, and overall motor proficiency will increase.

Most of us expend considerably less than maximum effort when we exercise. First, as an activity becomes more and more aerobic (performed in the presence of oxygen, such as jogging), the likelihood of sustained maximal effort decreases proportionately. Maximal effort can be sustained for only very brief periods of time. But explosive movements such as those found in shot putting, weightlifting, or high jumping may occur at extremely high levels of effort. If you don't exert maximal effort in these activities, your achievements, measured in the traditional fashion (feet, yards, inches), will be less than impressive. In endurance activities you cannot afford to prolong maximal effort; you won't last if you do.

Many of the exercise forms in which we engage are not entirely aerobic or anaerobic (performed in the absence of oxygen), but somewhere in between. When this is the case, the idea is to find a level of performance intensity that provides the greatest amount of "efficiency." *Pace* is the term we use to control rate of performance. When you shovel snow in the driveway, you intuitively select a pace you can maintain until the job is completed. You make observations about certain of your responses to the demands of the exercise (heart rate, breathing rate, and overall feeling of comfort or difficulty). Then you use this feedback to adjust your performance rate. If you work too fast, you will be obliged to quit early. If you shovel too slowly, you'll never get done.

Your target heart rate indicates how hard you should work during exercise in order to build heart-lung endurance. To obtain the best cardiorespiratory training effect, exercise so your heart beats that fast.

The psychological facts we discussed earlier also enter our present analysis. Motivation, aspiration, self-esteem, and body image are instrumental in determining the amount of effort we expend during exercise. If you are well motivated to exercise—that is, if you attach considerable importance to what you are doing and have a good understanding of your reasons for doing it—your effort may very well be maintained at comparatively high levels of intensity. You will be able to do more, when and if you think of yourself as a competent performer whose body is well suited to the demands of the activity. And, of course, training will produce organic changes that support your self-confidence. When you are fit, and you know it, you begin to behave like a fit person. When this happens, you can exercise more. See Appendix D for a position statement by the American College of Sports Medicine (ACSM) on the *Recommended Quantity and Quality of Exercise for Developing and Maintaining Fitness in Healthy Adults*. Some of these recommendations with regard to intensity of exercise are included in Chapter 3.

CONCLUSION

In this chapter we have discussed important decisions you must make about your exercise program. The extent to which your program will yield beneficial results depends upon a number of factors.

Choosing an activity you like is an important primary step. Enjoyment, previous experience, and your level of readiness are additional considerations, as are frequency and duration of exercise. Avoiding and managing fatigue and stress are particularly important. The degree of effort you should expend during exercise is yet another important consideration in making good choices.

SUMMARY

1. Choices regarding the activity you choose to incorporate into an exercise program need not be etched in stone. If you find that choice was a mistake, select a different activity using the feedback you learned from your original choice.
2. Choose an exercise activity that can be done by observing other people and asking them questions; with the help of books from the library; or by contacting your local recreation department, YMCA, Boys Club, or other similar organization.
3. Criteria for selecting an exercise activity include the amount of enjoyment it can provide, its cost, any previous experience you have with it, its social aspects, your level of readiness, and the amount of time necessary for participation.
4. The amount of time you should exercise relates to your exercise goals. If you are exercising for social reasons, participate as often as you can. If you are exercising for competition, then time must be set aside regularly and training should be highly structured.
5. When selecting an exercise, you should evaluate that exercise's fatigue- and stress-generating aspects.
6. There are two kinds of fatigue: physiological and psychological. Physiological fatigue involves internal and biological changes. Psychological fatigue involves perceptions and intellectual awareness of physiological fatigue states.

7. The buildup of waste products due to muscular contraction and depletion of fuel supplies in the muscle needed for contraction causes inhibition of further muscular contraction.

8. When your reactions to exercise become bothersome or overwhelming—that is, stressful—it may be time to modify or stop the exercise.

REFERENCES

BORG, G. "Physical Performance and Perceived Exertion." *Studia Psychologia et Paedogogica*, Series Altera, Investigationes. Gleerup, Lund, Sweden, 1962.

LAMB, D.R. *Physiology of Exercise.* New York: Macmillan, 1978.

FOX, E.L. *Sports Physiology.* Philadelphia: W.B. Saunders, 1979.

NOBLE, B.J. *Physiology of Exercise and Sport.* St. Louis: Times Mirror, 1986.

6

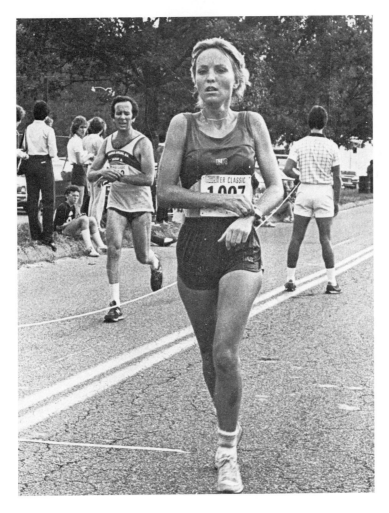

Planning Your Individualized Program and Keeping It Going

When you phone for flight reservations, the airline agent asks a lot of questions before he or she can confirm your arrangements, such as how and when you will reach your destination. When you seek to modify your level of fitness, you must first be sure to have a clear understanding of your starting point and your goal. We're serving as your travel agents; we'll show you how to fly first class. But you must get things going by providing information: who you are; your strengths and skills; how you look; how well you function physiologically; how efficient, graceful, and accurate your body movements are. You need this information to put together your personal plan for fitness and wellness. You need to know your point of departure.

In previous chapters you responded to various checklists and questionnaires that enabled you to gather information about your abilities, personality, ways of looking at problems, social relationships, and perceptions of your physical characteristics. Now this wide array of observations must be organized, synthesized, and put into perspective. This is the time to conduct an assessment review. In this chapter we ask you a lot of questions, and you've got to provide a lot of honest answers.

LIFE-STYLE ASSESSMENT

First, what have you learned about your life-style? Can you characterize it as being easygoing to hectic? Do you blitz through your day? Race from one commitment to the next? Is your day highly structured and organized? Or are your daily activities only vaguely interrelated? Do they follow in reckless and arbitrary order and yield little or insignificant accomplishment at the day's end? Are you pleased or bothered by the end product of your day's efforts? The answers to these questions lie in the information you provided earlier.

Now, take a close look at your answers. Try to zero in on your life-style. Do you like it? Is it good for you? Do you want to change it? What level of wellness can you precisely claim? Complete the Life-Style Assessment Review box to help you make sense of your exercise program.

The type and content of the exercise program you design for yourself is contingent upon your answers to these kinds of questions. If your life-style is low-key and subdued, perhaps your exercise program should provide a good deal of mental as well as physical stimulation. If your typical day is already overloaded with excitment and arousing experiences, you may select a program that emphasizes sustained, rhythmic, endurance types of activities. Can a carefully planned program of exercise done sometime during your day serve as a link between other activities? Can it help you ease out of one kind and into another?

LIFE-STYLE ASSESSMENT REVIEW

Directions: Complete the items below by reviewing your responses to questions in earlier chapters.

1. My life is
   - _____ a. too hectic   or _____ easy going
   - _____ b. too disorganized   or _____ structured
   - _____ c. boring   or _____ exciting

2. My daily activities
   - _____ a. are not well integrated   or _____ are coordinated
   - _____ b. result in significant   or _____ yield little
     accomplishments
   - _____ c. make me pleased   or _____ bother me

3. When I evaluated my health behaviors, I found I needed to improve

   _____

   _____

   _____

   _____

4. To improve my health behavior, I need to

_____

_____

_____

_____

5. I determined my strongest component of health to be _____

and my weakest component of health to be _____

6. To use my strongest component of health, I can engage in the following types of physical activity:

_____

_____

_____

_____

7. To strengthen my weakest component of health, I can

_____

_____

_____

_____

PSYCHOSOCIAL ASSESSMENTS

How about the perceptions you hold of yourself as an achieving, competent, productive individual? Now's the time to look yourself squarely in the mirror and formulate a profile of yourself from the psychosocial point of view.

What are the ways in which you react to environmental stressors? Are your mechanisms for managing stress reactions effective? Does exercise now figure prominently in your stress management strategy? Are you able to relax when you know it is important to do so? What kinds of stressors seem to cause relatively acute reactions, and what kinds of stimuli rarely seem to bother you, although they tend to disturb others?

You've already provided information about your personal reactions to stress, and we've discussed the nature of stress and its physiological and behavioral manifestations and ramifications. Now we want you to relate what you know and have learned to planning your fitness/wellness program. Start thinking not only about the potential exercise has for stress management, but specifically about how a particular program, conducted at a certain time during the day, might be helpful in coping with some of your personal stress reactions. Remember, the purpose of this chapter is to encourage you to begin utilizing information and observations for yourself to formulate an exercise program that works for *you*.

Now, put your reading aside. Take pencil and paper and make a list of physical activities that make sense for *you*. Just write down words like swimming, badminton, dancing, basketball. Rely on the assessments you've made about yourself, and the insights into your needs, goals, strengths, and weaknesses you've developed as a result of your reading and thinking so far. As you proceed, edit the list: cross out activities or add to them.

1. MOTIVATION

What is motivating you to begin exercising regularly? Do you want to prevent illness and disease, lose weight, be more physically attractive, develop confidence, have fun, make friends, manage stress? Are there other reasons for your wanting to begin a fitness program? Whatever your motivation, you would be wise to understand it. To develop the best program for you, you must know what purpose you want that program to serve. In this way you will select exercise activities and locations most likely to meet your needs; and, if your needs are being met, you will be more likely to maintain a habit of regular exercise. To help you rank your motivations for exercising regularly, since it is likely that several motivations are important to you, we have listed some motivations below. Place a number 1 alongside the motivation most important to you, a number 2 alongside the second most important reason you want to begin exercising, and so on until you get to the least important (number 7).

_____	To prevent illness/disease	_____	To have fun
_____	To lose weight	_____	To make friends
_____	For physical attractiveness	_____	To manage stress
_____	To develop confidence		

2. LOCUS OF CONTROL

Before discussing this topic, circle the following answers that best describe your beliefs.

1. a. Grades are a function of the amount of work students do.
   b. Grades depend on the kindness of the instructor.
2. a. Promotions are earned by hard work.
   b. Promotions are a result of being in the right place at the right time.

3. a. Meeting someone to love is a matter of luck.
   b. Meeting someone to love depends on going out often so as to meet many people.
4. a. Living a long life is a function of heredity.
   b. Living a long life is a function of adopting healthy habits.
5. a. Being overweight is determined by the number of fat cells you were born with or developed early in life.
   b. Being overweight depends on what and how much food you eat.
6. a. People who exercise regularly set up their schedules to do so.
   b. Some people just don't have the time for regular -exercise.
7. a. Winning at poker depends on betting correctly.
   b. Winning at poker is a matter of being lucky.
8. a. Staying married depends upon working at the marriage.
   b. Marital breakup is a matter of being unlucky in choosing the wrong marriage partner.
9. a. Citizens can have some influence on their governments.
   b. There is nothing an individual can do to affect governmental function.
10. a. Being skilled at sports depends on being born well coordinated.
    b. Those skilled at sports work hard at learning those skills.
11. a. People with close friends are lucky to have met someone to be intimate with.
    b. Developing close friendships takes hard work.
12. a. Your future depends on whom you meet and on chance.
    b. Your future is up to you.
13. a. Most people are so sure of their opinions that their minds cannot be changed.
    b. A logical argument can convince most people.
14. a. People decide the direction of their lives.
    b. For the most part, we have little control of our futures.
15. a. People who don't like you just don't understand you.
    b. You can be liked by anyone you choose to like you.
16. a. You can make your life a happy one.
    b. Happiness is a matter of fate.
17. a. You evaluate feedback and make decisions based upon it.
    b. You tend to be easily influenced by others.
18. a. If voters studied nominees' records, they could elect honest politicians.
    b. Politics and politicians are corrupt by nature.
19. a. Parents, teachers, and bosses have a great deal to say about one's happiness and self-satisfaction.
    b. Whether you are happy depends upon you.
20. a. Air pollution can be controlled if citizens would get angry about it.
    b. Air pollution is an inevitable result of technological progress.

You have just completed a scale measuring locus of control. Locus of control is the preception of the amount of personal control you believe you have over events that affect your life. People with an *external* locus of control believe they have little control of such events, whereas people with an *internal* locus of control believe they have a good deal of control of these events. To determine your locus of control, give yourself one point for each of the following responses:

ITEM	RESPONSE	ITEM	RESPONSE
1	a	11	b
2	a	12	b
3	b	13	b
4	b	14	a
5	b	15	b
6	a	16	a
7	a	17	a
8	a	18	a
9	a	19	b
10	b	20	a

Scores above 10 indicate internality and scores below 11 indicate externality. Of course there are degrees of each, and most people will find themselves scoring near 10.

You will have great difficulty engaging in exercise regularly if you possess an external locus of control. It stands to reason that when you believe what you get is the result of fate, luck, chance, or of some decisions of powerful others, there is little if any reason to do something yourself. So if you scored external on this scale, you need to work on viewing your world differently. You have to realize that you are in control of you and the events that affect your life--perhaps not totally, but certainly to a great extent. If you scored internal, you are well on your way to assuming responsibility for the achievement of your fitness goals, or their lack of achievement. You view what you get or accomplish as dependent mostly, though not completely, on your own actions and can therefore take the credit as well as the blame for your successes and failures.

3. ASSERTIVENESS

Assertive behavior requires interaction with others. And you're not likely to modify your assertive or nonassertive inclinations while doing situps alone on the living room floor. Team or group activities that require planning and cooperative decisions are fertile experiences for assertiveness training.

You have just completed a scale to measure how assertively you usually act. Several definitions are necessary at this point:

1. *Assertive behavior:* Expressing yourself and satisfying you own needs. Feeling good about this and not hurting others in the process.

To determine how assertive you are, indicate how characteristic or descriptive each of the following statements is of you by using the code given.

+3 = very characteristic of me, extremely descriptive
+2 = rather characteristic of me, quite descriptive
+1 = somewhat characteristic of me, slightly descriptive
−1 = somewhat uncharacteristic of me, slightly nondescriptive
−2 = rather uncharacteristic of me, quite nondescriptive
−3 = very uncharacteristic of me, extremely nondescriptive

_____   1. Most people seem to be more aggressive and assertive than I am.
_____   2. I have hesitated to make or accept dates because of "shyness."
_____   3. When the food served at a restaurant is not done to my satisfaction, I complain about it to the waiter or waitress.
_____   4. I am careful to avoid hurting other people's feelings, even when I feel that I have been injured.
_____   5. If a salesperson has gone to considerable trouble to show me merchandise that is not quite suitable, I have a difficult time in saying no.
_____   6. When I am asked to do something, I insist upon knowing why.
_____   7. There are times when I look for a good, vigorous argument.
_____   8. I strive to get ahead as well as most people in my position.
_____   9. To be honest, people often take advantage of me.
_____   10. I enjoy starting conversations with new acquaintances and strangers.
_____   11. I often don't know what to say to attractive persons of the opposite sex.
_____   12. I will hesitate to make phone calls to business establishments and institutions.
_____   13. I would rather apply for a job or for admission to a college by writing letters than by going through with personal interviews.
_____   14. I find it embarrassing to return merchandise.
_____   15. If a close and respected relative were annoying me, I would smother my feelings rather than express my annoyance.
_____   16. I have avoided asking questions for fear of sounding stupid.
_____   17. During an argument I am sometimes afraid that I will get so upset that I will shake all over.
_____   18. If a famed and respected lecturer makes a statement that I think is incorrect, I will have the audience hear my point of view as well.
_____   19. I avoid arguing over prices with clerks and salespeople.
_____   20. When I have done something important or worthwhile, I manage to let others know about it.
_____   21. I am open and frank about my feelings.
_____   22. If someone has been spreading false and bad stories about me, I see him or her as soon as possible to "have a talk" about it.
_____   23. I often have a hard time saying no.

_____ 24. I tend to bottle up my emotions rather than make a scene.
_____ 25. I complain about poor service in a restaurant and elsewhere.
_____ 26. When I am given a compliment, I sometimes just don't know what to say.
_____ 27. If a couple near me in a theater or at a lecture were conversing rather loudly, I would ask them to be quiet or to take their conversation elsewhere.
_____ 28. Anyone attempting to push ahead of me in a line is in for a good battle.
_____ 29. I am quick to express an opinion.
_____ 30. There are times when I just can't say anything.

Source: (1973) Spencer A. Rathus. "A 30-Item Schedule for Assessing Assertive Behavior," _Behavior Therapy_ 4:398-406.

2. _Nonassertive behavior:_ Denying your own wishes so as to satisfy someone else's. Sacrificing your own needs to meet someone else's needs.
3. _Aggressive behavior:_ Seeking to dominate or to get your own way at the expense of others.

To score this scale, first change (reverse) the signs (+ or -) for your scores on items 1, 2, 4, 5, 9, 11, 12, 13, 15, 16, 17, 19, 23, 24, 26, and 30. Now total the plus (+) items, total the minus (-) items, and subtract the minus total from the plus total to obtain your score. This score can range from -90 through 0 to +90. The higher the score (closer to +90), the more assertively you usually behave. The lower the score (closer to -90), the more nonassertive is your typical behavior. This particular scale does not measure aggressiveness.

4. ALIENATION

For each of the following statements, place one of the following letters in the blank spaced provided:

A = strongly agree
B = agree
C = uncertain
D = disagree
E = strongly disagree

I _____   1. Sometimes I feel all alone in the world.
P _____   2. I worry about the future facing today's children.
I _____   3. I don't get invited out by friends as often as I'd really like.

N____ 4. The end often justifies the means.

I ____ 5. Most people today seldom feel lonely.

P____ 6. Sometimes I have the feeling other people are using me.

N____ 7. People's ideas change so much that I wonder if we'll ever have anything to depend on.

I ____ 8. Real friends are as easy as ever to find.

P____ 9. It is frightening to be responsible for the development of a little child.

N____ 10. Everything is relative, and there just aren't any definite rules to live by.

I ____ 11. One can always find friends, if one is friendly.

N____ 12. I often wonder what the meaning of life really is.

P____ 13. There is little or nothing I can do toward preventing a major "shooting" war.

I ____ 14. The world in which we live is basically a friendly place.

P____ 15. There are so many decisions that have to be made today that sometimes I could just blow up.

N____ 16. The only thing one can be sure of today is that one can be sure of nothing.

I ____ 17. There are few dependable ties between people anymore.

P____ 18. There is little chance for promotion on the job unless a person gets a break.

N____ 19. With so many religions abroad, one doesn't really know which to believe.

P____ 20. We're so regimented today that there's not much room for choice even in personal matters.

P____ 21. We are just cogs in the machinery of life.

I ____ 22. People are just naturally friendly and helpful.

P____ 23. The future looks very dismal.

I ____ 24. I don't get to visit friends as often as I'd like.

Source: Dwight G. Dean, "Alienation: Its Meaning and Measurement," *American Sociological Review* 26 (1961):753-758.

You have just completed an alienation scale. To score this scale, award yourself the number of points indicated for each response you made:

1.	4	A	3	a	2	U	1	d	0 D
2.	4	A	3	a	2	U	1	d	0 D
3.	4	A	3	a	2	U	1	d	0 D
4.	4	A	3	a	2	U	1	d	0 D
5.	0	A	1	a	2	U	3	d	4 D
6.	4	A	3	a	2	U	1	d	0 D
7.	4	A	3	a	2	U	1	d	0 D

8.	0	A	1	a	2	U	3	d	4	D
9.	4	A	3	a	2	U	1	d	0	D
10.	4	A	3	a	2	U	1	d	0	D
11.	0	A	1	a	2	U	3	d	4	D
12.	4	A	3	a	2	U	1	d	0	D
13.	4	A	3	a	2	U	1	d	0	D
14.	0	A	1	a	2	U	3	d	4	D
15.	4	A	3	a	2	U	1	d	0	D
16.	4	A	3	a	2	U	1	d	0	D
17.	4	A	3	a	2	U	1	d	0	D
18.	4	A	3	a	2	U	1	d	0	D
19.	4	A	3	a	2	U	1	d	0	D
20.	4	A	3	a	2	U	1	d	0	D
21.	4	A	3	a	2	U	1	d	0	D
22.	0	A	1	a	2	U	3	d	4	D
23.	4	A	3	a	2	U	1	d	0	D
24.	4	A	3	a	2	U	1	d	0	D

Alienation consists of three factors:

1. *Social isolation.* The lack of significant others (friends, relatives, etc.) in whom one can confide.
2. *Normlessness.* The lack of rules, regulations, and standards by which one chooses to live.
3. *Powerlessness.* The feeling of not being in control of one's own destiny.

To determine your scores on each of these three factors, add up separately the points for all the items preceded by an I (social isolation), an N (normlessness), and a P (powerlessness). The higher your score, the more you possess this factor.

When this scale was administered to male undergraduates, they averaged 36.64, with the following subscores:

- Social isolation—11.76
- Normlessness—7.62
- Powerlessness—13.65

Undergraduate women averaged 36.25, with these subscores:

- Social isolation—14.85
- Normlessness—7.63
- Powerless—12.73

How did you score on the alienation factors? Did you learn that there is a lack of trusted friends, acquaintancces, and relatives in your world? Is *social alienation* a problem for you? If it is, you can structure your program so that it contributes to the reduction of alienation. Your circle of acquaintances may be enlarged by membership in an exercise club, health spa, or YMCA. Participation in organized sports (at a level that suits your skill and experience) provides opportunity to befriend teammates as well as opponents. Playing in leagues and tournaments (team as well as individual sports) also encourages this outcome, since you will meet and interact with many competitors on and off the playing fields.

A second aspect of alienation we identified earlier is *normlessness*. Organized sports impose rules, regulations, and standards on participants and can therefore encourage the acceptance of rules that have meaning and relevance. If normlessness is one of your vulnerabilities, activities such as racket sports, basketball, softball, and flag football can provide an opportunity to abide by regulations. In these activities, much of what you do, and when you do it, is *externally regulated*. That is, in large measure you respond to cues, signals, and the behavior of others. This may be just what you need to help you modify your normlessness. Distance running, rope skipping, and similar self-regulated activities will not contribute very much to this end. But they may very well have an impact on another form of alienation, *powerlessness* (the feeling of not being in control of your destiny).

Standing atop a mountain, ready to ski down, finds you in a position laded with opportunity for control. It's you and the mountain. Your downhill excursion begins when you are ready. You stop for a rest and resume the descent when you decide to do so. Skating, calisthenics, weight training, gymnastics, and diving also permit self-initiation. And when you cycle, swim, or jog, you determine how far and how fast you will go. You are in control.

5. SELF-ESTEEM

Using the scale below, place the number alongside each body part listed that represents your feelings about that part of yourself.

Scale:
1. Have strong feelings and wish a change could somehow be made
2. Don't like, but can put up with
3. Have no particular feelings one way or the other
4. Am satisfied
5. Consider myself fortunate

Body:
_____ 1. hair   _____ 4. hands
_____ 2. facial complexion   _____ 5. distribution of hair
_____ 3. appetite   over body

_____	6. nose	_____	27. digestion
_____	7. fingers	_____	28. hips
_____	8. elimination	_____	29. skin texture
_____	9. wrists	_____	30. lips
_____	10. waist	_____	31. legs
_____	11. energy level	_____	32. teeth
_____	12. back	_____	33. forehead
_____	13. ears	_____	34. feet
_____	14. chin	_____	35. sleep
_____	15. exercise	_____	36. voice
_____	16. ankles	_____	37. health
_____	17. neck	_____	38. sex activities
_____	18. shape of head	_____	39. knees
_____	19. body build	_____	40. posture
_____	20. profile	_____	41. face
_____	21. height	_____	42. weight
_____	22. age	_____	43. sex (male or female)
_____	23. width of shoulders	_____	44. back view of head
_____	24. arms	_____	45. trunk
_____	25. chest	_____	46. breathing
_____	26. eyes		

Now add up all the point values you assigned to the parts of your body and divide the sum by 46. Your score should fall between 1 and 5.

Next, use the same scale for the following components of your self:

_____	1. first name	_____	18. self-consciousness
_____	2. morals	_____	19. generosity
_____	3. ability to express self	_____	20. ability to accept
_____	4. taste in clothes		criticism
_____	5. sense of duty	_____	21. thoughts
_____	6. sophistication	_____	22. artistic and
_____	7. self-understanding		literary taste
_____	8. life goals	_____	23. memory
_____	9. artistic talents	_____	24. thriftiness
_____	10. tolerance	_____	25. personality
_____	11. moods	_____	26. self-respect
_____	12. general knowledge	_____	27. ability to concentrate
_____	13. imagination	_____	28. ability to take orders
_____	14. popularity	_____	29. sensitivity to opinions
_____	15. self-confidence		of others
_____	16. ability to express	_____	30. ability to lead
	sympathy	_____	31. last name
_____	17. emotional control	_____	32. impulses

_____	33. manners	_____	45. ability to meet people
_____	34. handwriting	_____	46. self-discipline
_____	35. intelligence level	_____	47. suggestibility
_____	36. athletic skills	_____	48. neatness
_____	37. happiness	_____	49. vocabulary
_____	38. creativeness	_____	50. procrastination
_____	39. strength of conviction	_____	51. will power
_____	40. conscience	_____	52. self-assertiveness
_____	41. skill with hands	_____	53. ability to make
_____	42. fears		decisions
_____	43. capacity for work	_____	54. dreams
_____	44. conscientiousness		

Once again, add up all the point values you assigned to the parts of your self, and this time divide the sum by 54. Your score should fall between 1 and 5.

The first scale you completed measures your body esteem; that is, in how high a regard you hold your body. Put another way, this scale measures the degree of feeling of satisfaction or dissatisfaction with the various parts or processes of your body. The second scale measures your self-esteem; that is, in how high a regard you hold your self. What you think of your body and what you think of your self can have tremendous significance for the development of your fitness program. If you have body parts with which you are dissatisfied, perhaps your program can be designed to improve those body parts. If you have parts of your self with which you are dissatisfied, perhaps your program can be designed to improve those parts. For example, if you stated you wanted to improve your back, you might consider exercises to strengthen your abdominal muscles. Or, if you stated on the self-esteem scale that you wanted to improve your capacity for work, you might consider endurance-type exercises when designing your training program.

6. STRESS

Circle all the following events you have experienced within the last year. If you are a typical college student, use the first list. If you are older than the typical college student, circle the items on the second list.

Mean value	Event
(50)	Entered college
(77)	Married
(38)	Had either a lot more or a lot less trouble with your boss
(43)	Held a job while attending school

(87)   Experienced the death of a spouse

(34)   Experienced a major change in sleeping habits (sleeping a lot more or a lot less, or a change in part of the day when asleep)

(77)   Experienced the death of a close family member

(30)   Experienced a major change in eating habits (a lot more or a lot less food intake, or very different meal hours or surroundings)

(41)   Made a change in or choice of a major field of study

(45)   Had a revision of your personal habits (friends, dress, manners, associations, etc.)

(68)   Experienced the death of a close friend

(22)   Have been found guilty of minor violations of the law (traffic tickets, jaywalking, etc.)

(40)   Have had an outstanding personal achievement

(68)   Experienced pregnancy, or fathered a child

(56)   Had a major change in the health or behavior of a family member

(58)   Had sexual difficulties

(42)   Had trouble with in-laws

(26)   Had a major change in the number of family get-togethers (a lot more or a lot less)

(53)   Had a major change in financial state (a lot worse off or a lot better off than usual)

(50)   Gained a new family member (through birth, adoption, older person moving in, etc.)

(42)   Changed your residence or living conditions

(50)   Had a major conflict in or change in values

(36)   Had a major change in church activities (a lot more or a lot less than usual)

(58)   Had a marital reconciliation with your mate

(62)   Were fired from work

(76)   Were divorced

(50)   Changed to a different line of work

(50)   Had a major change in the number of arguments with spouse (either a lot more or a lot less than usual)

(47)   Had a major change in responsibilities at work (promotion, demotion, lateral transfer)

(41)   Had your spouse begin or cease work outside the home

(74)   Had a marital separation from your mate

(57)   Had a major change in usual type and/or amount of recreation

(52)   Took a mortgage or loan *less* than $10,000 (such as purchase of a TV, school loan, etc.)

(65)   Had a major personal injury or illness

(46)   Had a major change in the use of alcohol (a lot more or a lot less)

(48)   Had a major change in social activities

(38)   Had a major change in the amount of participation in school activities

(49)   Had a major change in the amount of independence and responsibility (for example, for budgeting time)

(33)	Took a trip or a vacation
(54)	Were engaged to be married
(50)	Changed to a new school
(41)	Changed dating habits
(44)	Had trouble with school administration (instructors, advisors, class scheduling, etc.)
(60)	Broke or had broken a marital engagement or a steady relationship
(57)	Had a major change in self-concept or self-awareness

Source: G.E. Anderson, "College Schedule of Recent Experience, "Master's Thesis, North Dakota State University, 1972.

If you are older than the typical college student, determine which of the following events you have experienced within the past year:

Mean value	Life event
(100)	Death of spouse
(73)	Divorce
(65)	Marital separation
(63)	Jail term
(63)	Death of close family member
(53)	Personal injury or illness
(50)	Marriage
(47)	Fired at work
(45)	Marital reconciliation
(45)	Retirement
(44)	Change in health of family member
(40)	Pregnancy
(39)	Sex difficulties
(39)	Gain of new family member
(39)	Business readjustment
(38)	Change in financial state
(37)	Death of close friend
(36)	Change to different line of work
(35)	Change in number of arguments with spouse
(31)	Mortgage or loan for major purchase (home, etc.)
(30)	Foreclosure of mortgage or loan
(29)	Change in responsibilities at work
(29)	Son or daughter leaving home
(29)	Trouble with in-laws
(28)	Outstanding personal achievement
(26)	Wife begin or stop work
(25)	Change in living conditions
(24)	Revision of personal habits

(23)	Trouble with boss
(20)	Change in work hours or conditions
(20)	Change in residence
(19)	Change in recreation
(19)	Change in church activities
(18)	Change in social activities
(17)	Mortgage or loan for lesser purchase (car, TV, etc.)
(16)	Change in sleeping habits
(15)	Change in number of family get-togethers
(15)	Change in eating habits
(13)	Vacation
(12)	Christmas
(11)	Minor violations of the law

Source: Thomas H. Holmes and Richard H. Rahe. "The Social Readjustment Rating Scale," *Journal of Psychosomatic Research* 11:(1967):213-18.

To obtain your score on the first scale, multiply the number of times an event occurred by its mean value. Then total all the scores. For the second scale, just total your points.

Your score is termed your *life change units* (LCU). This is a measure of the amount of significant changes in your life to which you have had to adjust. In other words, your LCU is a measure of the stressors you have encountered this past year. The original research in this field was conducted by Holmes and Rahe, who developed the Social Readjustment Rating Scale. They argued that if stress resulted in illness and disease, then people experiencing a great deal of stress should report more illness than people reporting only a little stress. Their theory was supported when they found that people who scored 150-199 LCU in one year showed a 37 percent chance of those stressors leading to illness or disease the following year; those scoring 200-299, a 51 percent chance; and those scoring over 300, a 79 percent chance. The first scale we presented, the one developed by Anderson, is an adaptation of Holmes and Rahe's scale. The relationship to illness and disease on the Anderson scale is not as explicit as on the Holmes and Rahe scale, but the higher the score on this scale, the greater the chance of illness or disease developing.

If you've dealt with a large number of stressors during the past year, then you should consider exercise as a way to reduce harmful reactions to stress (Bartley and Belgrave, 1987). In Chapters 2 and 3 we described psychological responses to stress and tried to indicate how exercise and training may be beneficial. In Chapter 12 we will discuss the management of stress reactions in greater detail.

The particular form of stress-reducing exercise one chooses varies from person to person. Know what works best for you. Perhaps physical activity that must be performed in a special environment would be wise; it might enable you to be removed physically from the sources of stress. Sometimes something as simple as a change of location alleviates much of a stressor's impact. For some, exercise that is particularly physically demanding and stressful itself is beneficial. For others, physical activity characterized by low degrees of stress might be best (they're already saturated with stressful stimuli).

Just as stimuli are perceived as stressful or nonstressful on individual bases, so are the various forms of exercise. If other persons appear in some manner to be causally related to your stress reactions, perhaps an individual activity performed privately might be helpful. If, on the other hand, a sense of alienation appears to be the source of your stress reaction, exercise involving social interaction might be indicated.

PSYCHOSOCIAL ASSESSMENT REVIEW

Directions: Refer to your scores in Psychosocial Assessments 1-6 to complete the following items.

1. I have an _____(external or internal)_____ locus of control. _____

2. I have a _____(high, medium, low)_____ self-esteem. _____

    The part of my body I need to work on to improve my self-esteem is my

    _____ .

3. My <u>assertiveness</u> score indicated I was _____

    (assertive or nonassertive).

4. I have a _____(high, medium, low)_____ level of alienation·

    The factor of alienation I scored best on was _____

    (social isolation, normlessness, powerlessness)

5. My <u>stress</u> score (life change units) indicated I have a _____

    _____(high, medium, low)_____ degree of stress.

6. Considering my psychosocial assessment results, a good physical fitness

    activity for me to engage in regularly is _____(high, medium, low)_____ .

OTHER ASSESSMENTS TO CONSIDER

Medical Evaluation

Be sure to check out your overall readiness for exercise by having a medical examination if your reading of Chapter 4 indicates you need one. Don't make any assumptions about your status if the information in Chapter 4 leads you to question your preparedness for fitness activities. Visit your physician. If deficiencies are uncovered, take action to remedy them. If vulnerabilities are observed, consult with your physician about ways to overcome them. It may be necessary to do this before beginning your exercise program.

Fitness Appraisal

Examine the fitness profile you constructed in Chapter 4. You've got a pretty good notion of what you look like in terms of cardiorespiratory health, body composition, muscular strength, endurance, and flexibility. Now, what form of exercise seems to be consistent with your characteristics? As you attempt to answer this question, remember that your choice can be a response to fitness strengths *or* weaknesses. You might, for example, select calisthenics, yoga, or tumbling because you happen to be very flexible, *or* because you know you are particularly low in flexibility and wish to do something about it. People who enroll in automotive training classes may usually be classified into one of two groups: (1) Those who love to tinker under the hood and who know quite a bit about how the car engine and parts function and (2) those who know very little but who are upset at the prohibitive cost of professional auto repair and service costs. The same kind of motivational issue may be involved in selecting your physical activity.

Take a look at the list of exercise activities you've started to compile. Examine it now in terms of your physical and mental strengths and weaknesses. Try to consider exercise options that will work for *you*. Be rational. Think about who you are, and what you need. Begin to cross out activities that don't fit your life-style, your medical and fitness profiles, and your interests and social needs. Be straightforward in your deliberations, for your ultimate goal is wellness, which is contingent on honest self-appraisal and a serious desire to adjust to or overcome personal limitations.

WELLNESS THROUGH AN INDIVIDUALIZED PROGRAM

For most of us, purchasing customized products is prohibitively expensive. When the item we want is standard, its cost is usually considerably lower than if it is in any way distinctive. You pay extra for anything that departs from the mass-produced model. This is true when you shop for a new automobile, a suit of clothes, or even when requesting a restaurant meal through special order. If the menu says the fish is served fried and you want it broiled, you pay more. Often, this added expense not only deters you from getting what you really want, but it may make you decide to forget the item entirely. You conclude: "If I can't have what I want, then the heck with it."

Not so with what we're selling in this book—fitness and wellness. You can have precisely what you want and need, at no extra cost (just a little initiative). Step forward and take what works best for *you*. Design an exercise program that suits *your* time schedule, satisfies *your* social interests, is responsive to *your* personal physiological, anatomical, and psychological vulnerabilities and strengths. Organize a physical activity regimen with *your name on it*.

Build a prototype program and try it for a week or two. If it needs modification, take it back to the drawing board. You've acquired a solid foundation of information about exercise and training, and you've gathered some very direct information about yourself. You've got a handle on who you are, what wellness means, and how to pursue it through exercise. Now let's see how you can keep it going.

Keeping It Going

We won't hide the truth; maintaining an exercise program when that is not your style is very difficult. It seems that no matter how well motivated you are or how much will power you're able to muster up, sooner or later your best intentions are shattered, and so is your program. Those of you used to exercising will have an easier time of it. All that's required of you is to adjust what you normally do to be more consistent with what is known about effective exercise. It is the rest of you, the more sedentary ones, to whom this section is devoted. We'll present a number of effective behavior change techniques and show you how you can use them to achieve your goals, to maintain your program under normal circumstances, and to exercise even under trying circumstances.

These techniques have been made specific to exercise, but they can be used for other behaviors as well. Those of you who do exercise regularly and feel you have no need for this information should apply this material to other behaviors; for example, cigarette smoking, dieting, studying, or making it to appointments or classes on time. To help you make this application, we have used some nonexercise examples to illustrate some of the techniques.

Achieving Your Goals

Many hints and skills can help you achieve your exercise goals. Here are some to consider.

Being Realistic.   One of your authors was playing tennis with a friend one pleasant summer day. The sun was out, the birds were chirping, a slight breeze rustled the leaves, and the water in the creek alongside the tennis courts was gently caressing the rocks as it moved downstream. All in all, the day couldn't have been any better. That is, unless you were Don. You see, his game was off and he was serving long and netting too many backhands.

Enough was enough, Don thought; when he next netted his favorite cross-court forehand, his temper got the best of him. Before anyone realized what was happening, Don's tennis racket flew clear over the fence, above the trees beyond, and smack into the middle of the creek. All we could do was watch as the racket kept pace with the water heading downstream, never to be seen again by Don, his friends, or his relatives.

Some of you may know a Don, and some of you may be one. The problem is in being realistic. Sometimes has-beens think they should be as talented as when they were at their peak. Usually, though, they are no longer devoting as much time to that activity, or they have passed the age when physiology allows them to give a superior performance. In other cases it's not so much a matter of a has-been, but rather a never-was. Some people believe they should perform like the athletes they see on television; so a golf shot 190 yards from the green that lands short and to the left ruins their day. But the fact is that they never were any good at golf.

So be realistic in setting goals. If you set unobtainable goals or don't allow yourself enough time to achieve them, you may be frustrated and give up. All that may be required, in fact, is an adjustment to make your goals reachable. At the beginning, set goals you know are all within your reach. Make them easy to achieve. In this way you will be reinforcing your exercise behavior with a feeling of success. Remember, where you are starting from will in large part determine where you can go, and how fast. Don't ignore that information when establishing fitness goals.

On a sheet of paper, write the fitness goals you would like to achieve and the date by which you want to achieve them. Since we believe strongly that you should choose your goals and the time you are willing to commit to achieving them, we can't and won't set goals for you. To achieve high-level wellness, these goals must balance with other aspects of your life. So you are the best one to decide what these goals should be because you are the one who knows your life best.

Periodic Assessment.   Now that you've decided what your fitness goals are, you need to decide how you will determine if and when you've achieved them. To do that, you must periodically assess your accomplishment. For us to be specific about how to do this assessment is impossible, because we don't know what your goals are. However, we can offer some general advice.

First of all, your assessment should be consistent with your goal. For example, let's assume you've said you wanted to decrease your heart rate by 10 percent. You've decided to achieve that goal by running 3 miles every other day. It would be inappropriate to evaluate that goal by determining whether you've actually run 3 miles every other day. The running is the program. The decrease in heart rate is the goal, and that is what should be measured. However, if you haven't kept a record of your adherence to the exercise program, you will not know if you did not decrease your heart rate because you didn't exercise regularly or because the exercise itself was at too low a level. So it is necessary to keep a record of how intensely and how frequently you exercised. But the evaluation must be of the goal itself. If the goal was achieved, great. Then you might want to set another goal or establish a program to maintain that one. If the goal was not achieved, you should look at the record you've kept on the intensity and frequency of exercise to determine if your program needs adjustment; also look at the goal itself to decide if it is a realistic one.

Another point to remember is that assessment should be periodic. If you take your pulse twice a day to look for a decrease in heart rate, you may be frustrated to find no change for several measures in a row. This frustration may threaten your motivation. On the other hand, if you wait for three weeks to assess changes in your heart rate, you are giving up the reinforcement that accompanies goal achievement and may have waited longer than necessary to proceed toward another goal. Assessment should be done between when you begin your exercise program and when you expect to achieve your goal. It should not be too frequent, but not too infrequent. The actual timing will vary depending upon your goal, but make assessments periodic. Some of the measures we've used in Chapters 3 and 4 could be a good beginning for assessing your fitness goals. Take a few moments now to write down how you will assess the achievement of the goals you specified earlier.

Achievement Techniques

At this point you have identified your fitness goals and how you will periodically assess your program toward or accomplishment of them. Now we will develop additional components of the exercise program, apart from the exercise itself, that will help you achieve your goals. One of these components is social support.

Social Support and Contracting.   Social support is just another way of saying "other people to encourage and help you." It is much easier to adopt a habit of regular exercise, or any habit for that matter, if you are encouraged by others (Cairns and Pasino, 1977). Even the difficulty of losing weight by dieting has been shown to be affected by social support (Brownell et al., 1978), and when families lent support to other family members who were ill, these patients were more apt to comply with the medical regimens prescribed for them by health care providers (Becker and Green, 1975).

To use social support effectively, you should choose a significant other—someone close and important to you—who is willing to participate in a program to get you started in regular exercise (Feldman, 1986). This person should periodically inquire how you are doing, should congratulate you or reward you somehow if you are doing well, should work with you to adjust your program if you are having difficulty, and should even be prepared to participate with you on occasion.

One way to use social support is to make a *contract* with your supporter. In this contract you will specify how frequently and how intensely you intend to exercise. You may even specify a physiological change you expect to occur by a certain date; for example, you might state that you expect to lose 6 pounds in 2 weeks. This contract should also specify the reward for meeting your goal and the punishment for not meeting it. The reward can consist of something material, such as a new article of clothing; or it can consist of something intangible, such as a walk under the stars. Whatever you choose should actually be rewarding and something you would not obtain or do otherwise. Likewise, the punishment should be punishing—within limits, of course. For example, you might choose to punish yourself by not watching TV for one week or not eating a favorite food. Take a moment now and list 5 rewards and 5 punishments you could use in your contract.

REWARDS   PUNISHMENTS

1. _____   1. _____
2. _____   2. _____
3. _____   3. _____
4. _____   4. _____
5. _____   5. _____

You're now ready to write your contract. Use the Fitness Control box as a model.

FITNESS CONTRACT

I _____ desire to improve my physical
              (your name)
fitness because _____ . I have decided I
                        (the reason)
intend to _____
                        (your goal)
by _____ . If I achieve this goal, I will reward
            (date)
myself by _____ . If I do not achieve my
                    (the reward)
goal, I will punish myself by _____ .
                                    (the punishment)

_____   _____
(Your signature)   (Today's date)

_____   _____
(Witness signature)   (Today's date)

A contract need not involve other people; you can make a contract with yourself. When developing a contract, keep the following principles in mind (Mahoney and Thoreson, 1974):

1. The contract should be fair.
2. The terms of the contract should be clear.
3. The contract should be systematic and consistent.

    4. Procedures should be systematic and consistent.

    5. It is preferable, though not necessary, for at least one other person to be involved.

Reminder Systems.   One way to remember things is to make a note of them. Reminder notes will help you remember to exercise, especially if you leave the notes in places where you can't miss them. The doors of the bathroom and refrigerator are good spots. The bathroom mirror is another.

A Gradual Program.   Too often, people who have never exercised regularly or have not exercised regularly for some time, expect to be able to run a mile in under 4 minutes. Less obvious, but no less unrealistic for many people, is the goal of exercising every other day when they have been sedentary for years; or of exercising intensely when they haven't done that for a while. Giving up the sedentary life "cold turkey" may be extremely difficult for you; if it is, don't fret. Instead, use a graduated plan in which you start slowly and gradually increase both frequency and intensity. Graduated plans have been used successfully with a number of behaviors (Dunbar et al., 1979); you

---

LESLIE'S INDIVIDUALIZED PROGRAM

When Leslie assessed her life-style, she found her daily activities were hectic and disorganized, resulting in dissatisfaction with her accomplishments. Her psychosocial assessment found Leslie to have an external locus of control, low self-esteem, high assertiveness, high alienation (in particular, social isolation), and high stress. A medical examination cleared her for exercise, and an evaluation of her fitness determined she was quite flexible but needed improvement in muscular strength (in particular, her lower body) and cardiorespiratory endurance.

With this information, Leslie began to plan her individualized exercise program. She decided to jog and set a goal of running 3 miles, 4 days a week, within 3 weeks. Since jogging would develop lower body strength while at the same time developing cardiorespiratory endurance, it was a fine choice for improving her physical health.

However, after 3 weeks Leslie could only run 1 mile at a time and was bored with jogging. It was time to assess her progress and adjust her program. What Leslie found was that she had neglected her life-style and psychosocial assessments when she developed her program. Her social isolation was not lessened as a result of jogging alone, her high stress was actually worsened by her attempt and failure to run 3 miles, and her low self-esteem became lower when she viewed herself a failure at exercising. Furthermore, her weak legs began to hurt from jogging rather than feel stronger.

The adjustments Leslie made responded to the problems she identified by standing back and assessing her progress. She stopped jogging and began bicycling. In fact, she joined a bicycle club that organized short trips. Her legs began to feel better and stronger, since they were being exercised but relieved of the pounding of jogging. Her social isolation was lessened by her interacting with other bikers. And her self-esteem improved as a result of feeling more fit and being accepted as a member of the club.

Without periodic assessment, exercise plans cannot be adequately revised.

could use one to study more, to change your eating habits, or to decrease your use of alcohol, as well as to start a program of regular exercise.

Tailoring.   No two people are alike. Not the most provocative statement—in fact, so obvious it's absurd to even have to mention it. And yet we sometimes act as though we don't know this fact. When people adopt wholesale an exercise program designed for a group, without adjusting that program to their own needs and circumstances, they are increasing the likelihood that they will soon stop exercising regularly. Some people are free to exercise in the mornings; others in the evenings. Some people are in better physical condition than others. Some people eat their meals at different times than some other people. Some are more committed to exercise than others. Some have a heavier travel schedule than others. We could go on and on, but the point is that any program of regular exercise must be tailored to the individual exerciser. We present exercise activities for you in later chapters, but you must choose which to do, when to do them, how frequently, and how intensely.

The Health Beliefs Model.   A model describing why people act as they do regarding health-related behavior has been proposed by Becker (1974). This model states that people will be most apt to adopt a healthy behavior, such as regular exercise, if:

1. They consider it likely they will contract a disease or illness if they don't (susceptibility).
2. The illness or disease they may contract is severe enough to be of serious concern (severity).
3. The health behavior, if adopted, can prevent the serious illness or disease (prevention).
4. The barriers to performing the health behavior are not too difficult to overcome (removal of barriers).

You can use this model to increase the likelihood of your starting a program of regular exercise. To do so, think of exercise as a means of preventing obesity, since regular exercise in conjunction with dietary changes can control your weight. Furthermore, consider obesity a severe condition, since it is related to hypertension, stroke, and coronary heart disease—our society's major killers. So far, then, you have susceptibility, severity, and prevention. Next, you'll need to identify barriers that are preventing you or have the potential to prevent you from exercising regularly.

When developing your fitness program, pay attention to barriers to your exercising regularly. Try to devise ways to lessen the effect of these barriers. For example, if transportation is a barrier, develop a program that includes activities you can do in your home or near where you live, such as jogging or riding a stationary exercise bike. Awareness of these barriers will allow you to lessen their impact and thereby increase the likelihood that you will actually begin and maintain a physical fitness program.

Professional Help.   The reason so many people enroll in classes, join clubs and spas, and buy books about fitness is because they recognize the need for professional help in developing, beginning, and maintaining a program of regular exercise. Training in exercise physiology, behavior modification, physical education, and health education are some examples of the kinds of professional help available. Private health clubs, YMCAs and YWCAs, and adult education courses should all offer this expertise. Professionals will be able to help you determine the frequency and intensity of your exercise, and recommend behavior modification techniques to ensure that you stay with your program. Furthermore, these experts will be able to help you decide on fitness goals, on the means of assessing their achievement, and on the kinds of activities most conducive to your personality and appropriate to your goals.

You can achieve physical fitness and high-level wellness on your own, without professional help or any other kind of assistance. This book is designed to help you do that. However, professionals can relate the contents of this book to you specifically and can serve as another reinforcer of your behavior once you begin your program. Be sure, though, that these experts are really qualified. With any profession that has become popular to the point of being a fad—and professions concerned with physical fitness meet this criterion—there seeems to be an influx of people who often lack the qualifications to be effective. Check the training of the professionals you choose to help you with your program. Big muscles are not enough; neither is the completion of several marathons. Rather, find out if they have a degree in a related area (for example, physiology, medicine, exercise physiology, sports medicine, physical education, health education) and what their experience is in developing, conducting, and evaluating fitness programs.

Chaining.   In chaining, one behavior is linked to a previous one and that to a previous one, and so on. You can use chaining to help achieve your fitness goals. The point to remember here is that you want to have as few links as possible between the decision to exercise and actually engaging in a fitness activity. To demonstrate this point, let's look at two people. U.R. Wrong and I.M. Right.

U.R. Wrong decides to exercise after school and work, at about 5:30 P.M. So U.R. rushes home and starts gathering exercise clothes. In one drawer are gym shorts and socks. A shirt is in another drawer; the sneakers are under the bed in another room; the car keys have been left in the foyer, and warm-up suit and gloves in the closet. On the way to the track U.R. finds the car needs gas and stops to get some. At the school where the track is, U.R. parks the car, gets out, and locks the door behind. A short walk to the track, and U.R. is ready to exercise.

I.M. Right also decides to exercise after school and work. However, I.M. prepares beforehand. Left on the bed in the morning are all the clothes needed for later—including sneakers, warmup suits, and gloves. I.M. decides to run around the neighborhood instead of the track, so all that is required at 5:30 P.M. is to come home, dress, step outside the front door, and exercise.

If we consider each behavior needed to exercise as a link in a chain, we can see tht U.R. Wrong had many more links. The more links, the more difficult it is to exercise, and the more likely it is that you won't. The trick is to decrease the links for a behavior you want to adopt and increase the links for a behavior you want to give up. If you want to give up cigarette smoking to improve cardiorespiratory fitness, for example, you can increase the links by wrapping the pack of cigarettes in a sock, wrapping tape around the sock, taking it to a room in which you seldom smoke, locking it in a cabinet, taking the key and wrapping it in a sock with tape, and then keeping the key in a different room from the cabinet. Now, to smoke, you must go to the room with the key, unroll the tape, take the key out of the sock, go to the room with the cabinet, open the lock, remove the sock in which the cigarettes are located, unravel the tape, remove the cigarettes, get a match, and light up. After doing all that a couple of times, you will be less apt to smoke cigarettes.

Covert Techniques.   Some of you may be so inactive or busy that you have difficulty engaging in regular exercise. Three techniques have been shown to be helpful regarding behavior change that initially requires no changes whatsoever. These are called *covert* techniques.

- *Covert Rehearsal.* This procedure requires you to imagine yourself exercising regularly. Your image must be extremely vivid: Notice all the details (what you're wearing, the weather, the location), smell the atmosphere, feel the bodily sensations, and so on. Being able to imagine yourself in this manner will make it more likely that you will actually put yourself in that situation. You will have desensitized yourself to the image of you exercising, so that seeing yourself exercising will not seem foreign. It will then be easier for you to actually exercise.
- *Covert Modeling.* For some of us, even imagining ourselves exercising is difficult. It is just not us! If that is the case with you, there is still hope. First, identify someone else you *can* envision exercising. Next, imagine, as vividly as you can, that person exercising. Once that image is clear in your mind, substitute yourself for that other person in that situation. Model the image of you exercising after the image of the other person exercising.

  In other words, have yourself do and feel everything in your image of yourself exercising as you had the other person do and feel when you imagined him or her exercising. After a while, it will be easier for you to think of yourself as a potentially regular exerciser, and it will be more likely that you will become one.
- *Covert Reinforcement.* When you can imagine yourself exercising, it is a good idea to reward yourself for that. The use of another image as a reward is called *covert reinforcement*. Usually a pleasant image is used as a reward and is allowed to surface and be focused on only after the "goal image" is successfully accomplished.

MAINTAINING YOUR PROGRAM: GUIDELINES

Once you've begun a regular program of exercise, the trick is to maintain it. In addition to the methods already described, here are some specific guidelines.

Material Reinforcement

Behavior that has as its consequence a reward tends to be repeated (Feldman, 1985). Consequently, if you want to exercise regularly, you should reward yourself when you do. Material rewards can take many forms, but they must be rewarding. Your rewards, though, should not counteract the benefits of the exercise. We know a professor who used to jog along the Charles River in Boston and stop every mile at a different bar for a beer. The ingestion of alcohol may have been unhealthier than not jogging.

Social Reinforcement

Peer group pressure need not be limited to negative influences. We can use such pressure to encourage and reward desirable behavior. Take a moment to list five people whose opinions you value. Then enlist these people as social reinforcers to inquire about your exercise behavior and pat you on the back if you report engaging in it regularly. They will boast about your fitness to others in front of you. They will express envy of you and admiration of your persistence. All this will make you feel good, and result in your wanting more such rewards. You will then be more likely to continue exercising. After a while, exercising will become a part of your life-style, and you will no longer have to be rewarded for continuing to do it.

Joining a Group

One of the reasons Weight Watchers, Inc., is so effective in helping people lose weight is that it employs group support and positive peer pressure. It is often easier to accomplish your goals if you are working with others in a group. To help maintain your program of regular exercise, you can commit yourself to a group of exercisers. This can be accomplished in several different ways. For example, you can commit yourself financially by joining a health spa or fitness center. Or you can commit yourself socially by scheduling a regular time when you and several friends meet to exercise together. You can even enroll in a fitness class at a local Y or community college. Any group involvement will increase the likelihood of your keeping at your training program.

Boasting

We have known students who have taken two tests a day and done well in one and poorly on the other, and who have complained about the poor grade for days. In and of itself, this might not be all that terrible, but when they forget about how well they did on the other exam, one begins to wonder about their health in terms of balance and perspective. Many of us are like this. We relive negative experiences by repeatedly thinking about them, being embarrassed about them all over again or in other ways feeling inadequate. About situations in which we did well, we say: "Aw, shucks, it was nothing," in our best false-modesty voice, and then proceed to forget about them. We certainly should learn from our mistakes, but we shouldn't dwell on them unnecessarily. Likewise, we should learn from our successes. In this case, we *should* dwell on them. Such a habit will significantly and positively affect our self-esteem and make us healthier.

Regarding exercise, how often have you heard someone ask, "How far do you usually run?" only for the other person to reply, "Oh, only 3 miles." A better reply might be, "Well, I'm proud that I run 3 miles regularly!" Boasting like this, in a nonoffensive way, will make you feel good and thereby serve to reinforce your exercise behavior. Wellness will be better served by a tactfully boastful reply than by a falsely modest one.

Self-monitoring

Self-monitoring is the process of observing and recording your own behavior (Taylor, 1986). It is helpful to know that your exercise program is having a positive effect, that it is taking you down the road toward your goal. One of the problems dieters experience is that the scale tells them they've lost a lot of weight at first, but then weight loss seems much less rapid. What is happening is they are losing water at first, rather than body fat. Afterward, their water balance is maintained and the weight loss reported is really fat. However, not recognizing what is occurring, many dieters become excited at first and then so discouraged that they eventually stop dieting. Don't make the same mistake. Assuming that your exercise goal is realistic, don't expect miracles. Don't expect more rapid change than is warranted by our knowledge of the effects of exercise and training upon the body. However, do make periodic assessments of where you are in terms of your starting point. When you see slow but steady progress toward your goal, you will be encouraged to maintain your program.

Making It Fun

In this discussion of beginning and maintaining a program of regular exercise, we should not overlook one of its significant potential benefits—it can be fun. In fact, we argue that if it is not fun, you've selected the wrong activities for your exercise program. You see, if it is not fun most of the time, you will not continue it for very long. We present so many options in this book that you should be able to find activities that will accomplish your goals while at the same time providing your enjoyment. All you need to do is be selective. Think about your choices carefully, and seek help from others when appropriate.

EXERCISING UNDER DIFFICULT CIRCUMSTANCES

If you maintain your training program long enough, you will invariably encounter obstacles. We have selected five such obstacles to discuss and to demonstrate how, if you're serious about training, your program need not be interrupted. These obstacles are travel, work, injury, being busy, and having visitors.

When Traveling

If you travel often, you should consider that circumstance when developing your program. For example, rather than join a local health club, you would be wise to join one with facilities throughout the country so you can exercise when you are in a different city. The YMCA and YWCA, Jewish Centers, and some nationally franchised health clubs have facilities throughout the United States. In addition, you should select activities that take into consideration regular travel. You would be better off jogging, for example, than playing tennis. Jogging requires little by way of equipment or facilities and does not entail obtaining a partner. Tennis requires a racket that may be bulky to travel with and means that you'll be able to exercise only if you can find someone with whom to play. The factors to consider then, if you travel often, are equipment, facilities, and dependence on other people.

If you travel infrequently you have even less of a problem, although you still may need to make special arrangements. You might be able to make prior arrangements with someone so you'll have a partner with whom to exercise; you might be able to rent facilities (racketball court time), and you might take advantage of exercise opportunities not usually available to you (snow for skiing). Viewed in this way, travel can be a pleasant enhancement to your exercising, providing you with new partners, new settings, and new activities.

If you find travel regularly interfering with your exercise program, you should think about whether or not you are making excuses not to exercise. If that is the case, then you haven't chosen an activity enjoyable enough so that when you're not able to do it, you feel deprived. If this describes your situation, reconsider the activities you've chosen to achieve your goals and choose others.

When Confined to a Limited Space

If you are confined to your office or some other indoor place, that too need not interrupt your fitness program (Liebman, 1982). Figures 6.1 and 6.2 depict two exercises you could do in an office to develop or maintain flexibility. The neck exercise in Figure 6.2 is particularly relevant, since being confined to an office with a lot of work (or a lot of studying) can lead to tense neck muscles and may result in tension headaches. Maintaining flexibility in the neck muscles will help prevent these headaches.

Figures 6.3 and 6.4 show two exercises to improve and maintain muscular strength, one of which involves a partner. You'd be surprised how many

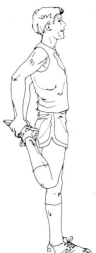

FIGURE 6.1   Front leg flexibility (quadriceps)

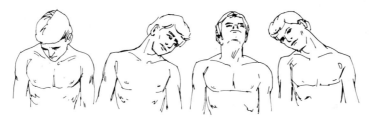

FIGURE 6.2   Neck rotation exercise stretching neck muscles

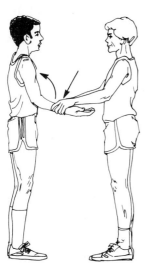

FIGURE 6.3   Improving muscular strength with a partner

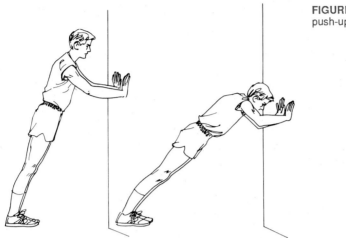

FIGURE 6.4 Standing push-ups

co-workers or other students would be willing to participate in fitness activities with you if you ask them.

To improve and maintain cardiorespiratory endurance while confined to an office takes some ingenuity, but it is possible. If you are fortunate enough to be able to afford an exercise bike, you can keep one in your office and ride it even while doing work. If not, you can always purchase a rope and skip rope in your office during "downtime." There are many ways to adapt the exercises presented throughout this book to confined areas. The point is that limited space or facilities need not interrupt your fitness training.

When Injured

As with the other obstacles presented in this section, you can use an injury as an excuse not to exercise. On the other hand, in many cases an injury need not interrupt your training; it can just alter it. For example, an injury to your leg may preclude jogging, but not swimming. An injury to your shoulder may disqualify squash, but not jogging. For most minor injuries, common sense will dictate what you can and cannot do. We will discuss care of these injuries in Chapter 13, but remember that most minor injuries do not mean you have to stop exercising.

Most serious injuries—those requiring consultation with professional health care providers—have a greater potential for interfering with regular exercise. However, even with serious injuries, some form of exercise is usually possible. Before proceeding with any exercise, however, consult the professional caring for you. After seeking and obtaining advice, you must decide what you will do and what you will not do.

When Very Busy

"I don't have any time to exercise. I'm too busy." It rings out almost like a battle cry. Let's assume that someone actually believes he or she is too busy to exercise regularly or that his or her schedule necessitates an interruption in training. In other words, the person is not just using the schedule as an excuse. Closer examination of this statement, however, indicates a fallacy. Everyone has the time; some of us just choose to use our time for other purposes. Some of the uses of our time, when we scrutinize them carefully, are actually appropriate. That is, based on our values, it makes sense to use our time in that fashion. However, other uses of our time are often inconsistent with our professed values.

We may say we value health and fitness, but we take a long lunch instead of a short workout and a short lunch. Or we meet our friends for a drink at the local watering hole instead of exercising. It is our belief that most of us would find the time to exercise, even during finals week or when the annual report is due, if we really valued fitness. What is required is for us to take some time to examine our schedules and to adjust them so the time for regular exercise is found. In some instances, that will mean shorter workouts or maximizing exercise time by being ultraselective about activities. But in no instance does it mean we cannot have an exercise program.

When You Have Visitors

Suppose a friend comes to stay for 2 weeks. What happens to your program? Visits from friends or relatives may actually encourage exercise, but they often interfere. There are several strategies you can use to help you maintain your training program in such situations. If your visitors are also regular exercisers, there's no problem. Just exercise at the same time, even if you are all doing different activities. In that way, no one will feel deprived of anyone else's company. If your visitors are not exercisers, plan short trips they can take when you are exercising. Sightseeing trips are ideal. If relatives are also nearby, perhaps they can entertain your visitors. What is required is some planning prior to the visit and some ingenuity as a part of that planning. What is not required is an interruption in your training.

CONCLUSION

Well, there it is. You have the assessments you need to *develop* your own exercise program and you have the strategies with which to *maintain* that program. Some of us will find particular strategies more useful than others; and some of us will need to use more of this arsenal than others. With proper planning, however, all of us can adopt a life-style that includes regular exercise—exercise that contributes to our wellness as well as to our physical health.

SUMMARY

1. To organize a physical fitness program requires knowing the present fitness status and the fitness goal.
2. In assessing one's life-style to relate a physical fitness program to it, determine the pace of life and the daily activities in which one engages.

3. Psychological and sociological characteristics are important considerations in developing a physical fitness program.

4. The following psychosocial factors should be considered in developing a physical fitness program: motivation, locus of control, assertiveness, alienation, self-esteem, and stress. A medical examination (if indicated) and a fitness appraisal should be additional inputs into the development of a fitness program.

5. Techniques for achieving physical fitness goals include social support, contracting, reminder systems, beginning gradually, tailoring, utilizing the health beliefs model, obtaining help from professionals, chaining, and using the covert techniques of covert rehearsal, covert modeling, and covert reinforcement.

6. Techniques to help improve the chances of maintaining the program once it has been started include material reinforcement, social reinforcement, joining a group, boasting, self-monitoring, and making the program fun.

7. In spite of obstacles to exercising regularly such as traveling, being confined to a limited space, being injured, being very busy, or having visitors, there are means and strategies by which regular exercise can continue uninterrupted.

REFERENCES

BARTLEY, DIANNE A. R., AND FAYE Z. BELGRAVE. "Physical Fitness and Psychological Wellbeing in College Students." *Health Education* 18 (1987):57–60.

BECKER, MARSHALL H. "The Health Belief Model and Personal Behavior." *Health Education Monographs* 2 (1974): 326–473.

BECKER, MARSHALL H., AND LAWRENCE W. GREEN. "A Family Approach to Compliance with Medical Treatment—A Selective Review of the Literature." *International Journal of Health Education* 18 (1975): 1–11.

BROWNELL, K. D., ET AL. "The Effects of Couples Training and Partner Cooperatives in the Behavior Treatment of Obesity." *Behavior Therapy* 16 (1978): 323–33.

CAIRNS, D., AND J. A. PASINO. "Comparison of Verbal Reinforcement and Feedback in the Operant Treatment of Disability due to Chronic Low Back Pain." *Behavior Therapy* 8 (1977): 621–30.

DUNBAR, JACQUELINE M., GARY D. MARSHALL, AND MEL F. HOVELL. "Behavioral Strategies for Improving Compliance." In R.B. Haynes, D.W. Taylor, and D.L. Sackett (eds.), *Compliance in Health Care*. Baltimore, MD: Johns Hopkins University Press, 1979.

FELDMAN, ROBERT H. L. "Modifying Stressful Behaviors." In Jerrold S. Greenberg, *Comprehensive Stress Management*, pp. 223-243. Dubuque, IA: Wm. C. Brown, 1986.

FELDMAN, ROBERT H. L. "The Assessment and Enhancement of Health Compliance in the Workplace." In George S. Everly and Robert H.L. Feldman,

Occupational Health Promotion: Health Behavior in the Workplace. pp. 33–46. New York: John Wiley, 1985.

LIEBMAN, SHELLEY. *Do It at Your Desk: An Office Worker's Guide to Fitness and Health.* Washington, DC: Tilden, 1982.

MAHONEY, M. J., AND C. E. THORESON. *Self-Control: Power to the Person.* Monterey, CA: Brooks/Cole, 1974.

TAYLOR, SHELLY E. *Health Psychology.* New York: Random House, 1986.

7

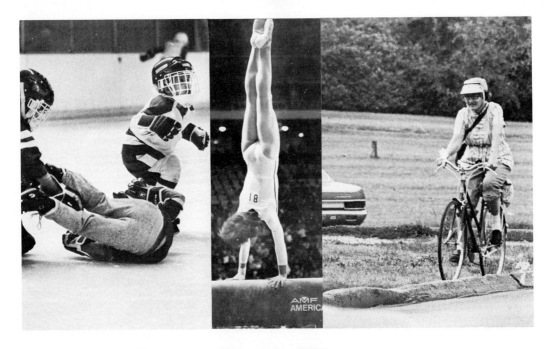

Physical Fitness
Throughout Life

Sounds of tinkling glasses and loud talking fill the air. The room is crowded with middle-aged men and women caught up in ritualized handshaking and affected laughter. Occasionally a kiss or embrace of dubious sincerity is exchanged. Although neither style nor quality of dress is uniform, it's obvious that they've tried to look as fine and stylish as possible. Movement is guarded; eyes look everywhere; body language bespeaks nervousness and hesitancy. Many are animated and excited:

> Oh my God, Harry Sloan, is that *really* you? I thought it might be you! Just look at you, Harry—so prosperous looking, so distinguished with your gray hair. I really didn't think you'd be here. Come on, I want you to meet my wife.
>
> Rebecca—Rebecca Colter, you haven't changed at all—not one iota in thirty years. It's amazing, you look just the same as when I last saw you. Don't you remember me? I'm Carol Pritcher, that is, the former Carol Pritcher—now I'm Mrs. Carol Toller, mother of two sons in college, a married daughter, a deaf Siamese cat, a cocker spaniel and two parakeets. You—look—terrific!

The thirtieth reunion of the old high school senior class brings the classic confrontation with the proverbial ravages of time. The old grads stand in front of faces with added wrinkles; heads with hair of different color (and less of it) than they remember; bodies with more girth. They've seen these changes in their own mirrors over the years, but they've been able to rationalize them. The encroachments occur gradually. They can be blamed on a poor night's sleep, a tough day at the office, or an argument with a spouse or a disobedient child. But the class reunion has the capacity to lay reality painfully on the line. And for some of us, the awareness that we're moving on in years, that we're indeed undergoing physical change, is a real problem. Others take it in stride.

Ironically, casual acceptance of aging, in and of itself, is not necessarily a desirable thing. The important issue is in what way(s) the acceptance is occurring. Is the individual giving up activities that have provided pleasure and reward for years because of society's insistence that "people of a certain age should no longer be doing that?" Are chronological milestones (rather than biological age) being used arbitrarily to cause cessation of certain activities?

No doubt about it. There are true, apparent, and measurable physical differences between 18- and 48-year-olds. Many of these differences go beyond gray hair and added inches around the waistline. In this chapter, we'll look at physiological, structural, and performance changes along the chronological continuum from childhood to old age, and at the fitness programs appropriate to various stages in the life cycle.

You should be able to benefit from this review for a number of reasons:

1. You were once a child, and what we point out in this chapter may help clarify observations you've made about your own childhood, and about your interest or lack of interest in physical activity or sport; your self-confidence level as a child; your relationships with other kids. You may currently be working or planning to work with children in the capacity of coach, youth leader, or camp counselor. Perhaps you live at home with younger brothers or sisters. And perhaps you have children of your own.

2. It will be beneficial to you in your search for a better understanding of your environment and your quest for personal wellness to learn about changing physical capacities as you age. As you look at older people, remember that some day *you will be where they are now*. And what you do now about fitness and wellness can affect your life later.

Let's start this review where we all start: in childhood.

EXERCISE FOR CHILDREN

Much of what occurs in adult life is influenced by childhood experiences. An appreciation for physical activity, sport, and exercise (or for that matter, aversions toward these experiences) is partially implanted in us when we are very young. And as children grow and develop, their values are further shaped and modified.

As the women's movement, electronic technology, and other social changes affect our system of values, what we convey to kids also changes. Today, adults are transmitting messages about exercise and sport far different from those of 40 or 50 years ago. Today, little resistance is offered a child who wishes to exercise or play.

Kids love to run, kick, tumble, and jump. Teachers of young children usually find it easy to capitalize on the natural eagerness of kids for physical activity. The challenge often faced by teachers in the school setting is to get children to appreciate proper and improper times for exercise. In addition, kids must develop an understanding of how to exercise safely. For the most part, sport is the mode in which the majority of American children express their need or desire to participate in physical activity. Let's look now at how exercise affects children who participate.

Cardiorespiratory Fitness

For a long time, authorities were convinced that strenuous exercise was harmful to children. It was believed that the arteries near the heart increased in size at a slower rate than the heart muscle itself. Books published as late as 1967 included this misconception. Consequently, an unnecessary and ill-advised overprotection of children prevailed. Fortunately, we now know that exercise is not only something that children can deal with physiologically, but something profitable and positive. But it's difficult to assess the positive effects of exercise upon cardiorespiratory fitness in children because we often tend to overlook the fact that natural growth and developmental factors are also important contributors to physiological improvement. More and better research studies should recognize and control for these factors.

Up until the age of approximately 13, maximum oxygen intake improves. In fact, if we correct for body size, children have scores that are very comparable to, or even exceed, those of adults. After age 13, the intake values of males begin to exceed those of females (see the section on male-female differences). This means we can expect children to perform at least respectably and safely (as far as cardiorespiratory factors are concerned) in activities that are basically *aerobic* (in the presence of oxygen). Maximum oxygen intake is our best available measure of readiness for aerobic exercise.

Not surprisingly, children who participate in rigorous exercise programs show relatively higher functional (physiological) capacities than those who do not exercise. And although the evidence is not yet conclusive, observations by Saltin and Grimby (1968) suggest that in adults who for years trained heavily as kids, some forms of physiological superiority linger in comparison to adults who did not train as children. But despite what we've so far said about the physiological capacities of children and how they are enhanced through exercise, there remains an unavoidable observation that we would all do well to appreciate: *Children are not scaled-down adults.* Although training has enabled many young performers to produce outstanding athletic achievements, we should not overlook the important cardiorespiratory differences between young children and adults. For example, their size (shorter limbs) places them at mechanical disadvantages that have to be overcome by expending greater physiological effort. They have to move their legs more often over a distance when competing in a foot race with adults to cover the same ground. More energy is therefore needed, and the activity therefore becomes more taxing for children.

Strength, Muscular Endurance, and Flexibility

As we noted, most children who train or exercise regularly in our society probably do so in sport programs. Therefore, research on the effects of exercise on kids is restricted to youth sports activities, and to subjects who fall within the age range of about 9 to 16. We know relatively little about adaptation to exercise in children who run around the backyard or neighborhood park, or who play in the street (Ridenour, 1978). With this limitation in mind, let's look at muscular strength, endurance, and flexibility as they relate to exercise and children.

Muscular Strength.   One striking difference between children who participate in sport programs and those who do not is in muscular strength. The strength of children will typically improve substantially in response to strength training. This is due to children's infrequent participation in activities requiring muscular strength. However, weight training is a questionable activity prior to puberty. Pediatricians are concerned about the possible harmful effects of joint overload on the ends of long bones. And a study by Bloor, Pasyk, and Leon (1970) suggests that severe exercise stress at young ages may have detrimental effects on subsequent muscular development. It's important to remember this when advising children about strength training.

Muscular Endurance.   The ability of children to deal with lactic acid (a waste product of muscular activity) is considerably lower than is that of adults. Therefore, children and youth tend to quit much earlier than adults in endurance-type activities. But as is always the case, motivation and other psychological factors influence the performance of children perhaps even more than of adults. Parents and coaches learn how to press the right buttons in children to stimulate great effort and terrific athletic feats. Sometimes this borders on exploitation and abuse and leads to what we call "overachievement injury."

Flexibility.   Flexibility begins to decrease in children at about age 12, after increasing steadily from approximately age 6. After puberty, females have a greater potential for flexibility than males because their centers of gravity are lower and their legs are shorter. It's not surprising, therefore, that activities such as dancing, tumbling, gymnastics, and springboard and platform diving have always been popular with girls and women.

Obviously, movements that emphasize stretching and/or strengthening joints will improve flexibility. So, when designing activity programs for children or advising them about what to include in their exercise routines, give attention to stretching movements. Irrespective of what the child's activity preference is, try to incorporate some flexibility work. Children tend to be more flexible than adults, but this ability still requires attention. Exercise programs for youth that emphasize flexibility yield improvements rather quickly.

In addition, improved flexibility will help prevent many types of exercise-related injury. The flexible performer will move with greater efficiency through a wider range of motion. And the stretching exercises employed to increase flexibility will prepare the muscles and joints for the demands of strenuous activity (warmup).

Body Composition

A great deal of what we know about exercise and body composition in children derives from animal studies. The embarrassing fact is that we probably have more information about what treadmill or wheel running does to bone, body fat, and muscle tissue in young rats than we have about these relationships in children. Scientists find it difficult to gather conclusive information about exercise and body composition in children for several reasons.

First, very significant changes in growth and maturation occur quite normally (but not evenly or proportionately) during various stages of childhood, independent of physical activity patterns. Heredity and growth and sex hormones, in combination with nutritional and environmental factors, apparently influence increases in body muscle and fat (Figure 7.1). Studies that focus on exercise relative to these kinds of changes should therefore take into account (or control for) these important influences (Parizkova, 1973). Unfortunately, many of them do not.

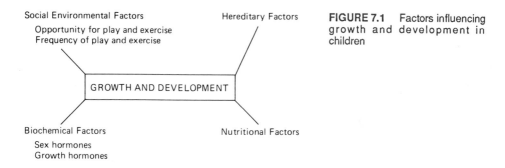

Social Environmental Factors
    Opportunity for play and exercise
    Frequency of play and exercise

Hereditary Factors

GROWTH AND DEVELOPMENT

Biochemical Factors
    Sex hormones
    Growth hormones

Nutritional Factors

FIGURE 7.1   Factors influencing growth and development in children

Another problem with many of the research studies is that they tend to use as subjects middle- or upper-class children who are *already* involved in sport programs. Such biased sampling tends to prevent an objective and honest examination of exercise's effect on *all* children. Children who *are* participating in youth sport programs may very well be taller, more muscular, and better nourished than those who are not involved, particularly if tryouts have weeded out the less tall, less muscular, and less well nourished.

But despite these drawbacks in our understanding, certain observations are worth reporting, considering, and remembering.

1. Exercise of the endurance kind, done fairly rigorously and regularly, does not seem to have any negative effect on growth and/or body composition in children. However, many experts have expressed concern over the *possible* harmful long-term effects of competitive athletics on physical growth. Of course, precise interpretations of words such as "prolonged," "intensity," and "stressful" are necessary before we can satisfactorily understand the relationship of exercise to growth and body composition. Also, the age at which exercise is begun is a critical factor.

2. Elementary school-age children participating in regular exercise programs tend to be leaner (less fatty), according to some studies (Sobolova et al., 1971). (In Chapter 11, you'll read about the many ways in which exercise interacts with the storage and burning of body fat.)

3. Older male children (high school age) who participate in athletics tend to be taller, stronger, and leaner than nonathletes. Once again, these differences probably reflect training effects, but they may be a function of selection of the tallest, strongest, and leanest to make the team.

4. No evidence exists which suggests that the body height attained in adulthood is related to physical activity in childhood.

So, although we might be intuitively ready to doff our hats to exercise in acknowledgement of the numerous benefits it offers youthful participants, more and better research is really needed.

Fitness Programs for Children: Guidelines

We've tried to provide a helpful overview of some of the effects of exercise during childhood. Our hope is that much of this material will assist you in preparing, leading, or evaluating exercise programs for kids. But perhaps the most meaningful and important information of all takes the form of caution. We want to emphasize the need to select physical activities for children wisely, with an eye toward possible injury. Distinctive structural, mechanical, and physiological characteristics of children mean their responses to exercise are different from those of adults. These reponses must be carefully considered when organizing fitness programs for children (Micheli, 1979).

For the most part, culture, climate, and available facilities determine, or at least heavily influence, the kinds of physical activities children select. Kids will tend to translate their natural desire for play into activities compatible with their geographical location, as well as the fields, courts, and play areas to which they have access. But despite the practicality of their selections, there often exists a need to moderate or temper their enthusiasm for an activity with regard to potential injury. When performing sport skills, children tend to emulate the form and style of their athlete heroes and heroines. They frequently adopt positions or stances to which they are biomechanically poorly suited. And because of this, they benefit from wise counsel from teachers, coaches, or more experienced older friends or leaders. Children's susceptibility to certain kinds of injury deserves consideration by all who work with them in physical activity settings.

Growth Plate Injury.   At the end of the skeleton's long bones are columns of cartilage cells, which in children are in various stages of development. Ultimately, this site on the bone becomes hardened and resilient to injury. But in childhood it is especially vulnerable to damage when traumatized. A blow or acute wrenching movement of a long bone may result in a fractured growth plate (see Figure 7.2). The consequences of this kind of injury may be extremely serious, for example, stunted growth or uneven development of the joint.

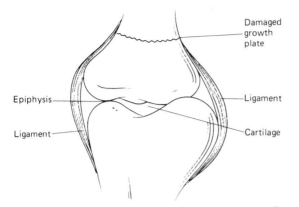

Damaged growth plate

Epiphysis

Ligament

Ligament

Cartilage

FIGURE 7.2   The growth plate and other aspects of two long bones where they interface

Epiphyseal Injury.   The ends (epiphyses) of the long bones and the cartilage that is supposed to protect and lubricate this area are far more susceptible to injury in childhood than in adulthood. Elbow, knee, hip, and ankle joints are common places that can suffer this kind of injury in physical activities. Damage to the protective cartilage where long bones articulate (meet) may lead to premature arthritis.

Elbow Injury.   Baseball, along with apple pie, is said to be symbolic of America. One of its fundamental skills, pitching, is the source of frequent injury to the elbow joints of young players. Although any of the throwing sports carries this liability, curveball pitching, which involves usual compressing of the outer side and stretching of the inner side of the joint, is particularly stressful. Throwing is not a natural activity for humans, and children should not be expected to repeat this kind of movement for long periods of time. This caution also holds true for activities such as javelin and football throwing.

Lower Back Injury.   Physical exercise that involves much bending of the spine can result in stress fracture to the lower spinal vertebrae, which involves a slow loss of bony substance at a particular site. If the activity that caused the stress fracture continues, a complete fracture may result. Young female gymnasts may experience this condition. Youth are also vulnerable to injury of the cartilage in the vertebral bodies, where damage to the growth plate may occur. Frequent compression of the spine, like that experienced by high school football players, may also cause this condition.

If children persist in participating in activities originally designed for adults and adult bodies, then rule changes and equipment and facility modification should be considered (as they often are in the case of Little League baseball and Pop Warner football). However, modification of some activities still does not make them entirely appropriate or safe for children. As we've indicated previously, children are vulnerable to injury in certain parts of their bodies (particularly between the ages of 8 and 14), and special protective equipment, although helpful, does not free them from that vulnerability.

Just as adults sometimes do, kids may seek satisfaction of psychological needs through exercise. It is very likely that youth also use sport and physical activity to satisfy a need for friendship (affiliation), a need to do something well (excellence), a need to subdue or dominate others (aggression), a need to do things on their own (independence), a need for excitement and tension (stimulus seeking), and a need for recognition, status, and prestige (success). And in their quests to fulfill their needs, they deserve guidance, leadership, and teaching from patient, caring adults.

FITNESS PROGRAMS FOR THE ADULT YEARS

Adulthood covers a broad chronological span in which many organic, structural, and functional changes occur. The range of physical fitness is also wide in adulthood, and readiness for vigorous physical activity is considerably less homogeneous than in childhood. Therefore, it's inappropriate to even try to write an exercise prescription for all adults. What we can do is provide a number of guidelines, cautions, and good ideas that should apply to many of you.

Kind, Amount, and Timing of Exercise

Three questions deserve immediate attention: (1) What kinds of exercise should adults do? (2) How much exercise should they do? and (3) How often should they do it? (American College of Sports Medicine, 1978).

Adults—or anyone seeking to elevate fitness levels—need activities that provide gradually increasing stress to the cardiorespiratory system. They also require incrementally increasing resistance to the skeletal muscles, performed with periodically increasing numbers of repetitions. Additionally, they would do well regularly to lengthen and stretch skeletal muscles as well as connective tissue around the joints. And of course, keeping stored fat within appropriate levels is a high fitness priority.

To stress cardiovascular systems, adults need rhythmic, enduring, repetitive activities that are fairly vigorous. Walking, cycling, rope skipping, swimming, or jogging are good examples. Swimming is good if the exerciser is particularly heavy, since the buoyancy provided by the water prevents the trauma to the knees and other joints that obese persons may experience when jogging or even walking. Some very heavy adults find it difficult to negotiate a bicycle. Swimming is therefore a particularly good exercise for those adults.

It's a good idea to provide variety for adult exercisers. Often the physical exuberance so common in childhood has faded. (Of course, we're counting on a retrieval of this enthusiasm once the program is begun.) But in the beginning, some adults with renewed motivation for exercise after years of abstinence need a little hoopla to sustain them. So periodic changes of environment are helpful, such as altering the jogging trail by running it in the opposite direction, doing calisthenics to music, dressing in different exercise

WHAT KINDS OF EXERCISE SHOULD ADULTS DO? HOW OFTEN?

Activities that emphasize large muscle groups and involve cardiorespiratory endurance are recommended. These may be incorporated in game and/or competitive situations. Rhythmic and aerobic experiences are particularly important for cardiovascular development and maintenance. Other types of activities (tennis, handball, racketball) may be incorporated into the regimen as additions, so to speak, for fun.

Healthy adults should try to participate in continuous aerobic activity for 15 to 60 minutes, depending on the intensity of the exercise. Beginning exercisers would do well to perform at low to moderate levels for relatively longer periods of time. A good criterion for determining how much exercise adults should do is sustaining a pulse rate of between 110 to 120 beats per minute or a little higher if the exerciser is already in pretty good shape.

Programs in which participation is 3 days a week at the intensities described above should fill the bill. Going beyond 3 days a week may be good or not so good, depending upon the exerciser and the exercise. Jogging and running for adults who are exercise beginners may produce orthopedic injuries when done in excess of three times per week. Swimming is not as likely to produce the same effect. Three times per week should be enough for calisthenics, stretching, and rhythmic-endurance exercises. Other game or recreational activities, such as racket sports, may be added on other days.

Combative, competitive activities such as tackle football (or even flag football) and basketball carry substantially high injury risks (particularly of the orthopedic kind) as biological age advances. It's presumptuous to identify precisely the age at which an adult should no longer pursue these kinds of experiences. Sometimes adults have difficulty disengaging from sports that have provided them a great deal of satisfaction for a long period of time. An alternative is lifetime or carryover sports, which can be continued for many years.

costumes or uniforms, varying the time of day when exercise is done, and so on.

The development of great muscular strength is probably not a high priority for most adults, unless they are engaged in professional athletic careers. So weight training with very heavy resistances is probably not appropriate for most adults, particularly those who are beyond their mid-thirties. Adults whose jobs require unusual muscular strength have probably already cultivated it, and its maintenance is likely to be achieved by the on-the-job demands. However, if an adult is interested in building greater strength, many of the available (but expensive) machines provide resistance in comparatively safe environments.

Muscular endurance training makes a good deal of sense for adults. Whether beating or mixing a batter in the kitchen, giving junior a lift on the shoulders at the zoo, raking the autumn leaves from the front lawn, or dancing all evening to your favorite music with your favorite partner(s), endurance demands are more frequent challenges for most adults than strength demands. Most daily strength demands are met satisfactorily, although it's probably wise to mention the importance of adequate lower back and abdominal strength.

And if inadequate strength levels in these or any other areas are diagnosed, remedial measures should be undertaken.

Flexibility exercises are very important ingredients of adult fitness programs. The collagen (fibrous material in connective tissue) undergoes chemical changes in adulthood and causes connective tissue to increase in density. Tendons and ligaments become more resistant to stretching (tight) and should be stretched regularly to be kept loose. Range of joint motion tends to decrease with aging, but flexibility training can counteract this tendency.

Changes in body composition accompany aging. Adherence to sensible dietary measures can diminish many undesirable alterations in muscle-to-fat ratios and bone tissue composition. There is evidence that regular exercise can retard some of the changes in body composition due to aging.

Lifetime Sports

Athletic activities that are learned during youth and engaged in during adult years are referred to as *lifetime* or *carryover sports*. If you are to benefit physically, socially, and psychologically from participation in activities such as tennis, swimming, dancing, and bowling as an adult, it is wise to acquire necessary skills early in life.

But not all activities are appropriate beyond youth. For most middle-aged (and older) adults, rigorous gymnastics, wrestling, and football are inadvisable. Sailing, racket sports, and golf *are* probably appropriate activities for many adults. Some sports, such as volleyball, soccer, and softball, are likely to be appropriate for some individuals. Skills for lifetime or carryover sports may be complex and require development over a long period of time. Therefore, an early start is a good idea.

Adult Fitness: Special Situations

Menstruation and Exercise.   Female sexuality in general is surrounded by more than its fair share of myths. But no area is shrouded in more misunderstanding than is the menstrual cycle. To be sure, important physiological menstrual effects may correlate with physical performance. However, these depend upon the individual. Young women vary much more with regard to these factors than women in their late twenties and thirties. In fact, there is evidence that *dysmenorrhea* (cramps associated with the menstrual cycle) appears to be less common in females who are physically active. According to testimony provided by women athletes, physical performance may or may not be hindered by menses. Apparently a number of important variables determine its effect: (1) the kind of activity, (2) the point in the cycle during which activity is being performed, and (3) the psychology of the performer.

Participation in endurance activities may be impeded somewhat by premenstrual retention of fluid. Obviously, this might be a problem in activities such as long-distance swimming or running. But sprintlike activities show no inhibited performance—in fact, Olympic records have been set by women in all stages of the menstrual cycle. Some athletes do, however, report a slightly less than optimal performance during the premenstrual phase. And there have been occasional reports of athletes who cease menstruating entirely during times of intense physical training.

The significance of any aspect of the cycle as a factor in physical performance is uncertain. In addition, every woman is not likely to be visited by all the premenstrual stressors at once. If you're in good overall physical shape, the negative aspects of the menstrual cycle may not affect you much, and they need not occur at all (Parlee, 1973).

Amenorrhea and Participation in Sport.   Some women experience menstrual irregularity as a result of strenuous physical activity. However, nonathletic women have as many menstrual problems as do athletes (Wells, 1985). Presently there is no conclusive evidence that suggests participation in endurance sport activities necessarily leads to amenorrhea (the absence of menstrual periods). However, amenorrhea may be related to a condition known as *osteoporosis*. This disorder involves a gradual increase in the fragility and thinness of the bones due to a loss of some of the bony tissue's essential minerals, in particular, calcium. Although the relationship of amenorrhea to this condition has not yet been entirely clarified, there is some evidence that production of the important hormone estrogen is inhibited in amenorrheic females. As a result bone mass decreases and women who are amenorrheic are predisposed to the development of osteoporosis (Cann et al., 1984; Drinkwater et al., 1984).

Pregnancy and Exercise.   One frequent series of questions women ask revolve around the issue of exercise and pregnancy. Should women stop exercising when pregnant? What effect can rigorous exercise have on the developing embryo or fetus? Let's have a look at these and related questions.

A number of gold, silver, and bronze medals have been won by pregnant Olympic athletes since 1952. In most cases, the women didn't even know about their condition, because it was early in the pregnancy. Apparently, there is little change in physical performance during the early months. During the first trimester (first three months of pregnancy), the *placenta* (a membranous filter through which the blood of the pregnant woman passes oxygen and nutrients to the fetus) produces an unusually high amount of the hormone progesterone. This may very well account for the relatively good feeling many women claim during this time. Some of the premenstrual stresses (backache, headache, and so on) are believed to be related to a progesterone shortage associated with the premenstrual phase of the cycle.

During the first three months, the incidence of miscarriage due to physical trauma is extremely small. The protective structure accommodating the developing fetus is incredibly effective. In well-trained, fit females, the probability of physical trauma to the fetus is extremely low. Unless some unusual gynecological problem is identified by a physician, regular participation in an exercise program may certainly be maintained, particularly among women who have always exercised. There are ample data to permit the conclusion that complications in pregnancy and childbirth are fewer in women who have been training (athletes) than in those who have not.

A 3-pound weight gain is typical during the first trimester of pregnancy, but a 10-pound gain is the average during the second. This extra weight, combined with a bulging abdominal area and fluid retention, is usually enough to cause withdrawal from high-level sport competition—but not necessarily from friendly games of tennis, or participation in swimming or jogging routines (Katz, 1983). Particularly strong blows to the abdominal area in the eighth or ninth month may start premature labor contractions, so activities such as basketball, flag football, or other contact sports are inadvisable during this phase.

Undoubtedly, one of the most important guidelines for both physician and pregnant patient to follow is how the woman feels. Again, we emphasize that the fetus is secure, protected, and safe in a well-cushioned sac of fluid. It is almost invulnerable as it resides in the healthy pregnant woman—and participation in a program of exercise before and during pregnancy can make her more fit for childbirth. After all, childbirth is in large measure a matter of powerful muscular contractions. Certainly, a physically sound, healthy individual whose musculature and connective tissues are toned and strong would be well prepared for an uncomplicated delivery.

Abstinence from Sex.   Sex, being the controversial and popular topic that it is, always seems to generate a vast array of myths and untruths. Many of them are as fascinating as they are ludicrous. For decades, for example, male boxers and football players were advised to abstain from intercourse for weeks prior to competition. They were told that sex would sap their strength—make them soft. Abstinence would supposedly create an enviable meanness or toughness that would serve them well in competition.

For most of us, meanness, toughness, and irascibility are generally not helpful styles in our day-to-day social interactions. If indeed this is what abstinence produces, then only in highly circumscribed situations might it be useful. In many forms of exercise and sport skill, relaxation rather than meanness or heightened arousal is likely to produce better performance.

But what about the physiological effects of sex prior to physically demanding exercise or athletic competition? Of course marathon bouts of intercourse might lower blood sugar (as participation in a vigorous exercise is prone to do) and induce overall fatigue, depending upon how fit you are for sex. If you're going to be swinging on chandeliers and sliding down banisters while indulging in sex, you're likely to feel tired afterward. And if shortly thereafter you are scheduled to play tennis or run a foot race, you may expect to perform a little less than optimally. But, on the other hand, you may have released a good deal of muscular tension, alleviated stress, reaffirmed or strengthened an emotional commitment, or simply enjoyed yourself.

Injury to Sex Organs.   Another question of a somewhat sexual nature has to do with injury to sexual organs during exercise. For example, some women have expressed concern about damage to the breasts. However, gynecologists report very few breast injuries—probably because most women do not participate in contact sports. And women who do participate in activities such as basketball, for example, usually wear protective covering. Breast volume may be a factor in certain kinds of physical activity such as running over long distances, where the breasts may move in opposition to the vertical motion of the chest wall. Specially designed brassieres can be used to contain breast tissue so that it moves with the chest wall, thereby avoiding soreness.

Rarely do injuries to the female genital organs occur during exercise—so secure and protected are the ovaries, fallopian tubes, and uterus in the pelvic area. Males, of course, are much more disposed to genital injury during exercise because of the externality of their sex organs.

FITNESS PROGRAMS FOR THE ELDERLY

The Andean village of Vilcabamba in Ecuador, a region in the Karakoram Mountain Range in Pakistani-controlled Kashmir, and the community of Abkhagia in the Georgian Soviet Socialist Republic in the Soviet Union all share an unusual reputation. They are places in the world where people supposedly live longer and remain more vigorous in old age than in most modern societies. What factors contribute to the unusual longevity of people in these communities, where men and women well beyond 100 years of age are common? According to the National Center for Health Statistics, life expectancy in the United States for males and females is 69.9 and 77.6 years, respectively. Only slightly more than 10 percent of our population is over 65, and there are roughly 3 centenarians per 100,000 people in the United States.

Clearly, genetic factors play an important role in longevity. Almost all the centenarians in the three communities had parents who lived to be 100 or more. But after careful study, researchers have also observed other factors present in all three societies. First is the esteem in which the elderly are held in these societies. They receive encouragement to work and to be productive community members. Their efforts are appreciated and valued. They continue to hold jobs and fulfill important responsibilities for their families. Second is the very low daily caloric intake of these 100-year-olds. They are reported to eat about 1800 calories a day, in comparison to the approximately 3300 calories eaten daily by the so-called "average American" (Food and Nutrition Board, National Academy of Sciences-National Research Council, 1979). The third factor has to do with the physical locations of these basically agricultural communities. All are situated in fairly remote and mountainous regions where mere locomotion involves arduous climbing or descending steep slopes. Thus, the elderly inhabitants of these places have spent years in hard physical work. Perhaps their cardiovascular functions have been strengthened. In addition, exercise may postpone deterioration in certain aspects of the central nervous system due to aging (Spirduso, 1983). Thus, excellent physical condition may contribute to longevity.

The 65th year is usually considered the benchmark for entry into old age—although researchers often operationally define this milestone a little differently (age 60 or 70). Recently there's been a flurry of research interest in

GOOD PHYSICAL ACTIVITIES FOR THE ELDERLY

Activity	How often (approximate)	Duration (approximate)
Walking	3 times per week	3/4 hour
Swimming	3 times per week	1/2 hour
Dancing	2 times per week	Sets of approximately 20 minutes with intervals of rest
Stretching calisthenics	every day	10-15 minutes
Golf	2 or 3 times per week	as long as necessary to complete 9 or 18 holes
Horseshoe pitching	according to desire	approximately 1/2 hour
Shuffleboard	according to desire	approximately 1 hour
Bocce	according to desire	approximately 1 hour
Croquet	according to desire	approximately 1 hour

this area, but to date the body of available information is rather meager, particularly with regard to exercise. Dr. John Holloszy (1983) of the Washington University School of Medicine has presented a number of reasons why information regarding the effect of aging is difficult to acquire. Among them are these: (1) Subjects would have to be followed for many years; (2) the number of subjects available to study who are over 65 is limited, and many will die soon after age 65; and (3) elderly persons in American society are disinclined to exercise regularly and rigorously.

A further complication is the relatively high degree of physiological and structural vulnerabilities of senior citizens. So, although caution is the keynote here, abstinence from exercise is not. There should be a way for people of every age to enjoy the benefits of some kind of regular exercise. In the case of the elderly, we simply may have to think and plan a little more carefully and creatively. Here are some factors to consider when planning exercise programs for the elderly.

1. The skeletal structures tend to be more prone to fracture in the elderly than in youth or middle ages.
2. Connective tissue is usually more dense, and ligaments and tendons less elastic. Range of motion may be significantly limited in some senior citizens.
3. Muscle mass is somewhat diminished, and reaction and reflex times are slower.

Those who do exercise regularly would, of course, be expected to demonstrate far lesser degrees of these signs of diminished prowess and ability.

So careful assessment of capacities is critical when developing exercise programs for the elderly.

Prudence dictates avoiding combative and contact activities. Wrenching and sharply twisting movements should also be avoided. So should sudden starting, stopping, or changing of direction. Slow rhythmic stretching activities are appropriate and desirable. Frequent rest intervals should be provided, and participants should not be too strongly encouraged to continue after professing fatigue.

Walking is an excellent activity for the elderly, especially in groups where exercisers can socialize and monitor the well-being of others. And, of course, supervised swimming is terrific (it appears that we are forever praising its virtues for exercisers of all types and ages).

Dancing is something many of the elderly are eager to incorporate into their exercise programs. They have done it at one time or another in their lives (or are still doing it), and are familiar with its demands. There is therefore little of the anxiety and trepidation that might accompany introduction to new activities. Folk, square, and social dancing can be rigorous, fun, and socially fulfilling. Fairly high levels of cardiorespiratory and muscular endurance requirements are also usually incorporated in these activities.

Duration and intensity of exercise for the elderly should be determined on an individual basis. Again, we emphasize how critical assessment of beginning levels of readiness for activity is. Personal needs and interests should also be evaluated. These considerations, along with medical input and a fair measure of discretion, should form the basis of the exercise prescription for the elderly.

EXERCISE AND LONGEVITY

Among health professionals, a number of important issues remain controversial. Clear-cut and definitive research findings that would resolve such questions as the role of dietary cholesterol in atherosclerosis and the specific effects of long-term, heavy use of marijuana are not yet available. Consequently, we are obliged to combine whatever information is available with personal experience, heresay, and intuition. Obviously, such decisions are difficult to make. But the person claiming or desiring wellness seeks to exercise as much control as possible over the forces that affect life-style and life itself. So we read, think, and listen to information about dietary cholesterol and marijuana and ultimately decide what we will do.

Longevity and exercise is another of these debatable issues. Quite frankly, sufficient and conclusive evidence in support of the case for enhanced longevity due to exercise has not yet been established. What a terrific thing it would be if we could fortify the attitudes we express in this book with such an assertion. Then we'd have little difficulty in persuading you to exercise. What greater motivation for exercise could there be than the promise of added years in which to enjoy the wellness you are striving to achieve? However, a recent study by Paffenbarger et al., (1986) provides such promise. They observed that exercise participation greatly enhanced the quality of life and extended life

AGING EFFECTS AND PHYSICAL ACTIVITIES THAT MAY POSTPONE OR REDUCE THEM

Effects	Physical Activities
1. Reduced cardiac output	Aerobic activities; jogging; swimming; cycling
2. Lowered pulmonary ventilation	Exercises that stretch rib cage joints; aerobic activities of moderate to high intensity
3. Elevated blood pressure	Aerobic activities; jogging; swimming; cycling
4. Decrease in muscular strength	Weight training (heavy resistance)
5. Decrease in muscular endurance	Aerobic dance; calisthenics
6. Decrease in flexibility	Stretching; bending
7. Increase in percentage of stored body fat	Jogging; running; swimming; cycling
8. Loss in skin elasticity	Weight training (to maintain muscle tonus and "fill out" skin)

span. In fact, "by the age of 80, the amount of additional life attributable to adequate exercise, as compared with sedentariness, was one to more than two years" (p. 605).

Paffenbarger and his colleagues studied the physical activity patterns as well as other life-style characteristics of 16,936 male alumni of Harvard University who had entered college between the years 1916 and 1950. Questionnaires were mailed to those who were alive. The Harvard Alumni Office provided a list of individuals who had died as well as underlying causes of death. The researchers' purpose was to examine the relationship between mortality rates and amount of physical activity done per week (expressed in terms of kilocalories used per week for exercise). Risk of death was found to be higher for those who smoked cigarettes or who had higher than normal blood pressure (hypertension). But perhaps the most meaningful outcome of this study was that as physical activity increased (habitual exercise) from less than 500 to 2,000 or more kilocalories per week, the death rate decreased.

Certainly, in view of the information presented so far in this book, you'd be hard pressed to conclude that exercise shortens life expectancy. After all, exercise has been shown to improve cardiovascular efficiency; change cardiovascular risk profiles; decrease low-density plasma cholesterol (the harmful kind); and increase high-density plasma cholesterol (the protective kind); decrease resting and exercising heart rate; and along with dietary control, play important roles in the management of obesity, hypertension, and diabetes.

What do you think? Will you live longer if you exercise regularly? And, what is just as important, will you live better?

Aging begins at the moment of conception. And concern over this inevitable process is experienced almost as soon as the developing child tentatively enters relations with others out of the home. Readiness for preschool; for kindergarten; for T-ball or Little League baseball; for Cub Scouts or Brownies; for the driving license (the great American puberty rite); for spending the night away from home or staying up or out late are all determined on the basis of age. You're either too young or too old for the armed services. In many states, you can't marry without parental consent until you reach a certain age. Awareness of age pervades our consciousness—it is an inescapable concern of all in our society.

Ironically, we're not sure what aging is. It is very difficult to separate this phenomenon from changes in habits and life-style in general. For instance, some individuals, at some time in their lives, stop dancing or playing tennis. Are subsequent changes in muscle tone or agility therefore due to aging or to stopping exercise? Aging involves a combination of organic buildup as well as breakdown. Let's take a look at some aspects of aging within the context of exercise and wellness.

Cardiorespiratory Fitness

Frequently throughout this book, we've bemoaned the inadequacy of research into some of the subjects we've discussed. Aging and cardiorespiratory fitness are unfortunately no exception. Since "old" subjects rarely train at the high intensities young and middle-aged adults do, comparisons of training programs as well as effects are difficult. From the evidence we do have, however, we are able to offer a number of conclusions.

First, cardiac output is somewhat reduced in elderly exercisers (Pollock, 1973; Saltin, 1969). For the same workload, they must function closer to their cardiovascular capacity than younger individuals. In persons 65 years of age and older, maximal *pulmonary ventilation* (the movement of air into and out of the lungs) is lowered. Stiffening of the rib cage joints and cartilage, as well as lung tissue deterioration, are the probable causes of this reduction in function (Shepherd, 1972).

Apparently, the years 15 to 20 represent the peak time for Max VO_2 (males). The average Max VO_2 at age 60 is approximately two-thirds the average value at age 20 (Robinson, 1938). Other studies by Grimby and Saltin (1966), Heath et al. (1981), and Pollock et al. (1974) conclude that men in their fifties who exercise regularly and vigorously have a maximum oxygen uptake capacity 20 to 30 percent higher than that of young men who do not exercise. Blood pressure, which rises during exercise in accordance with difficulty, tends to be higher in older subjects (exercise as well as resting blood pressures).

Strength, Muscular Endurance, and Flexibility

As individuals mature, greater numbers of muscle cells are probably stimulated into action during activities requiring strength responses. This would explain the observation that we tend to become stronger as we grow older, up until about age 25, when strength levels off for about five years before beginning a gradual decline (Montoye and Lamphlear, 1977). This observation is applicable to both men and women, although there are significant strength differences between the sexes after about age 11 or 12. But strength decrements may be postponed or avoided with training. Furthermore, the data collected and published by scientists typically represent mean or average values. This suggests that individuals who train for strength may be able to avoid sharp decreases in muscular strength due to aging.

Both kinds of tissue (muscle and nervous) undergo deterioration during aging. Endurance, therefore, as in the case with strength, typically diminishes after about the midtwenties. The decrease is gradual and may not even be noticeable unless measured carefully in the laboratory. Again, decrements in muscular endurance can be minimized with training.

To those of you who are anxious about declining muscular endurance and your ability to participate efficiently and pleasurably in exercise and physical activity after the midtwenties, we say: Don't panic! Again, we remind you of two important points. The changes are not really very perceptible for years after the decline begins, and then they're usually significant only at high levels of performance or competition. And perhaps even more important, strategic pacing and overall experience can override small strength and/or endurance decrements in most competitive sport activities.

During aging, changes occur to the joints as well as to the surrounding connective tissue. If joints are not regularly exercised, tendons, ligaments, and joint capsules become shortened and thick, and it is difficult to stretch them to regain lost range of motion. The stiffness and difficulty in stretching and bending often observed in elderly subjects can be prevented or at least significantly reduced by regular exercise. If you've ever been in a cast for weeks, you know how dramatically different joint movement is after its removal. Sometimes it requires weeks of special exercises to regain normal motion. Some of the protective and lubricating tissue within joints actually wears away as a result of years and years of use. Consequently, some forms of movement may be painful (arthritis). Swimming is often prescribed for arthritis victims, since the buoyancy provided by the water brings relief from weight-bearing stresses on the bones and joints.

Body Composition

Generally, at about age 25 there begins a slow and barely perceptible series of changes in the amounts and composition of fat, muscle, and bone tissue. Some of these changes usually become meaningful or even statistically significant only in middle and/or old age. Percentage of stored body fat tends to increase while percentage of muscle tissue decreases. These shifts may be postponed or reduced in severity through exercise and careful calorie counting. As these shifts occur, total body weight may remain constant (Sidney, Shepherd, and Harrison, 1977).

Other compositional changes are more difficult to inhibit, occur more slowly, and ultimately yield more dramatic observations. Among these are loss in skin elasticity (wrinkles, hanging skin or folds under the chin and backs of arms); loss of bone minerals (Womersley et al., 1976) and protein, which makes bones more susceptible to fracture and postural defect; and skeletal height reduction (Parizkova and Eiselt, 1980), partly caused by wearing away of connective tissue between the vertebrae of the spine.

SEX DIFFERENCES AND EXERCISE

What do we really *know* about performance capacities according to sex? Do important differences exist across the board—differences worth talking about? Are they small and easily overcome with extra effort, or are they formidable obstacles?

It has only been during the last 10 years or so that researchers have explored these questions. Passage of Title IX of the Education Amendments of 1972 and the hotly debated Equal Rights Amendment to the U.S. Constitution have undoubtedly stimulated a good deal of public interest and subsequent scientific inquiry into these issues. Scientists have begun to look at the female as she works, performs physically, and plays and competes on the athletic field (Harris, 1975). Manufacturers of sport and exercise equipment have also jumped on the bandwagon. All sorts of fitness and athletic paraphernalia especially designed for women are available now. Jogging bras and special shoe sizes are but two examples.

Approximately 10 years' worth of research falls considerably short of providing answers with the quality and depth necessary to clarify many fuzzy areas dealing with gender and physical performance. Much more well-conceived and methodologically sound research is needed before we may speak confidently and definitively about human physical and motor sex differences. But let's have a look at what is available. Let's review what is presently known about the body, and the way it functions during exercise, with an eye toward sex differences.

Cardiorespiratory Fitness

The ability to continue in certain physical activities, such as soccer, basketball, distance running, swimming, and cycling, is basically dependent upon the capacity of the heart, blood vessels, and blood (the circulatory system) to distribute blood to working muscles. The lungs (respiratory system) must provide the oxygen that makes it way from environmental air to the blood. In addition, chemical waste products must be removed by the blood and brought to special organs to be excreted or changed chemically. The greater the intensity of exercise, the greater are the demands upon the circulatory and respiratory systems. In fact, in some activities, circulatory and respiratory efficiency determine performance quality (success) to a much greater extent than muscle strength.

No differences according to sex have been noted in responses to training programs that attempt to improve cardiorespiratory fitness (Flint, Drinkwater, and Horvath,1974). However, most of the research that reports this conclusion has used healthy and young male and female subjects. We really don't know much about middle-aged or older men and women or very young boys and girls. But at least in normal, healthy females, the gains or improvements due to training are expected to be proportionately just about the same as for males. That is, the absolute size of a score on a test of cardiorespiratory endurance for males is expected to be greater than for females after training, since it was probably greater before training; but the *amount of gain* is expected to be equal.

However, males are advantaged in that their average ability to bring in air from the environment and distribute it is greater than that of females. Therefore, males are benefited in certain kinds of activities that emphasize cardiorespiratory efficiency. Some scientists believe that the natural difference in aerobic capacity between males and females is due to the greater amounts of hemoglobin and greater percentage of red blood cells found in men. The volume of blood pumped by male hearts and in circulation in the male body is also greater. Men have larger hearts and lungs (Drinkwater, 1973).

But two additional pieces of information bear upon our discussion of this topic, and each has the capacity of tilting the scale in a direction favorable to women. First, the age at which females peak cardiorespiratorily is lower than that for males. Women demonstrate their highest aerobic or endurance scores between the ages of 9 and 14, whereas men do not peak until around age 15. Second, factors such as strategy, skill, motivation, and experience may further decrease the size of any innate endurance gap between the sexes when physical activity takes place within a competitive sport.

But (and this is quite an important "but"), *trained females* will demonstrate cardiorespiratory endurance superior to that of *untrained males*. The level of physical fitness a female attains may override the aerobic gender gap. Women are constantly redefining their performance boundaries and are now shattering Olympic track and swimming records previously held by men. Clearly, a substantial part of the endurance differential due to sex is of social and cultural origin.

Strength, Muscular Endurance, and Flexibility

Pound for pound, males are stronger than females. They simply have about twice as much muscle mass in relation to total body weight (Wilmore and Behnke, 1970). Their muscular endurance (repetitive capacity of muscular contraction) is also superior. Some studies report that women's leg strength is much closer to men's than their arm strength.

At young ages, muscular strength and endurance differences between the sexes are slight. They increase significantly from puberty onward. Evidently, male hormone productivity influences the functional capacities of skeletal muscles. So in activities requiring the expression of absolute strength, such as weightlifting, it is expected that men will do better than women. But women store considerably more body fat than men and therefore may be advantaged in other physical activities. Women hold a number of national and international long-distance swimming records, and this may be due to the added buoyancy and insulation against cold provided by fatty tissue. Women may also be advantaged in marathon running, where it is beneficial for participants to switch to fat as a source of energy as early in the run as possible to conserve carbohydrates to be used as fuel in the later stages. Women apparently are able to make this change earlier and more efficiently than men. In all probability, top female marathon times will soon be very close to those of males.

Women enjoy a clear and uncontested supremacy when it comes to flexibility (the range of motion around a joint). Females consistently score higher than males, at all ages, on tests of flexibility. Since practice and training have marked influence on flexibility, it stands to reason that cultural factors may account for this sex difference. Girls, for example, traditionally engage more in activities that enhance flexibility, such as ballet, modern dance, acrobatics, tumbling, and gymnastics. But perhaps structural (skeletal) differences also account for greater flexibility among females, particularly in certain joints. Females have narrower shoulders and broader hips than do men. Adult males have longer leg and arm lengths (relative to upper body length) than females. Females also have weaker joints and less dense bones, so there is less resistance to muscular tension. Joints are therefore more extensible. Structural differences in the pelvis as well as a lighter chest cavity provide for a comparatively lower center of gravity in women. This probably contributes to their superiority in balancing activities.

Body Composition

When attempting to understand performance capability in physical activity, it is important to distinguish fat and lean weights from *total body weight*. Total body weight, usually expressed in pounds or kilograms, does not provide us with enough helpful information. Two individuals may be comparable in height, weight, and skeletal construction, and yet because the proportions of their body weights devoted to fat storage and muscle tissue differ, their performances in physical activity would be expected to vary. The performer with more fat and less muscle (but same total weight as the other person) would probably perform less efficiently or effectively in an activity requiring strength.

There are body composition differences between males and females (see Figure 7.3). Females store significantly more body fat than males and have considerably less muscle tissue. These differences contribute to advantages and disadvantages in certain physical activities, but in some sport contexts they are virtually meaningless: archery, rifle and pistol shooting, bobsledding, bowling, golf putting.

The hormone estrogen, which is present in much greater amounts in females after puberty, accounts for their greater quantity of stored fat. But women who train very heavily, such as marathon runners who may run in excess of 100 miles per week, can approach the fat and lean weight values for male runners. This is due to the tremendous caloric expenditure involved in

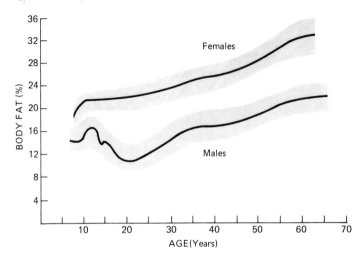

FIGURE 7.3   Body fat during growth and aging. Shaded areas represent one standard error above and below the means.

Reprinted with permission of Macmillan Publishing Company from *Physiology of Exercise: Responses and Adaptations* by David R. Lamb. Copyright © 1978 by David R. Lamb.

long-distance running, which accounts for a good deal of fat metabolism. Heavy training may also result in increases in muscle size. So physical activity, when organized into an extended and vigorous training program, may result in changes in the relationship between fat and lean body weight, even though total body weight may remain substantially unchanged.

CONCLUSION

We believe that the concept of wellness, when correctly interpreted, should be applied to all persons of all cultures, of all ages, and of all types. In our particular framework, the notion of wellness helps establish the importance of exercise and the condition of readiness for exercise known as fitness. Wellness is for all who live.

The concept of wellness applies at any age. The elderly as well as youth, and those whose biological or chronological age falls in between, can enhance life's quality—can mobilize their strengths, vulnerabilities, passions, and aversions to form a mantle that can be worn with comfort and security.

In this chapter we have looked at specific effects of exercise in relation to age and sex. We have concluded that although certain physical capacities vary as we get older, fitness programs tend to benefit us at all ages. However, the kind, amount, and timing of exercise should be compatible with the needs, interests, and capabilities of children, adults, and the elderly.

We have also observed that some differences in cardiorespiratory fitness, strength, muscular endurance, flexibility, and body composition exist between males and females.

SUMMARY

1. Differences in physical capacities (muscular strength, muscular endurance, flexibility) and body composition distinguish children from adults.

2. Authorities used to believe that strenuous exercise for children was harmful due to a disparity between the growth rate of the heart's arteries and heart itself. However, more current and accurate information has been acquired and it is now known that children can exercise without harm to the heart.

3. For the most part, culture, climate, and available facilities determine, or at least heavily influence, the kinds of physical activities children select.

4. Guidelines for children participating in physical activity should be followed to prevent growth plate, epiphyseal, elbow, and lower back injuries.

5. Adults selecting a physical fitness program need to determine what kinds of exercises to do, how much exercise to do, and how often to exercise.

6. Women exercisers may develop a cessation of menstruation—amenorrhea. The decrease in estrogen resulting from amenorrhea or from menopause can lead to a decrease in the calcium in the bone making the bones brittle and weak. This weakened condition of the bone is known as osteoporosis.

7. There are physiological and structural vulnerabilities associated with older age. These should be considered prior to engaging in physical activity.

8. In the elderly, skeletal muscles tend to be more prone to fracture, connective tissue is usually more dense with ligaments and tendons being less elastic, and muscle mass is somewhat diminished.

9. There are gender differences related to exercise. These gender differences include the following variables: cardiovascular endurance, muscular strength and endurance, flexibility, and body composition.

REFERENCES

AMERICAN COLLEGE OF SPORTS MEDICINE. "The Recommended Quantity and Quality of Exercise for Developing and Maintaining Fitness in Healthy Adults." *Medicine and Science in Sports and Exercise,* 10 (1978): vii.

BLOOR, C. M., S. PASYK, AND A.S. LEON. "Interaction of Age and Exercise on Organ and Cellular Development." *The American Journal of Pathology* 58 (1970): 185–99.

CANN, C. E., M. C. MARTIN, H. K. GENANT, AND R.B. JAFFE. "Decreased Spinal Mineral Content in Amenorrheic Women." *Journal of the American Medical Association* 251 (1984): 626–29.

DRINKWATER, B.L. "Physiological Responses of Women to Exercise." In J.H. Wilmore (ed.), *Exercise and Sports Sciences Reviews*, Vol. 1. New York: Academic Press, 1973.

DRINKWATER, B .L., K. NILSON, C.H. CHESNUT, W. J. BREMNER, S. SHAIN-HOLTZ, AND M.B. SOUTHWORTH. "Bone Mineral Content of Amenorrheic and Eumenorrheic Athletes." *The New England Journal of Medicine* 311 (1984): 277–81.

FLINT, M. M., B.L. DRINKWATER, AND S. M. HORVATH. "Effects of Training onWomen's Response to Submaximal Exercise." *Medicine and Science in Sports and Exercise,* 6 (1974): 89–94.

FOOD AND NUTRITION BOARD, NATIONAL ACADEMY OF SCIENCES—NATIONAL RESEARCH COUNCIL. *Recommended Dietary Allowances,* 9th ed. Washington, DC: National Academy of Sciences, 1979.

GRIMBY, G., AND B. SALTIN. "Physiological Analysis of Physically Well Trained Middle-Aged and Old Athletes." *Acta Medica Scandinavica* 179 (1966): 513–26.

HARRIS, D. "Research Studies on the Female Athlete—Psychosocial Considerations." *Journal of Physical Education and Recreation* 46 (1975): 33.

HEATH, G. W., J. M. HAGBERG, A. A. EHSANI, AND J. O. HOLLOSZY. "A Physiological Comparison of Young and Older Endurance Athletes." *Journal of Applied Physiology* 51 (1981): 634–40.

HOLLOSZY, J. O. "Exercise, Health and Aging: A Need for More Information." *Medicine and Science in Sports and Exercise* 15 (1983): 1–5.

KATZ, J. *Swimming through Pregnancy.* Garden City, NY: Doubleday/Dolphin, 1983.

LAMB, D. R. *Physiology of Exercise.* New York: Macmillan, 1978.

MICHELI, L. J. "Sports Injuries in Children and Adolescents." In R.H. Strauss (ed.), *Sports Medicine and Physiology,* Philadelphia: W. B. Saunders, 1979.

MONTOYE, H. AND D. LAMPHLEAR. "Grip and Arm Strength in Males and Females, Age 10 to 69." *The Research Quarterly* 48 (1977): 109–20.

PAFFENBARGER, R. S., JR., R. T. HYDE, A. L. WING, AND C. C. HSIEH. "Physical Activity, All Cause Mortality and Longevity of College Alumni." *The New England Journal of Medicine* 314 (1986): 605–13.

PARIZKOVA, J. *Body Composition and Exercise during Growth and Development.* New York: Academic Press, 1973.

PARIZKOVA, J., AND E. EISELT. "Longitudinal Changes in Body Build and Skin-folds in a Group of Old Men over a 16-Year Period." *Human Biology* 52 (1980): 803–09.

PARLEE, M. B. "The Premenstrual Syndrome." *Psychological Bulletin* 80 (1973): 454-465.

POLLOCK, M. L. "The Quantification of Endurance Training Programs." *Exercise and Sport Sciences Reviews* 1 (1973): 55–188.

POLLOCK, M. L., H. S. MILLER, AND J. WILMORE. "Physiological Characteristics of Champion American Track Athletes 40-75 Years of Age." *Journal of Gerontology* 29 (1974): 645–49.

RIDENOUR, M. (ed.) *Motor Development, Issues and Applications.* Princeton, NJ: Princeton Book, 1978.

ROBINSON, S. "Experimental Studies of Physical Fitness in Relation to Age." *Arbeitsphysiologia* 10 (1938): 251–323.

SALTIN, B. "Physiological Effects of Physical Conditioning." *Medicine and Science in Sports and Exercise,* 1 (1969): 50–56.

SALTIN, B., AND G. GRIMBY. "Physiological Analysis of Middle-Age and Old Former Athletes: Comparison with Still Active Athletes of the Same Age." *Circulation* 38 (1968): 1104–15.

SHEPHERD, R. J. *Alive Man! The Physiology of Physical Activity.* Springfield, IL: Charles C. Thomas, 1972.

SIDNEY, K. H., R. SHEPHERD, AND J. HARRISON. "Endurance Training and Body Composition of the Elderly." *The American Journal of Clinical Nutrition* 30 (1977): 326–33.

SOBOLOVA, V., V. SELIGER, D. GRUSSOVER, J. MACHOVCOCA, AND V. ZELENKA. "The Influence of Age and Sports Training in Swimming on Physical Fitness." *Acta Paediatrica Scandinavica* 217 (1971): 63–67 (supplement).

SPIRDUSO, W. "Exercise and the Aging Brain." *Research Quarterly for Exercise and Sport* 54 (1983): 208–18.

WELLS, C. L. *Women Sport and Performance.* Champaign, IL: Human Kinetics, 1985.

WILMORE, J. H., AND A. R. BEHNKE. "An Anthropometric Estimation of Body Density and Lean Body Weight in Young Men." *Journal of Applied Physiology* 27 (1969): 25–31.

WILMORE, J. H., AND A. R. BEHNKE. "An Anthropometric Estimation of Body Density and Lean Body Weight in Young Women." *American Journal of Clinical Nutrition* 23 (1970): 267–74.

WOMERSLEY, J., J. V. G. A. DURNIN, K. BODDY, AND M. MAHAFFY. "Influence of Muscular Development, Obesity, and Age on the Fat-Free Mass of Adults." *Journal of Applied Physiology* 41 (1976): 223–29.

8

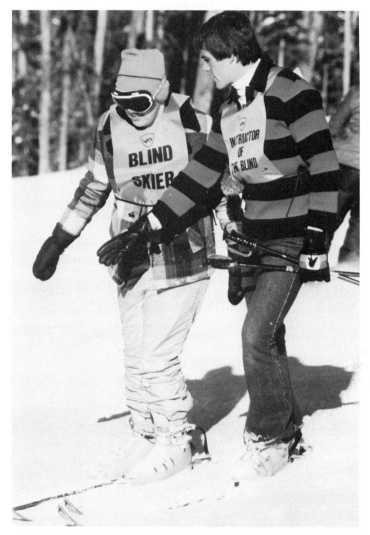

Your Exercise Environment

CHAPTER OBJECTIVES
1. To be able to discuss the outdoor environment factors in relation to exercise.
2. To be able to select proper clothing and equipment for exercise participation.
3. To be able to choose and maintain exercise equipment effectively.

Alberto Salazar had just won the 1982 Boston Marathon in a record-breaking 2:08:51. Incredibly, after having already raced more than 26 miles, he fought off a desperate surge by challenger Dick Beardsley. Moments later, he lay prostrate in a medical tent, not far from the finish line he had just crossed. The heat had gotten to him.

Despite his physiological strength, extensive training, and experience, world-class middle-distance and marathon runner Albert Salazar succumbed to the power of the sun. And it almost cost him his life. Had his body temperature fallen a little more, and had physicians not been on hand to administer an intravenous remedy, he might have died. Clearly, the physical environment is a force to be reckoned with during exercise.

The quality of our performance frequently depends on the physical environment. Our attitudes about our activity's pleasure are shaped by the elements. If we dislike heat or cold, wind or rain, then we may do less well if these conditions prevail in our exercise environment. Competitions are won or lost because of the environment, so environmental controls become important factors in the planning and construction of indoor sport, exercise, and recreation facilities.

Sometimes when you plan to exercise, you find yourself in a situation where heat, altitude, and air quality cannot be electronically or mechanically regulated—that is, outdoors. But you can modify your dress and equipment to suit the environment and perhaps choose a time of the day in which it's best to work out.

An understanding of typical human physiological responses to various environmental conditions will make your adjustments sensible and helpful. You'll be able to plan wisely and safely for exercise. And that's what this chapter is all about. We'll discuss performance responses to heat, cold, high altitude, and polluted air. We'll also discuss how to choose the proper clothing and equipment.

THE OUTDOOR ENVIRONMENT

Exercise in the Heat

Humans are warm-blooded animals; our body temperatures remain fairly constant. Cold-blooded creatures like lizards undergo wide internal temperature shifts in accordance with environmental conditions. We do not. The human body temperature hovers very close to 98.6 degrees Fahrenheit. If it deviates from this level by as little as a few degrees, the consequences can be serious, even fatal. The skin contains temperature sensors that inform the *hypothalamus* (an information-processing center in the brain) of the body's temperature status, and the hypothalamus then adjusts our internal temperature.

Vigorous exercises causes the body's temperature to rise. Some of the clothing and protective equipment you wear during certain kinds of physical activity may prevent the body's attempt to cool itself naturally by the evaporation of sweat from the skin(see Figure 8.1a). So be sure to attend to what you

---

WHAT THE ENVIRONMENT MEANS: A LITTLE EXPERIMENT

Let's try a little experiment. Read the following instructions. When you're finished, put the book down and follow them.

Instructions: Sit back comfortably in your chair, or if you're on the floor, stretch out fully. Close your eyes and try to relax completely. Focus on your slow and rhythmical breathing for about a minute. Now, in your mind's eye, return to the most exciting, most enjoyable, most fulfilling exercise or sport experience you can recall. Reconstruct as much of the event as possible. Include as many details as you can. Remember, this is the most gratifying, the *best* physical activity happening you've ever had.

Describe this event to a fictitious listener. Tell what you have remembered. Say it aloud, or write it if you wish.

Chances are that among the very first remarks you made was a reference to the weather or temperature on this special day. Early in your description you probably said something like this:

The day was gorgeous—it was bright and sunny. I was on the lake water skiing.

It was early autumn, brisk and clear, and I couldn't help noticing the changing colors of the leaves as I jogged into the park.

The beauty of the snow falling on this cold and isolated place was breathtaking. I looked down the trail, gripped my poles and prepared to push off on my skiis.

So you see, the environment is quite important to us when we are striving for high-level wellness through physical activity.

are wearing when exercising in warm weather or in a warm environment (England et al., 1982).

Appendix D contains ACSM guidelines relative to heat injuries experienced during distance running.

Perspiration During Exercise.   Although sweat may be a very troublesome by-product of exercise (it gets in your eyes and can make your hands lose their grips on bats, rackets, and clubs), it really is a desirable physiological response to an increase in internal temperature.

We have about 3 million sweat glands located throughout the body. As muscles contract, they produce heat that enters the blood through the tiny vessels (capillaries) surrounding skeletal muscle. (*Shivering* is an involuntary response to cold that generates heat due to muscular contraction.) Ultimately, heated blood is carried throughout the body. Some of the heat is lost through the lungs as it is removed through the vessels that nourish them. But most body heat is lost through the skin. You interfere with cooling if your cover too much skin.

High humidity also makes cooling difficult because sweat takes longer to dry. Drying sweat produces the desired cooling effect. According to Haymes and Wells (1986), "It is apparent that cardiovascular fitness is more important than gender in heat tolerance. There are some differences in how men and women respond to heat stress. While cardiovascularly fit women are as heat tolerant as men, they generally sweat less, and have higher heart rates and skin temperature" (p. 41).

Heat Disorders.   If and when exercise generates more heat than the body's safety mechanisms can handle, heat injury may occur (American College of Sports Medicine, 1975). You know you have a heat injury problem when you feel nausea, dizziness, and have difficulty in thinking clearly while exercising. This condition, known as *heat exhaustion*, is also characterized by heavy sweating.

HOT WEATHER TIPS

When Exercising in Hot Weather
Drink water frequently.
Wear light-colored, loose-fitting clothing.
Don't hesitate to stop if you feel unwell.

Symptoms of Heat Stroke
Extremely high body temperature.
Hot, dry skin.
No sweating.
Headache, nausea, confusion.
Unsteady gait.

In heat exhaustion, body temperature is likely to be fairly normal, but profuse sweating results in a loss of body water and a decrease in blood volume (blood is mostly water). The remedy is withdrawal from activity, rest, and *replenishment of water.* You can't get into trouble from drinking too much water. So if you suspect heat exhaustion, drink profusely or administer as much fluid as you can get a victim to take.

Heat stroke is far more serious and can be a real medical emergency. Rising body temperature and hot, dry skin are the major symptoms. When a lot of water has been lost because of elevated body temperature, the brain shuts down the sweating mechanism to prevent additional loss. This causes body temperature to rise dramatically. When this happens, temperature must be lowered *immediately.*

Lay the victim in a cool or shaded place and remove all clothing. Provide fluids and try to lower body temperature by dousing the victim with cold water or applying packs of ice or wet towels. Arrange for the victim to get to a hospital as soon as possible. Extremely serious and permanent damage can result if immediate action is not taken.

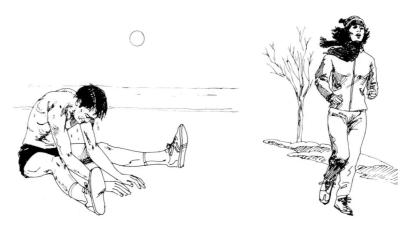

FIGURE 8.1a   An exerciser perspiring under a hot sun.

FIGURE 8.1b   An   exerciser shivering with cold

Exercise in the Cold

If mountain or winter sports are your preferred forms of exercise, then give special attention to this section. (See Figure 8.1b.) You really can't get into too much trouble in the cold as long as you continue to exercise vigorously. During sustained, vigorous activity, body temperature is greatly elevated. Heat production can increase as much as 20-fold, so even in terribly cold weather, appropriate body temperature can be maintained if you continue to exercise. That's why stranded hikers and back packers are encouraged not to sit down when waiting to be found in freezing or subfreezing temperatures.

WHEN EXERCISING IN COLD WEATHER

Keep extremities protected.
Wear layers of clothing.
Be alert to changes in color of unprotected extremities in others; warn them
   about frostbite.
Cover up after exercising in the cold.

Distance swimmers, cyclists, skiers, and runners generate a great deal of heat during exercise which enables them to feel comfortable in weather spectators find intolerably cold. In fact, you may very well prefer to exercise out of doors in cool or even cold weather. Many people find it invigorating. You can always put on another light sweater or T-shirt if you feel cold. For most of us, it's easier to add a layer or two of shirts or socks to become warmer than it is to cool off on a hot day while exercising. And woolen hats, gloves, or mittens (mittens will keep your hands warm because the heat generated by muscles in all fingers is trapped in one area) don't interfere with most sports or forms of exercise.

Covering the head is important if you want to keep the body warm. A great amount of heat is lost when the head is uncovered because the small blood vessels in the scalp are frequently dilated. A substantial blood supply is therefore always present in this area, and a lot of cooling is constantly occurring. If you're warm, remove your head covering; if you're cold, cover your head.

Cover up after exercising in the cold (you still perspire when you work out vigorously in cold weather), and be careful to check for frostbite. (In Chapter 13 we will go into more detail about training in cold environments so as to prevent injury.)

Exercise in High Altitudes

Some runners report experiencing a "high" during a particularly comfortable and extended run. And of course, there are highs that derive from drug use. Scientists have had difficulty in defining these phenomena precisely and in arranging methodologically sound research projects that would explore them adequately. We really don't have sufficient information about the so-called runner's high or chemically induced highs (in exercise or sport contexts) that has withstood the test of scientific scrutiny. However, we know quite a bit about another kind of high and its relationship to sport performance and exercise—*altitude.*

When altitude is much above sea level (about 5,000 feet), the reduced ability of the body to transport oxygen to organs and tissues becomes noticeable. *Hypoxia* is the name of this condition. When this happens, quite obviously, difficulty in physical work is a consequence.

VO_2 max decreases in both trained and untrained athletes as elevation increases (Buskirk et al., 1967). Therefore, endurance activities are most difficult to perform at high altitudes. Sprinters and field event participants and those whose bouts of activity are short-lived are not likely to be adversely affected by moderate altitude.

If you live in an area of relatively high elevation, you're likely to be *acclimatized* (adjusted) to the altitude. You would be expected to perform well in relation to your training efforts in this environment. But if your home is at sea level and you wish to backpack, climb, ski, or run at high altitudes, you're going to feel a real difference (Daniels, 1972). Probably the first symptom you'll recognize is the *hyperventilation* or breathlessness that accompanies exertion.

But there are other consequences of hypoxia that result in impairment to physical activity. Brain tissue is particularly sensitive to decreased oxygen availability. Therefore, many mental tasks become more difficult. Errors in judgment may increase. If you're out on a remote hiking trail or alone on the face of a mountain, you can't afford diminished mental alertness or sharpness. You need your brain to be functioning at full capacity. And this kind of deficit is also serious if you're not alone, but part of a team practicing or competing at high altitude. Vision is also affected by hypoxia. You will not see as well in dim light (sundown) when your oxygen supply is low. This is a serious liability to the downhill skier or backpacker who is homeward bound at the end of the day (McFarland, 1969).

We'd like to believe that when the tired climber or skier finally makes it back to camp, lodge, or tent, the problems caused by exercising in high altitude would be at an end. Not so. Sleep becomes a problem due to hypoxia, and therefore rest may be hard to come by. Breathing rate is supposed to decrease during sleep, but since distribution of oxygen throughout the body is impaired in high altitudes, the brain directs the breathing mechanism to compensate for the hypoxic effects by increasing its rate. This usually results in disturbed sleep (frequent waking up) and interference with much-needed rest for the weary exerciser (Weil et al., 1978).

Physical work at high altitudes may result in physiological responses that not only inhibit performance, but endanger the performer as well. An additional factor to bear in mind is the decreasing temperature that accompanies increasing altitude. Some type of training or preparation is indicated if high-altitude environments are to be the locations for your exercise.

To begin with, if you are going to train at high altitudes, you'll be incapable of maintaining the distance or effort with which you performed at sea level. In other words, if you arrive at the mountainous area a few days or a week prior to a planned climbing or hiking excursion after having trained at a significantly lower altitude, you'll be obliged to decrease the intensity of your workouts. You may lose some of the training edge you've acquired at sea level. On the other hand, most of your physiological functions will be stressed during altitude training. If you're just beginning to train, although physical work will be difficult, there should be some worthwhile training outcomes. So, there are trade-offs.

Most purely recreational hikers, climbers, backpackers or skiers don't really have the time necessary for special altitude training. Often such people have only a week or two of vacation time in which to satisfy their interests. But, if mountain sports are your thing, by all means give careful consideration to all the factors we've just noted.

Air Pollution

In our efforts to promote the physical benefits of exercise, we've emphasized the trained person's enhanced capacity to bring in environmental air and distribute its oxygen to the body's cells. We've noted that exercise-trained persons can do this with considerable efficiency. We've also observed that the demand for oxygen on behalf of muscle tissue increases during vigorous exercise. Without adequate distribution of oxygen by the blood, support of life processes becomes difficult and the quest for wellness obviously impossible.

But what happens if you are breathing in adequate amounts of environmental air, but all of it is foul as can be? What happens when the oxygen your blood is distributing to body cells is combined with harmful pollutants that can poison tissues? Moreover, how might such phenomena affect physical work performance?

What Is Air Pollution?   Oxygen, although the most essential of all human needs (without it, nothing else really matters), is not the only ingredient of environmental air. The air we breathe contains all sorts of gases, many of which, in certain conditions, are potentially harmful. And short of not breathing at all, we are at times hard pressed to prevent these pollutants from entering our lungs. The more polluted air we breathe and the longer the duration during which we do this, the greater are the harmful effects.

If you exercise in physical environments not controlled by artificial means (air filtration, cooling and heating), you have to be concerned with four types of pollutants: carbon monoxide, oxides of nitrogen, oxides of sulfur, and ozone. (The term *oxide* refers to the combination of particles of these gases with oxygen.) When you play tennis on an air-conditioned indoor court, you're not likely to have to worry about oxides, ozone, or pollutants. But if you are an inner-city jogger or cyclist, read on, take heed, and be concerned.

Carbon monoxide is a by-product of burned gasoline. Where there is heavy automobile traffic, there is a lot of carbon monoxide. Remember what we said about the function of hemoglobin in the blood (Chapter 3)? Hemoglobin combines with oxygen and transports it throughout the body. But hemoglobin combines much more readily with carbon monoxide. So, when and if it is available, carbon monoxide will displace oxygen as the preferred traveling companion of hemoglobin.

Carbon monoxide in significant quantities is poisonous. Too much of it, and too little oxygen, will cause death (suicide victims arrange for this to happen when they sit in their automobiles with the engine running, in a closed garage). Large doses of carbon monoxide can make you ill. Heavy inner-city traffic (rush hour in New York City or Los Angeles, California) produces terrifically high quantities of carbon monoxide—amounts that dramatically exceed levels prescribed as "good" by the Environmental Protection Agency (1978). According to a study by Hage (1982), daytime levels of carbon monoxide often rise to 25 to 30 parts per million, which has the equivalent effect upon the body as smoking two packs of cigarettes per day. So don't always assume that by stepping out of the house you're guaranteed a "breath of fresh air" (Committee on Medical and Biological Effects of Pollutants, 1977).

Ironically, most of the formidable pollutants with which we must contend are the results of our hunger for energy with which to fuel machines that supposedly make our lives more "civilized" and comfortable. Communities that contain a great number of motors and machinery (factories) are likely to have high levels of nitrogen oxides. This yellowish stuff, which coats buildings in urban areas having a lot of factories, is caused by nitrogen dioxide. Fossil fuel (coal), when burned, produces oxides of sulfur. Under normal conditions this substance is not particularly harmful. But when it comes in contact with water it forms sulfuric acid, which has the capability of penetrating deep into the respiratory tract (Jones, 1983).

Ozone is a valuable layer of gas that occurs naturally in the atmosphere. Without it, many of the sun's harmful rays would reach us. It serves as an important protective filter. But another layer of ozone has formed much closer to the earth's surface as a result of the mixture of nitrogen oxides and other pollutants in combination with sunlight. Inhaling large quantities of ozone can be harmful.

Exercise and Pollutants.   Exercise imposes additional demands on your cardiovascular and respiratory systems. And during vigorous physical activity, the increased loads upon these mechanisms can be substantial, or formidable (depending upon your fitness level).

When oxygen transport is inhibited by the presence of pollutants in the air, cardiorespiratory function is inhibited. VO_2 max, for example, declines (Ekbolm and Huot, 1972). Because carbon monoxide is a tasteless, odorless, and colorless gas, you receive no indication that it is creating havoc with your respiration. And carbon monoxide remains in the blood for hours after exposure, so its harmful effects are fairly long-lasting.

When you exercise, your rate and depth of respiration is increased. In addition, you tend to switch from nose to mouth breathing, thereby preventing the filtering mechanisms in the nose from doing their job. So, during exercise problems caused by air pollutants can be worsened.

Well, what can you do about this? You're certainly not going to abandon plans to exercise regularly! If possible, schedule your walk, jog, or cycle on the road or in areas near a thruway or major intersection for early morning—before traffic builds up or the sun gets too high. There is evidence that air pollutants in combination with heat can produce an even more potent harmful effect (Drinkwater et al., 1974). Heat stimulates the production of ozone and nitrogen dioxide. Ozone causes your rate of breathing to increase and severely irritates the mucus membranes in your nose and mouth (Adams et al, 1981).

If you are a smoker, the effects of ozone during physical activity will cause even more irritation.

Try to select the trails, roads, or locations for your exercise carefully. Don't exercise near sources of pollution. Stay away from places where factory exhausts fill the air. When you exercise with heavy pollutant concentration in the air, your performance will suffer. It will be relatively more difficult for you to exercise. Do not smoke cigarettes, and stay away from the smoke of others, especially during and immediately prior to working out. Cigarette smoke significantly raises the carbon monoxide level in your blood.

Another thing you can do which should give you greater control over the effects of pollutants is to learn to monitor regularly published air quality indexes. If you live in or near a large city, you can usually learn when air pollution reaches harmful levels. Reports with such information are broadcast over radio or appear in the daily newspapers. Sometimes, when things really get bad and your options for choosing an exercise location for the day are severely limited, you may be obliged to call off your workout. But be sure to make better plans for the next day. When the Pollution Standard Index (PSI), which has been developed by the Environmental Protection Agency (Savin and McCleary, 1983), exceeds 200 for any of the pollutants we've mentioned, give serious thought to skipping your exercise or moving indoors for the workout.

EXERCISE CLOTHING AND EQUIPMENT

Part of your exercise environment includes the clothing, shoes, and equipment (if any) that are needed.

Clothing That Fits You, the Situation, and the Exercise

Since each activity, environment, and person is different, it is difficult to be specific in recommending what to wear. However, there are some general guidelines you should follow:

Nylon vs. Cotton.   When exercising in the heat, your body cools itself by evaporation of perspiration. Nylon clothing will interfere with this process and should therefore be avoided in warm weather. Cotton clothing is light and allows the air to evaporate perspiration. In addition, several layers of cotton clothing worn in cold weather allows you to shed clothing as your body heats up.

Loose vs. Tight Fitting.   When the activity requires speed for some length of time, tight-fitting clothing is desirable. For example, when bicycle racing or swimming, loose fitting clothing may create too much resistance against air or water to allow for maximum performance. In other instances, however, comfortable, loose-fitting clothing allows for unencumbered movement. Of course, you don't want the clothing so loose that it interferes with your exercise.

Sports Bras.   It is advisable for women to wear a bra when exercising to avoid injury to ligaments. There are many sports bras on the market. Choose one that provides good upward support; limits the motion of the breasts; is made of absorptive, nonallergenic, and nonabrasive material; has all fasteners (hooks and eyes) covered on both sides; has wide straps; and has a wide cloth or metal underwire at the base of the bra to prevent it from riding up. You also can get a bra without fasteners that you slip into.

Athletic Supporters.   Men should wear jock straps when exercising to prevent injury to the testes and penis. Any athletic supporter on the market that provides support will suffice.

Rubberized Sweatsuits.   We've mentioned before that plastic or rubberized sweatsuits are dangerous! This point deserves repeating here. These suits do not allow the body to cool itself and can result in heat exhaustion and death. Although death is a sure way to lose weight, most exercisers don't have that strategy in mind. Avoid rubberized sweatsuits and other such clothing.

Designer Clothing.   People exercise for all sorts of reasons. In fact, when they integrate and coordinate those reasons, we say they are achieving high-level wellness. Those who exercise to improve their social lives are naturally concerned with their appearance. For them, the clothes they wear must be attractive as well as functional. To meet this need—and some would say to generate this need in the first place—well-known clothing designers have created all sorts of exercise clothes. These "designers clothes" are color-coordinated, show just the right amount of skin, and are outrageously priced. They make a statement: I am attractive, healthy, active, and well worth getting to know.

Needless to say, such expensive clothing is not necessary to exercise or to look attractive. There are many options to color coordinating your exercise clothing at a more reasonable fee; and some clothing stores sell expensive exercise clothing with minor defects at relatively low prices. Shop around; look for sales. It feels good to look nice at all times, even when exercising, so expensive clothes which make you feel that way are great if you can afford them. If not, with some ingenuity, you still can look and feel good if that's important to you.

Taking Care of Your Feet

Many forms of exercise involve your feet, so caring for them becomes an important consideration. In this section we will discuss how to choose shoes and socks for exercising as well as other factors related to the care of your feet.

Choosing Running Shoes.   To walk or jog, you should purchase a good pair of running shoes that fit well. The shoe should provide shock absorption with a multilayered spongelike sole, have a sturdy heel counter fitting snugly around the heel, and be flexible and lightweight. Purchasing inexpensive running shoes is not advisable. Since there are many shoe stores that specialize in athletic footwear, you will be able to obtain advice readily. In addition, *Runner's World* annually evelutes running shoes. You might want to consult these sources before spending upwards of $40 on a pair of running shoes.

Some of the characteristics of good running shoes that are evaluated by *Runner's World* are these (see also Cavanagh and Williams, 1981):

1. *Rearfoot and forefoot impact.* The ability of the shoe to absorb shock is necessary, since the force with which you hit the ground is three times your weight. Because many runners run on asphalt streets, the need for shock absorption is evident. The midsole cushioning (see Figure 8.2) is predominantly responsible for the shoe's shock absorption capabilities.

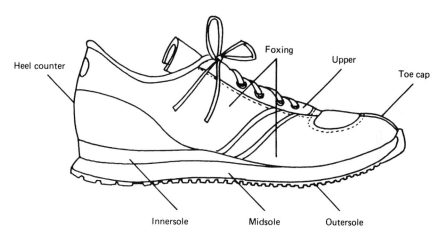

FIGURE 8.2   The running shoe

2. *Flexibility.* The shoe must be flexible enough so that it bends when you push off with your toes.

3. *Rearfoot control.* When your foot lands on its heel and rolls inward, you need stability in the heel region. The heel counter makes the major contribution to this stability. It should be rigid, and your heel should fit snugly in the shoe.

4. *Outersole wear.* At the price of running shoes these days, you'd like not to have to replace them too frequently. Consequently, rapid outersole

wear make a running shoe undesirable. Shoe stores often make a resoling service available to replace the outersole when the rest of the shoe is fine. In addition, you can purchase a synthetic rubber compound in a tube that can be squirted on the worn-out areas. It soon hardens to cover these areas. One of the most popular brands of this compound is Shoo-Goo, but there are others as well.

5. *Shoe Weight.* The more weight you carry, the more difficult it is to run. Consequently, the weight of the shoe is important.

6. *Traction.* It's no fun to slip while running. Therefore, a good running shoe should provide good traction on wet pavements.

7. *Permeability.* The upper material of the shoe should help control the temperature and the humidity within the shoe. It does this by transmitting water vapor out of the shoe. The degree to which it can serve this function is termed its degree of permeability.

Here are some other hints in selecting a running shoe:

1. Look at the foxing and the amount of added support it provides.
2. Look for a sturdy toe cap that does not cramp your toes.
3. Try the shoes on by standing and walking around in them. Your feet will swell from the pressure of standing on them. If you try them on while seated, they may not feel comfortable once you stand up.
4. Try the shoes on late in the day, after your feet have swelled from standing on them.

Choosing Other Sports Shoes.   Employees in most reputable athletic shoe stores can advise you on the selection of shoes for your sports interest. Generally, the more expensive the shoe the better it is. For instance, shoes with metal eyelets (holes the laces go through) and with soles sewn to the uppers rather than glued are usually more costly. However, your major concern should be support, and most brand-name athletic shoes provide adequate support for basketball, tennis, and the like. Try on the shoe and make sure it is comfortable. Flex it to see if it is flexible enough without being too flexible.

One word of caution: Do not use running shoes for these other sports activities. Running shoes are constructed mostly for straightforward movement. Tennis, basketball, and racketball require lateral movement as well, and shoes designed for those sports are made to provide support for these lateral movements. By the way, you do not need special shoes for aerobic dancing. A good tennis shoe will provide all the support and cushioning you will need.

Choosing Socks.   The important consideration in socks, as with shoes, is the fit. Socks that do not fit well can lead to blisters and short-circuit your exercise program. Tube socks fit a variety of sizes and generally shrink very little. Consequently, they tend to stay fitted even after laundering. However, regular wool or cotton sweat socks that fit well and do not shrink appreciably when laundered will do fine.

Orthotics.   Some people have problems with their feet and need these corrected when exercising. They may have leg imbalances or overpronate, for example. Orthotic devices can be placed in their athletic shoes to allow them to exercise in comfort and to diminish the risk of injury. Orthotics come in rigid or soft forms. The rigid orthotic made of plastic is usually recommended for joggers, but a podiatrist or orthopedic physician may have reason, in any particular case, to advise one or the other.

Ready-made inserts are available in drugstores or through ads in sports magazines and may be helpful in some cases. However, since each foot is slightly different from each other foot, if you have a problem you would be well advised to consult an expert. An examination and an orthotic insert generally costs approximately $100 to $300.

Preventing Athlete's Foot.   A bane to exercisers is the extreme itching on the soles of the feet and between the toes caused by a fungus and known as athlete's foot. We discuss this condition later when we consider fitness injuries. For now, it is enough to say that you should care for your feet by wearing clean, dry socks, and that your feet should be liberally powdered after showering.

Choosing and Maintaining Your Equipment

Some fitness activities require no equipment. Runners and swimmers, for example, can just get out and do it. Other activities, such as tennis, racketball, and bicycling, do require equipment. In this section we discuss some considerations relative to that equipment.

Bicycling.   To begin a bicycling exercise program, you obviously need a bicycle. A good 10-speed bike will cost approximately $300. However, you can get an adequate 10-speeder for about half that cost if you shop around or buy a secondhand one (consult the personal ads in your local newspaper). You'll also need a helmet (approximately $45) and gloves with padded palms (about $10). Of course, you can exercise with any bike—it need not have 10 speeds—if you choose. A good bike, though, will allow you to take trips that add to the enjoyment of biking (remember our wellness concept).

New cyclists often make mistakes that sometimes lead to injury, or that in any case make biking less enjoyable. Here are some of these mistakes (Edwards, 1983, pp. 66-67).

1. Spinning too slowly in too high a gear.
2. Riding too fast too soon.
3. Having an improperly set up bicycle.
4. Riding inefficiently.

Keeping your bike in good working order will also help prevent injury and will make your biking more enjoyable. Keep all moving parts well oiled, and remove dirt from the chain and gears. Wipe water from your bike to prevent rusting.

Stationary Cycling.   One excellent indoor conditioner is riding a stationary bicycle. Such machines have only one wheel, but you pedal it as you would a bicycle, and you get a similar workout on either.

In riding a stationary bicycle, you need to be careful about adjusting it properly. Two areas need to be given attention when adjusting your bike: the seat and the handlebars. To work your leg muscles properly, your knee should be just slightly bent when the pedal is in the fully down position (see Figure 8.3). Too great a bend or too little will result in inefficient use of the leg muscles. The handlebars should be adjusted so that you are relaxed and leaning slightly forward (see Figure 8.4). Last, you might consider wearing a pants clip if you will be pedaling while wearing long pants.

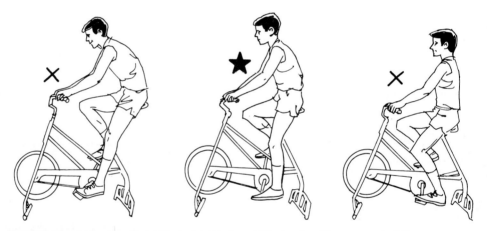

FIGURE 8.3   Correct seat height is depicted in the middle drawing. The seat on the left is too high and the one on the right is too low.

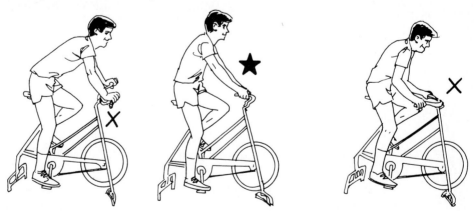

FIGURE 8.4   Correct handlebar adjustment is depicted in the middle drawing.

Racketball, Handball, and Squash.   In 1976 alone, there were a reported 3,220 eye injuries resulting from racket sports (U.S. Consumer Products Safety Commission, 1976). Although the indoor racket sports of racketball and squash, and the sport of handball, can be excellent fitness conditioners, they carry with them particular hazards. It should be obvious that participants in these activities need to wear eye protectors. Many people do not bother; others wear eye protectors which, for one reason or another, do not provide complete protection. When selecting an eye protector, do not choose the type with narrow bands and an opening between them. These might allow a ball hit hard to injure the eye in spite of the protector. Rather, choose a complete eye shield made of a strong material—polycarbonate is recommended.

There are many different kinds of rackets you can purchase for racketball. Most are metal or graphite. The graphite is more expensive and more sturdy. However, metal rackets are fine, and what feels comfortable to you is important.

Squash rackets are made of wood and, as with most athletic equipment, vary greatly in price. You can play an enjoyable squash game and become fit from it using an inexpensive racket. As you become more proficient, you might want to consider a more expensive racket.

Tennis.   Tennis rackets come in many shapes, sizes, and materials. There are regular-sized rackets, midsized ones, and oversized ones. There are wooden rackets, metal rackets, and graphite rackets. There are lightweight ones, regular weight ones, and heavy ones. And, of course, there are many sizes of grips. Your preference for size, shape, and composition should govern your selection. Larger-faced rackets decrease your power but increase your accuracy, and can do wonders for your net game. Regular-sized rackets can make your serve and ground strokes more powerful. Graphite rackets are more durable and flexible than wooden or metal rackets—and more expensive.

Selecting the proper grip size, however, should be a careful consideration, since a wrong-sized grip can increase your chance of injury. Figure 8.5 shows the way the fingers are positioned on a racket that fits. Notice that the thumb can cover the nail of the third finger. As with all rules, this one has its exceptions. In this case, make sure the size of the handle feels comfortable in your hand.

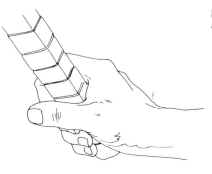

FIGURE 8.5   The properly fitted racket is one which allows the thumb to cover the nail of the third finger.

Tennis elbow is related to too large or too small a racket grip. If tennis elbow does develop, you can switch to a lighter racket to aggravate the elbow less. Also make sure your racket is balanced—not too top heavy or too light. Figure 8.6 shows how your racket should be balanced when supported at its throat.

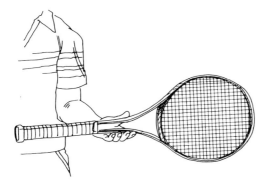

FIGURE 8.6   A way to test for proper racket balance

CONCLUSION

With the proper attention to your exercise environment, your program should be a healthy and effective one. Heed the advice we have provided for exercising in the heat, in the cold, at high altitudes, and where there is air pollution. Also pay attention to the environment factors you provide: clothing and equipment. With these factors accounted for, your exercise program will have the potential of helping you achieve high-level wellness.

SUMMARY

1. Great care should be taken when exercising in an outdoor environment. Specifically, necessary precautions should be taken when competing in extreme heat or cold conditions.
2. Vigorous exercise causes the body temperature to rise. As a result, the hypothalamus of the brain makes bodily changes to maintain the body temperature within normal limits.
3. Some clothing or protective equipment worn during physical activity can prevent the body from cooling itself naturally by preventing evaporation of perspiration from the skin.
4. Heat exhaustion and heat stroke are two of the dangers of exercising strenuously in an extremely hot environment.
5. Heat exhaustion is characterized by nausea, dizziness, and difficulty in thinking clearly. Treatment consists of ceasing the exercise, rest, and drinking plenty of water.
6. Heat stroke is characterized by extremely high body temperature, hot dry skin, no sweating, headache, nausea, confusion, and an unsteady gait. Treatment consists of cooling the body by being placed in a shady

area, removing clothing, drinking water, dousing the victim with cold water, or applying ice packs. Medical help also needs to be obtained quickly since heat stroke is a life-threatening condition.

7. When exercising in the cold, dress appropriately. That means wear a hat to conserve body heat, wear layered clothing, use gloves and scarves as needed, and always extra clothing (which can be removed) rather than too little clothing.

8. Exercising in high altitudes results in reduced ability of the body to transport oxygen to organs and tissue. This condition is termed hypoxia. After continued exercise over a period of time, a person will become acclimated to the altitude.

9. General guidelines for selecting exercise clothing include the following: choose cotton rather than nylon clothing, pay attention to the need for either loose- or tight-fitting clothing, women should wear a sports bra, and men should wear athletic supporters and avoid rubberized sweatsuits.

REFERENCES

ADAMS, W. C., W. M. SAVIN, AND A. E. CHRISTA. "Detection of Ozone Toxicity during Continuous Exercise via the Effective Dose Concept." *Journal of Applied Physiology* 51 (1981): 415–27.

AMERICAN COLLEGE OF SPORTS MEDICINE. "Position Statement on Prevention of Heat Injuries during Distance Running." *Medicine and Science in Sports and Exercise* 7 (1975): 7-9.

BUSKIRK, E. R., J. KOLLIAS, E. PICON-REATIQUE, R. AKERS, E. PROKOP, AND P. BAKER. "Physiology and Performance of Track Athletes at Various Altitudes in the United States and Peru." In R.F. Goddard (ed.), *The Effects of Altitude on Physical Performance*, pp.65-71. Albuquerque: Athletic Institute, 1967.

CAVANAGH, P. R., AND K. R. WILLIAMS. "Testing Procedure for the 1982 Runners World Shoe Survey." *Runner's World* 16 (1981): 26–33.

COMMITTEE ON MEDICAL AND BIOLOGICAL EFFECTS OF ENVIRONMENTAL POLLUTANTS. *Carbon Monoxide*. Washington, DC: National Academy of Sciences, 1977.

DANIELS, J.T. "Effects of Altitude on Athletic Accomplishment." *Modern Medicine*, June 26, 1972, pp. 73-76.

DRINKWATER, B. L., P .B. RAVEN, S. M. HORVATH, J. A. GLINER, R. D. RUHLING, N. W. BOLDRAN, AND S. TAGUCHI. "Air Pollution, Exercise and Heat Stress." *Archives of Environmental Health* 28 (1974): 177–81.

EDWARDS, S. "Cycling Minutes Off Your Time." *Runner's World*, April 1983, pp. 61–68.

EKBOLM, B., AND R. HUOT. "Responses to Submaximal and Maximal Exercise at Different Levels of Carboxyhemoglobin." *Acta Physiologica Scandinavica* 86 (1972): 474–82.

ENGLAND, A. C., AND OTHERS. "Preventing Severe Heat Injury in Runners: Suggestions from the 1979 Peachtree Road Race Experience." *Annuals of Internal Medicine* 97 (1982): 196–201.

HAGE, P. "Air pollution: Adverse Effects on Athletic Performance." *The Physician and Sports Medicine* 10 (1982): 126–32.

HAYMES, E. M., AND C.L. WELLS. *Environment and Human Performance.* Champaign, IL: Human Kinetics, 1986.

JONES, D. L. "The Effects of Sulphur Dioxide and an Aerosol during Exercise on Selected Pulmonary Function Measurements." Unpublished manuscript, 1983.

McFARLAND, R. A. "Review of Experimental Findings in Sensory and Mental Functions." In A.H. Hegnauer (ed.), *Biomedicine Problems of High Terrestrial Elevations*, pp. 250–65. Natick, MA: U.S. Army Research Institute of Environmental Medicine, 1969.

SAVIN, M., AND R. H. MCCLEARY. "Clearing the Air of a Clouded Issue." *Runner's World*, July 1983, p. 55.

UNITED STATES CONSUMER PRODUCT SAFETY COMMISSION. *Annual Report.* Washington, D.C. Government Printing Office, 1976.

UNITED STATES ENVIRONMENTAL PROTECTION AGENCY. *Information Documents on Automobile Emissions: Inspection and Maintenance Programs.* EPA 400/2-78-001. February 1978.

WEIL, J. V., M. H. KRYGER, AND C. H. SCOGGIN. "Sleep and Breathing at High Altitude." In C. Guilleminault (ed.), *Sleep Apnea Syndrome.* New York: Alan R. Liss, 1978.

9

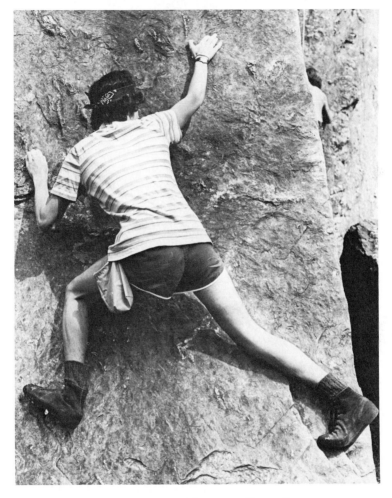

Weight Training:
Improving Your Physique

As you review your personal needs, goals, and interests, give some attention to whether they revolve around your body's general appearance. Are you motivated to improve your physical attractiveness? Is one of your primary objectives related to aesthetics or the grace with which you move? If these are among your paramount interests, then your list of exercise possibilities should include activities that yield meaningful weight loss, weight gain, or weight distribution outcomes.

For the most part, *physique*, or your body's appearance, depends on the amount and distribution of two kinds of tissue: muscle and fat. Exercise unquestionably modifies the quantity and location of each (Sonstroem, 1982).

Carefully planned heavy resistance training may yield desirable results if your goal is to enlarge certain skeletal muscle groups. This type of training need not necessarily involve weights. Many kinds of resistance against which the muscles must contract will serve equally well. Devices using springs, taut bands of rubber, or oil or water pressure may be employed. Cost, portability, availability, environmental demands, and preference will dictate the kind of mechanism you choose.

IMPROVING BODY PHYSIQUE

The legs, arms, shoulders, and abdominal area are the body parts that receive most attention when you set out to improve your physique.

Chest and Arm Muscles

Your own body weight may be used as resistance.

1. A sturdy horizontal tree limb can be used for pullups. (See Figure 9.1.) Make sure you have enough space between limb and ground to accommodate your body length with outstretched arms (you are going to hang before pulling up). Use a reverse grip, with palms pointing away from your face; grasp the limb with hands about shoulder-width apart.

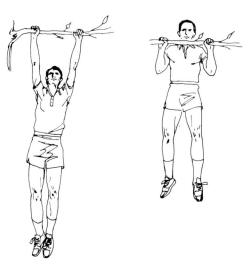

FIGURE 9.1   Pullups

From a hanging position, raise the body by flexing the biceps and triceps muscles. Record one pullup in your mind when your chin is even with the limb. Arm strength and endurance can be developed with this exercise. The training effect is like that produced by dumbbell or barbell curls.

2. Kitchen chairs can be arranged to train triceps (back of the arm) and chest muscles and increase strength and endurance. (See Figure 9.2.) Use three sturdy chairs. Place two adjacent to each other (facing in the same direction), with a space of about 2 1/2 to 3 feet between them. Directly opposite this space, about 4 feet away, place the third chair with its seat facing the seats of the other two.

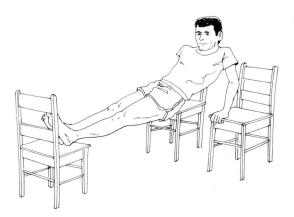

FIGURE 9.2   Rear dips

Now, with arms behind you, place the palm of each hand on each of the two adjacent chairs (knuckles toward the third chair standing alone). Palms are gripping the chairs' edges. The heels of your feet are placed on the edge of the third chair seat. Rear dips are done by lowering and raising the body while bearing weight on the heels and hands. Rear dips emphasize triceps strength and endurance. Be sure to have a soft surface (mat or carpet) underneath you in case you should fall to the floor.

3. Next you can do front dips. (See Figure 9.3.) Grip the seat edge of the odd chair with your toes and place one palm on each of the paired chair seats. Dips can be done by raising and lowering the straight body in the space between the chairs. Front dips emphasize triceps, chest, and shoulder (front part) strength and endurance. Be sure to have a soft surface (mat or carpet) underneath you in case you should fall to the floor.

FIGURE 9.3   Front dips

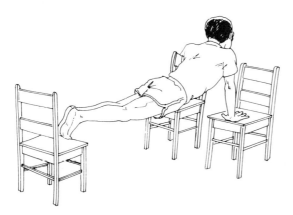

Abdominal Muscles

Situps and leg raisers can be done just about anywhere there is space to accommodate your body length. (See Figure 9.4.) A carpeted floor usually provides a good deal of comfort when doing these exercises. Tightened abdominal muscles help produce a streamlined appearance.

FIGURE 9.4   Bent-knee situp

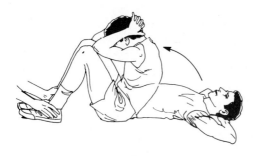

1. A situp is basically an exercise for the lower back, but it also brings abdominal muscles into action. Since it's difficult to isolate these muscles with a particular movement, sitting up is commonly used to strengthen the abdominal wall. You will derive a double benefit from this exercise in that both lower back and abdominal muscles are activated during its performance.

The starting position for the situp is lying on your back, knees bent slightly, and feet flat on the floor. Hands may be clasped behind your neck or placed by your sides. To do one situp, tuck chin to chest and curl upward, raising your trunk about 45 degrees from the floor.

2. Situps can be made easier to perform by hooking the toes under an object that will hold your feet down. This will permit your thigh muscles to help bring your torso from its reclining position to an upright or sitting position. Perhaps a partner can hold your ankles.

3. Clasping your hands behind your neck makes the exercise more difficult, since weight is added to the body part that has to be moved (upper body). Therefore, throwing the arms forward with each attempted repetition will make the situp easier to perform.

4. If you really want to give your abdominal muscles a run for the money, try sitting up with hands clasped behind the neck and heels drawn as far as possible toward the buttocks.

Leg Muscles

Calves can be strengthened and enlarged and their shapes more clearly defined by toe raisers.

1. Place the balls of your feet on a raised step, curb, or bench, leaving the rear part of your foot (heel) hanging free. You'll probably want to hold onto something to prevent losing your balance and falling. The action in this exercise calls for shifting the weight onto the balls of the feet and thereby rising onto the toes. Not only are the calf muscles affected by the exercise, but muscles located on the sides of the calves and muscles that control ankle movement are also activated.

2. Running also accomplishes these results, as does rope skipping.

3. Thigh muscles may be firmed and strengthened by side leg-raising exercises (inside of thigh) and partial squats (front of thigh). (See Figure 9.5.) To execute the side leg-raiser, lie on your side with head propped up by your hand (elbow and upper arm on the floor). One leg rests on the other. The top leg is raised as high as possible and then lowered to the starting position. The knee of the raised leg is kept straight. After a while, change position so that the top leg becomes the bottom leg, and vice versa.

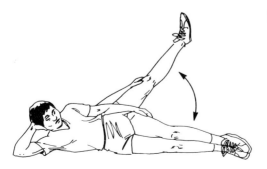

FIGURE 9.5   Side leg raises

4. Squats or knee bends will strengthen the front of the thighs as well as activate the muscles of the buttocks. But you should only go about one-third of the way down when squatting. This will prevent undue stress on the knees. To perform the squat, stand tall with heels about three-fourths of an inch apart, toes pointed slightly to the side. Hands may be placed on the hips or extended to hold onto a stable object that can support your weight (table top, doorknob). Lower your body slowly by bending your knees. Keep your back straight and the weight over your heels. Do not bounce, and do not go down to a full squat. (See Figure 9.6.)

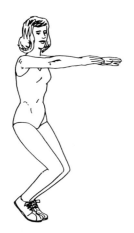

FIGURE 9.6   One-third squat

Overloading

Remember that in all these exercises it is important periodically to increase the number of repetitions or the amount of resistance against which the muscles contract. You may do this by strategically holding objects such as books or stones in your hands when you do squats; placing them on your tummy when doing rear dips on chairs; or wearing progressively heavier shoes (sneakers, shoes, hiking boots, ski boots) when doing leg-raisers and pullups. The number of repetitions will vary with your level of fitness and your goals. If your goals include increases in muscle strength and size, you should train two or three times per week. Three sets of 6 to 10 repetitions of each exercise are usually appropriate for most individuals.

Be sure to include exercises for all major muscle groups so that your training efforts yield a symmetrically developed body.

IMPROVING MUSCULAR STRENGTH AND ENDURANCE

Often the terms strength and endurance are used interchangeably to refer to skeletal muscle function. But they really refer to distinct muscle characteristics. *Strength* refers to the maximal pulling force of a muscle or muscle group, and *endurance* to the muscle's ability repeatedly to contract or sustain a contraction. Clearly, both functions are important in exercise. The degree to which they characterize muscle performance is a critical indicator of fitness for a particular activity. Lifting a load or moving an inanimate or animate object essentially depends on muscular srength. Chinups and situps are examples of muscular endurance. Chinups and situps are examples of muscular endurance. Since many physical activities have strength as well as endurance requirements, training for them should emphasize both types of muscular functions. Muscles that are high in endurance are likely to be fairly strong (Riley, 1977).

Types of Muscle Contraction

A large skeletal muscle such as the biceps brachi (the two-bellied muscle used to flex the arm) consists of thousands of small cells that shorten in unison to cause the muscular contraction necessary to bring your fist to your shoulder. Muscular contraction is involved in work. As noted in Chapter 2, our understanding of muscle contraction is incomplete. However we do know that when a motor unit shortens or contracts, all the muscle cells (fibers) that are stimulated contract.

Essentially there are four ways in which skeletal muscles contract: isometrically, isotonically, eccentrically, and isokinetically. The physical activity program you will design for yourself will undoubtedly contain many different kinds of movements that will entail all four types of muscular contractions.

When tension develops within a muscle but no change in its length occurs, the contraction is called *isometric* or *static*. When you try to lift an extremely heavy weight that is immovable, your muscle or muscles are moving isometrically. Few of the movements you are likely to engage in are perfectly isometric, but many are nearly so.

When the muscle shortens as it develops tension against a constant resistance (as in the case of most types of contraction), the contraction is known as *isotonic*, *dynamic*, or *concentric*. Although this type of contraction is perhaps better known to you than others, it has a serious drawback when used exclusively in strength training programs.

Consider the following factors when making decisions about the program you are designing for yourself. Imagine you are lifting a load by flexing the biceps muscles in your upper arm. You are attempting to bring a weight which you are gripping in your right hand toward your right shoulder. With your elbow extended, your upper and lower arms form a straight line (an angle of 180 degrees). As hand, weight, and lower arm begin their movement toward the shoulder as a consequence of biceps contraction, the angle between upper and lower arm decreases.

Research has shown that the greatest biceps strength or tension occurs at approximately 120 degrees and decreases as the angle becomes smaller. At approximtely 30 degrees, the muscle's tension is lowest. This means that the training effect varies throughout the range of movement, and that the maximum weight you can use for a particular biceps exercise is limited to the amount of resistance the muscle can overcome at its weakest strength point, 30-degree flexion. When special equipment is used to distribute the tension evenly throughout the *full* range of movement, the contraction is called *isokinetic*.

The fourth type of contraction typically observed in physical exercise is *eccentric*. In this kind of contraction, the muscle lengthens as it develops tension. When you struggle against gravity during downhill running or when you are lowering the weight you were hypothetically lifting in the previous example (hand to shoulder), the muscles are contracting *eccentrically*.

This information about muscle contraction is applicable to exercise programs that emphasize the use of weights or heavy resistances. If you are eager to increase muscular strength and endurance, you should consider this kind of training.

Developing a Weight Training Program

In the not so distant past, weight training environments were the exclusive domains of males. Countless numbers of adolescent boys expressed their developing sexuality and accompanying concern with physique by entering

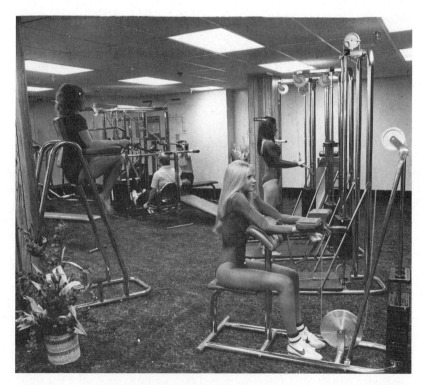

Although exercise such as weight training helps firm body parts, fat tissue cannot be changed to muscle tissue. It is only through a combination of proper exercise and reduced caloric intake that fat and weight reduction occurs.

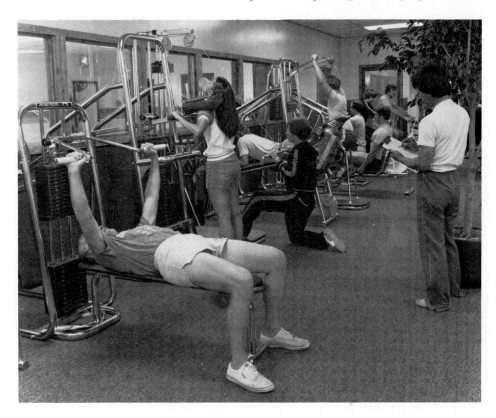

A single station circuit weight training facility

body building or weight training regimens. Many a barn, basement, or garage underwent conversion into a training facility to be used by an adolescent or young adult seeking the badge of manhood—a large and muscular body. This also holds true for untold numbers of today's young men.

But in the past, stereotypical characterizations of weightlifters tended to deter female participants, for weight training was believed to foster an exclusively male physique, characterized by bulging muscles. Recent research findings and resultant attitude changes have altered this stereotyped approach. Weight training has emerged from the basement and garage and entered the university gymnasium, the commercial health spa, and the corporate executive exercise room. Large numbers of contemporary females and males of almost all ages are attracted to well-lit, attractively decorated, air-conditioned environments where they often train side by side. Flexing and extending muscles, they move limbs against heavy resistance provided in carefully measured amounts by complex mechanized equipment. Today, many athletes in almost all sports, and fitness trainees of all levels, use weight training to increase strength and endurance.

Improving Health and Wellness Through Resistance Training. In addition to potential for improving absolute muscular strength and endurance and thereby improving your ability to lift, push, and carry heavy objects, weight training has other important contributions to make towards your health and wellness. Because your body shape and size can be altered through weight training, a change may occur in the ways in which you feel about your body. Thus, your personal evaluation of your physical self may be revised. Much of our overall self-perception (the view we hold of our entire selves) is contingent upon perspectives about the physical self. Therefore, by changing the physical appearance and changing personal evaluations about your body, you may very well be paving the way for changed and improved feelings about yourself, your health, and wellness.

A few basic principles underlie any successful weight training program.

Overload.   The weights or resistance should be greater than those typically encountered by the exercising muscle. Unless the muscle or muscle group is made to contract against resistance greater than normally encountered, the physiological response on behalf of muscle tissue will not yield strength increase. Heavier than normal resistance compels muscle tissue to contract with all or almost all of its fibers (maximal contraction), and this, over an extended period of time, encourages biochemical adaptations in the muscle that increase its strength.

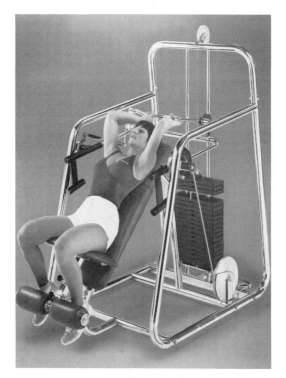

A pull-over machine

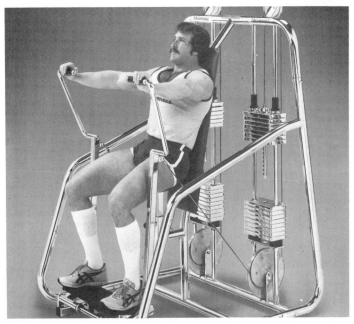

A seated chest press machine

The arm curl to work on the biceps

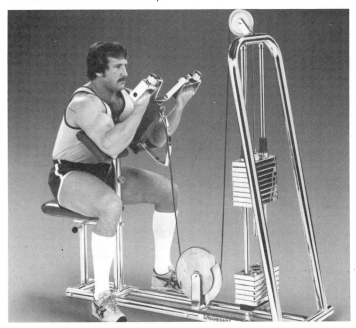

Progressive Resistance.   The resistance should be periodically increased. The muscles become accustomed to the resistance after a period of time, and you must therefore increase the resistance periodically in order for it to retain its overload character. If not, muscles will be contracting against an underload and not be experiencing strength increase.

Adjustments.   A good criterion to use for determining the appropriate time for adjusting the overload is fatigue, which begins to occur after a greater number of repetitions is performed with the same weight. If you've been able to do 10 repetitions with 60 pounds for a few weeks, then find that you can do 13 with the same weight, it's probably time to increase the load.

Sequence.   The sequence in which weight training exercises are performed will influence the effectiveness of training. Since smaller muscles fatigue sooner than comparatively larger ones, exercises involving predominantly larger muscle should come first. If not, smaller muscles may never experience overload. Training emphases should be varied from one muscle (or group) to another. Try to arrange your routine so that the large leg muscles, for example, are exercised before or after an arm exercise. Avoid consecutive exercise of muscles from the same or similar muscle group or body part.

Vary the order of the muscle groups you exercise just as you would different kinds of food on your dinner plate. You wouldn't load up on rice,

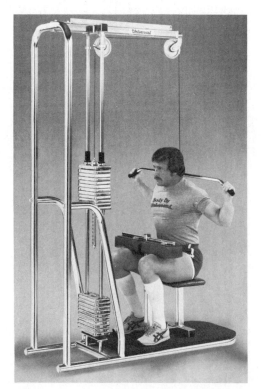

A high pulley machine

macaroni, and potato at one visit to the buffet table, but would most likely select a green vegetable, a potato or something high in carbohydrate, and fish or poultry. Arrange the order of your resistance exercises so that the muscles are activated in varied sequence on your weight training menu.

Specificity.   Weight training should include movements and movement patterns that predominate in the sports or activities for which preparation is being made.

If you are training with weights with the expectation of improving strength needed for a particular movement pattern (throwing, kicking, jumping), then your training program should emphasize the muscles or muscle groups that are to be used.

Try to use movements that stimulate the patterns you will use in particular sport or dance behaviors, since strength development is specific to muscle groups. This will also have a desirable training effect on joints, which play an important role in the execution of certain movement patterns.

Training Isotonically and Isometrically

Probably the most popular weight training program is of the isotonic kind. It appears to offer a few advantages over the isometric approach (or rather, isometric training offers some comparative disadvantages):

1. It produces strength over a wider range of motion than the isometric training program (but not as wide as isokinetic).
2. It more easily provides for self-testing and is therefore more highly motivating (mere observation of the amount of weight or resistance added is indicative of progress, whereas isometric training results must be assessed with special devices that measure tension).
3. It produces muscular endurance more effectively than the isometric approach because it provides for numerous repetitions (usually three sets of about six repetitions of each exercise), whereas isometric training involves maximal or near-maximal contractions held for approximately 2 to 5 seconds, 1 to 5 times each training session.
4. Isometric contractions produce high blood pressure, which can be dangerous in some trainees.

On the other hand, there are some very positive aspects of isometric training that may make it appropriate for you. Isometric training takes little time and requires no elaborate equipment, since resistance may be provided by body parts, walls, door frames, or readily available items in the environment. You can initiate a good isometric contraction by pulling against the interlocked fingers of both hands or by pushing vigorously against a parked automobile that you know to be immovable. Remember, an isometric contraction is one in which the muscle's length remains unchanged.

ISOTONIC GUIDELINES

Here are some cautions generated by research in exercise physiology designed to make your isotonic weight training safe and productive:

1. Determine the heaviest weight you can lift correctly one to six times. Perform 3 to 4 sets of the RM (repetition's maximum), with rests of about 5 minutes in between sets. RM should be determined for each exercise about once every two weeks of training.
2. Use correct form (no jerking of the weight), and don't increase the weight or resistance arbitrarily or too soon in the program.
3. If you wish to emphasize muscular endurance, do not increase the resistance even when your biweekly assessments suggest that you are ready to do so. Instead, increase the number of repetitions beyond 6 (perhaps to 8, 10, or 12). More repetitions tend to enhance the muscle's endurance function.
4. Training sessions held 3 to 4 times a week should do the job. Twice a week should be adequate for maintaining strength gained during previous training. Soreness and fatigue may result if training is done more frequently.

Here are some things to remember when planning an isometric training program:

1. You'll need to contract the muscle or muscle group at several different joint angles, since the physiological muscular response is specific to where the tension is created. If you contract isometrically at an angle of 75 degrees (such as biceps; forearm to upper arm), then that's the angle at which strength improvement will occur.
2. Try to make each contraction maximal.
3. It is not necessary to hold the contraction longer than 2 to 5 seconds.
4. Repeat each contraction 1 to 5 times during each training session on a daily basis.
5. One session of training per week will enable you to maintain (but not improve) your progress.

In addition, isometric training results in much less muscle soreness than isotonic training. Also (and certainly of no less importance to many of you), isotonic training requires frequent unloading or loading of plates from the dumbbells or barbells and consequently takes a comparatively longer time to complete than isometric training.

Table 9.1

Summary of Advantages of Isokinetic, Isotonic, and Isometric Training Methods

	Type of Training		
Criterion	Isokinetic	Isotonic	Isometric
Rate of strength gain	1	2	3
Strength gain throughout range of motion	Excellent	Good	Poor
Time per training session	2	3	1
Expense	2-3	2	1
Ease of performance	2	3	1
Ease of progress assessment	Expensive Equipment required	Excellent	Dynamometer required
Adaptability to specific movement	1	2	3
Probability of soreness	Little soreness	Much soreness	Little soreness
Probability of musculoskeletal injury	Slight	Moderate	Slight
Cardiac risk	Some	Slight	Moderate
Skill improvement	Some	Slight	None

Note: A rating of 1 is superior; 2, intermediate; 3, inferior

Source: David R. Lamb, *Physiology of Exercise* (New York: Macmillan, 1978). p. 141.

Although eccentric or isokinetic training methods are relatively new, there is a growing body of scientific observation which suggests that overall, isokinetic training programs may yield the most favorable results (see Table 9.1). But such programs require elaborate and expensive equipment. The Nautilus and Cybex equipment are examples of machines that provide for isokinetic contraction. They enable muscles to contract against the same level of resistance throughout a full range of motion.

IMPROVING FLEXIBILITY

If range of motion around a joint, or more simply the degree to which you can move your limbs with grace and efficiency is one of your important fitness focuses, then it's flexibility that interests you.

1. Dance, calisthenics, skating, and gymnastics would be appropriate to include on your list of activities.
2. Exercises that emphasize stretching fit the bill. But remember, whether it's resistance to training done with muscle size and shape in mind, or dance and gymnastics done with an eye toward flexibility, warming up and cooling down are important.
3. Prepare for your exercise and taper off after your activity in order to maximize training effects and to avoid injury.

There's no doubt that if you are to perform exercise efficiently, safely, and enjoyably, you must be able to move your body parts through as wide a range of motion as possible without straining or causing harmful stresses on tendons and ligaments. What we are unsure about is how much flexibility you actually require. The most prevalent opinion is that optimal degrees of flexibility are specific to particular activities engaged in and to individuals engaging in them. Some physical activities require rather high levels of flexibility in certain body parts. Diving, gymnastics, and certain swimming skills such as the dolphin kick used in the butterfly stroke are a few examples.

Another point to bear in mind is that flexibility is also specific to body parts. So it's more appropriate to speak of a person with good hip or ankle flexion (specific references to body parts or joints), rather than to assert that someone is "flexible."

Static and Ballistic Flexibility Exercise.   The terms static and ballistic refer to two kinds of movements that have relevance to improving flexibility. When a body part is moved slowly to the limit of its range of motion the movement or exercise is called *static*. This kind of stretching is less likely to cause muscle soreness. To improve flexibility, stretching should not be done with bouncing or jerking movements that rely on momentum to move the body part beyond its usual range of motion. This kind of flexibility exercise is referred to with the term ballistic..

It's also a good idea to warm up and relax muscles before stretching. Tissues around the joints should be activated and body temperature raised before stretching is begun. For example, you should walk a little before stretching your Achilles tendon (connects calf muscle to heel bone) to increase the temperature of surrounding tissue.

Yoga.   Yoga and other forms of meditation, although primarily designed as "relaxing" experiences, may also provide opportunity for flexibility improvement. By assuming certain prescribed positions (standing, sitting, etc.) while skeletal muscles are relaxed through breath and attentional control, a stretching or "loosening" effect may be achieved that results in enhanced range of motion in and around the joint.

CONCLUSION

The way you look is often a good indicator of your health and wellness. Muscle tone, strength, and endurance correlate well with level of physical fitness and appearance. Good muscle tone goes hand in hand with strength. Many muscles become more full and round as their strength increases. This kind of change may add shape and attractiveness to your body.

In this chapter we have attended to physique—your physical appearance. We have provided specific approaches and exercises for increasing strength and endurance in important muscle groups such as those in the chest, the arms, and the abdomen. The information provided should also be useful in developing programs for improving muscular strength and endurance. Specifically, we have dealt with isotonic, isometric, and isokinetic approaches to training.

Your ability to perform physical exercise and participate safely and enjoyably in sports depends on the degree to which your joints are flexible. In this chapter we have also recommended activities for improving flexibility.

Feeling good is certainly an important part of wellness; so is looking good.

SUMMARY

1. For the most part, physique depends on the amount and distribution of two kinds of tissue: muscle and fat.
2. Strength refers to the maximal pulling force of a muscle or muscle group and endurance to the muscle's ability repeatedly to contract or sustain a contraction.
3. When tension develops within a muscle but no change in its length occurs, the contraction is called isometric or static.
4. When the muscle shortens as it develops tension (as is the case in most types of contraction), the contraction is known as isotonic, dynamic, or concentric.
5. When the muscle lengthens as it develops tension, the contraction is said to be eccentric.
6. A well-developed weight training program will incorporate (a) overload, (b) progressive resistance, (c) adjustment, (d) sequence, and (e) specificity.
7. Isometric training results in less muscle soreness than does isotonic training.
8. Optimal degrees of flexibility are specific to particular activities engaged in and to individuals engaging in them.
9. Flexibility is specific to body parts.

REFERENCES

RILEY, D. P. *Strength Training: By the Experts*. West Point, NY: Leisure Press, 1977.

SONSTROEM, R. "Exercise and Self-Esteem: Recommendations for Expository Research." *Quest* 33 (1982): 124–34.

10

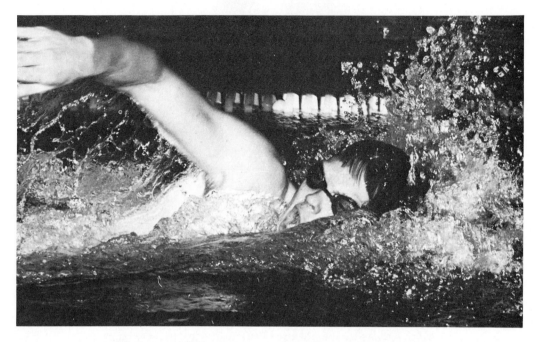

Cardiorespiratory Fitness

Many maladies claim significant numbers of American lives annually. But the leading killer today remains cardiovascular disease, which accounts for more than half of all deaths in the United States each year. Cardiovascular (heart and blood vessel) disease has been among the ten major causes of American deaths for decades. On an optimistic note, the American Heart Association reports a meaningful decline in mortality rate due to cardiovascular diseases— probably due to changes in the foods we eat, a decrease in cigarette smoking, and an increase in the number of people exercising regularly.

CARDIOVASCULAR DISEASES

Disorders resulting in impairment to arteries delivering blood to the heart muscle itself are known as *coronary heart diseases* (CHD). These account for most of all cardiovascular fatalities. Coronary heart diseases are of four types:

1. *Myocardial infarction:* death of muscle tissue resulting from inadequate supply of oxygen.
2. *Angina pectoris:* pain or tightness in the chest due to diminished blood (and oxygen) supply to the heart muscle.
3. *Atherosclerosis:* buildup of plaque (fatty deposits) or fibrin (causing clots) in arteries. *Stroke* occurs when these arteries service the brain.
4. *Arteriosclerosis:* hardening of the arteries, which causes them to narrow.

Medical research has produced an impressive amount of information that is helpful in preventing and reducing the severity of cardiovascular disorders. Although much more scientific inquiry into the causes of these diseases is needed, a number of *risk factors* have already been identified: obesity, diets high in animal fat and cholesterol, hypertension, tobacco smoking, and lack of physical exercise. Many researchers have concluded that coronary heart disease starts in childhood and that precautionary measures should begin long before the adult years, when these disorders usually strike.

Risk Factors for Cardiovascular Disease

Obesity.   The heart must provide blood flow to fat tissue, since fat cells require oxygen and nutrients for their metabolic function. The heart is therefore obliged to deliver blood for this purpose. Blood, carrying waste products from fat cell metabolism, must also be returned to the heart. These responsibilities impose an unnecessary burden on the cardiovascular system— unnecessary because excessive fat tissue, in typical circumstances, make no contribution to your health and well-being. Beyond an appropriate percentage of your total body weight, which varies with your age and sex (see Chapter 11), stored body fat is undesirable. It correlates highly with high blood pressure. A more detailed discussion of obesity as a health and wellness liability is provided in Chapter 11. Our purpose here is simply to indicate that obesity (grossly excessive storage of body fat) taxes the heart. Regular vigorous exercise is helpful in reducing stored body fat.

Diets High in Fat and Cholesterol.   Your body contains fatty/oily substances known as *lipids*. Lipids may be of high (HDL) or low density (LDL), meaning that they contain respectively high or low concentrations of oily materials such as cholesterol. The HDL/LDL ratio is linked by research findings to cardiovascular disease, particularly atherosclerosis. It is better to have more HDL than LDL. Cholesterol, a lipid containing a lot of saturated fat, is transported by HDL away from the lining of coronary arteries. LDL appears to deposit its cholesterol in the arterial walls, particularly at sites where the wall has been damaged. High blood pressure and smoking are associated with inner arterial wall damage and therefore contribute to an environment conducive to accumulation of cholesterol on arterial walls.

Platelets, substances normally found in the blood and involved in the process of blood coagulation, also tend to gather at these sites of injury. They create clots which, along with scar tissue from arterial wall lining, cause a buildup of plaque. The artery thus narrows and blood flow is hampered. There is also the danger that clots may break away and clog smaller blood vessels, causing stroke or heart attack.

The American Heart Association recommends that cholesterol intake be limited to 300 milligrams a day. Lowering dietary cholesterol does reduce heart attacks and related deaths, although most cholesterol (as much as 70 percent) is manufactured by the body naturally, no matter what you eat. Foods high in cholesterol include pork brains, beef kidney, beef liver, eggs, and shrimp.

Other Risk Factors

High Systolic Blood Pressure.   According to the Framingham study (Haynes, et al., 1978) findings, high systolic blood pressure is a leading cause of coronary heart disease. Additionally, "For CHD other than angina there is a strong relation to cigarette smoking for both younger men and women" (p. 10).

Glucose Intolerance.   Another risk factor associated with cardiovascular disease is a condition involving inordinately high amounts of sugar or glucose in the urine or blood. The result is diabetes which is significantly related to blood pressure. Clinical diabetes can be mediated through blood pressure and cholestrol control; as well as the administration of insulin.

Electrographic Evidence of Left Ventricular Hypertrophy (LVH). LVH (an increase in the size of the heart's left ventricle) is highly correlated with later development of CHD and with systolic blood pressure readings that exceed 140 mm Hg. However, even without this relationship to high systolic blood pressure, LVH remains an especially high risk factor in the onset of CHD.

Age. As one gets older, the risk of developing CHD increases. However, when age and gender are combined to predict the onset of CHD, the Framingham study has reported that women's risk of CHD increases as they get older while men's risk of CHD development increases to age 60 and then begins to decrease.

Two other risk factors bear mentioning: (1) *heredity* and (2) *psychosocial stress.* Heredity plays a role in the development of CHD in that your chances of developing CHD are greatly enhanced if family background suggests that CHD is prevalent in your family. Current theory suggests that holding anger "in" and becoming hostile causes an increased susceptibility to CHD (McDougall and others, 1985). However, additional research is needed for this to be established as an important risk factor.

Exercise has been shown to increase HDL in the blood, thereby making the HDL/LDL ratio more desirable. Serum cholesterol is also reduced. In fact, HDL may actually protect against atherosclerosis.

Therefore, the risk of developing cardiovascular disease is related to systolic blood pressure, serum cholesterol, cigarette smoking, glucose intolerance, electrographic evidence of left ventricular hypertrophy, age, and sex.

The Benefits of Exercise

In this chapter, we will deal with the relationship of exercise and heart disease. Although not by any means conclusive, there is considerable evidence that aerobic exercise, done regularly and with attention to important training principles such as overload, will reduce the risk of cardiorespiratory disease. Another aim of this chapter is to discuss exercise programs that are helpful in strengthening and rehabilitating cardiorespiratory mechanisms which have been damaged through disease.

The term *cardiorespiratory* suggests a relationship between your lungs, heart, and blood vessels. Essentially, the affiliation is as follows: Environmental air is breathed into the body and enters the lungs. Oxygen then diffuses from this volume of air into the tiny, thin-walled blood capillaries surrounding small air sacs (alveoli) in the lungs. Capillaries ultimately connect with arteries, which deliver oxygen and nutrients to your body's cells.

When the vital interaction of cardiac and respiratory mechanism falters or fails, the well-being of all your cells, tissues, and organs is undermined, and any of the four kinds of disease mentioned earlier is likely to occur.

Chapters 2 and 3 presented an overview of the structure and function of the cardiorespiratory system. Figure 2.8 shows the path of circulatory blood throughout the body. Review this material now to appreciate fully the emphasis in this chapter, which is *exercise and its benefits for the cardiorespiratory system.*

DEVELOPING CARDIORESPIRATORY FITNESS

We really cannot talk about cardiovascular and respiratory fitness without incorporating into our discussion the concept of maximum oxygen intake. Max VO_2 (as it is known by exercise physiologists) refers to the quantity of oxygen breathed in environmental air during strenuous exercise, in comparison with body weight (usually expressed in liters or milliliters). The higher your Max VO_2 value, the better your physiological readiness for exercise, or the higher your fitness level. Champion marathon runners, for example, have exceptionally high Max VO_2 values, and sedentary persons have very low values.

To determine your Max VO_2, you would ride a stationary bicycle or run on a treadmill while the volume of your inspired and expired air is measured. By the way, this is not something you typically do at home. A specially equipped laboratory, administered by trained technicians, is usually required.

The terms *cardiorespiratory endurance, cardiovascular endurance*, and *aerobic endurance* all refer to the same thing: persistence in continuing an activity. This ability differs from the endurance function of muscle (repeating or sustaining a contraction), which we have discussed previously. Cardiorespiratory endurance refers to the ability of the lungs to provide oxygen to the blood, and to the circulatory system's ability to transport it to the tissues of the body. Obviously, muscle endurance depends upon cardiorespiratory fitness, for without it sufficient oxygen would not reach working muscles.

Fitness training enhances cardiorespiratory endurance, and different kinds of training do this better than others. Endurance training is essential for sports and activities that require prolonged participation, such as distance running, cycling, swimming, skating, cross country skiing, wrestling, dancing, rope skipping, and gymnastics activities like the pommel horse (where a performer must stay up on the apparatus for an extended period). Training for such activities should emphasize performance for long periods of time. Remember, training effects tend to be specific to particular muscles as well as other systems. If you decide to select cycling as your mode of exercise, then you must stress aerobic, endurance-type activity (preferably riding a bicycle) during regular training. Your goal is to increase the capacity of the systems most often emphasized during cycling.

Cardiorespiratory endurance training therefore entails a greater number of sessions per week than muscle strength training, and each session will last longer. Begin your cardiorespiratory training with caution and patience. You'll need to train for about 6 to 10 weeks before you can observe substantial improvement in aerobic performance (activities sustained for a minimum of 5 minutes).

Target Heart Rate

Target heart rate, which we mentioned briefly in Chapter 5, should be calculated in order to determine the approximate degree of effort that best suits you for aerobic training. Try to gain proficiency in taking your pulse, since it is necessary for determining target heart rate. And remember to warm up and cool down thoroughly before and after each training session (this includes stretching). Consult the instructions in the accompanying box to determine your target heart rate. A rough estimate is provided. According to the ACSM guidelines, other factors such as resting heart rate and fitness level should be considered before commencing the exercise program.

Good Activities for Developing Cardiorespiratory Fitness

Almost any aerobic activity that is rhythmic, sustained for at least 25 to 35 minutes (perhaps a little less for certain categories of individuals such as the elderly), and rigorous in that it increases your heart rate is good for developing cardiorespiratory fitness. The more you train aerobically, the more efficient your energy systems become. Your ability to get rid of metabolic wastes also improves.

It's a good idea to train for improved cardiorespiratory fitness by using movements and movement patterns that are part of your preferred sport or activity. That is, if your aim is to improve cardiorespiratory fitness for swimming, do your training in the water. If you are a runner with a goal of increasing your maximum distance or sustaining a brisk pace throughout a road race, do your aerobic endurance training on the track, road, or cross country trail.

Although this type of specific training is an important consideration, there is also considerable training benefit to be derived from nonspecific activities. Therefore, if your primary interests are with swimming but your physician advises rest for a weakened shoulder, your cardiorespiratory endurance level may be sustained or even improved through running or cycling. Carryover benefits may occur from one aerobic activity to another if your target rate is maintained.

A good example of this is marathoner Joan Benoit, who had knee surgery weeks before the Olympic trials but maintained her cardiovascular endurance by lying on her back and pedaling a stationary bicycle with her hands. As all good stories should end, Joan Benoit won the marathon for women at the 1984 Olympics only several months after her surgery—an ending that would not have been possible had she not maintained her cardiovascular fitness while unable to run.

But because other systems of the body (muscular, nervous) must also be activated against progressively increased resistance (overload) for overall per-

---

ESTIMATING YOUR TARGET HEART RATE

To determine *your* approximate target heart rate, do the following:

1. Measure your heart rate by placing your first two fingers (pointer and middle finger) on the underside and thumb side of your wrist while seated. An alternative site is the lower neck just above your collar bone. You should feel pulsations of blood passing under your fingers and you should count how many pulsations occur in 30 seconds. Multiply that number by 2, and you have your heart rate per minute.
2. Then fill in the blank parts of this formula:

   a. 220 minus _____ = _____

         (your age)   (your maximal heart rate)

   b. .75 x _____ = _____

      (your maximal heart rate) (your target heart rate)

The interesting thing about the target heart rate is that as you improve your physical condition, you will need to work harder to get to your target heart rate. In other words, this method of determining the intensity of workouts is appropriate for people at all levels of fitness, and appropriate as their levels of fitness keep improving.

Obviously, you need to take your pulse during exercise to determine if the intensity of your workout is too light, too heavy, or just right. Take your pulse in the middle of exercising, if possible. A 10-second pulse count multiplied by 6, to arrive at your heart rate per minute, is recommended. However, if it is not possible to take your pulse while exercising, do so immediately upon the completion of exercising.

---

formance to improve, aerobic training programs should be structured around specific activities whenever feasible. Running seems to provide more carryover cardiorespiratory benefit than swimming or cycling (Fox, 1979).

Your total exercise time should be a minimum of about 25 to 35 minutes. A rough guideline to consider when determining how long you should exercise is that the number of minutes should equal 1 percent of your daily caloric consumption (Balke, 1974). Therefore, if you consume about 2,500 kilocalories per day, you should try to exercise for approximately 25 minutes. Three or four times a week should suffice.

Walking

Walking is among the simplest activities appropriate for cardiorespiratory training. Unless inhibited by structural or neuromuscular dysfunction, most people walk often and regularly. Once beyond the toddler stage, most of us do not have to be taught how to walk, although the mechanics of many of our walking gaits are far from perfect. In the human gait, left and right legs alternate as knees bend and feet push off the ground surface. Arms swing forward and to the rear in opposition to leg movement. Excessive bouncing and toeing out are walking errors that may cause inefficiency and early fatigue.

THINGS TO REMEMBER WHEN WALKING FOR CARDIORESPIRATORY FITNESS

1. Walk for about 2 to 5 minutes—then stretch—give particular attention to the Achilles tendons and calf muscles. It is best to warmup the muscles and connective tissue before stretching.
2. Have a pretty good idea of your course—its direction, terrain, and distance. Decide beforehand how far you'll walk.
3. Dress appropriately. Avoid garments that rub excessively against the skin. Select loose-fitting clothing. Wear layers of cotton fabric or light wool. Gloves or mittens and head covering are appropriate if you walk out of doors in cold weather.

Long walks satisfy our definition of aerobic activity. Walking is rhythmic, and the same mechanical pattern is repeated continually. Heart rate is elevated and kept elevated throughout the walk. The speed of walking will vary in accordance with motivation, level of fitness, distance to be covered, and cardiorespiratory fitness goals. It is an excellent aerobic training activity, particularly for obese individuals who might experience considerable difficulty with cycling or running. When done competitively in accordance with strict rules, race walking is a demanding athletic event. Walking may also be considered a fine recreational activity, since it permits social interaction and conversation when done with others. However, when used as a cardiorespiratory training regimen, walking requires a number of important considerations as described in the accompanying box.

If you are able to cover 3 to 4 miles in about an hour, your walking pace may be considered brisk. Your heart rate won't be as high as if you were running, and the amount of calories you will burn during this time will not be as great. However, the cardiorespiratory activation caused by such a walk will be substantial.

Jog-Walk

If you reach a point in your training when walking no longer provides the level of activation you desire or need, you should consider alternating jogging and walking. A good way to begin such a program would be to jog for 5 to 6 minutes at approximately 6 miles per hour, then walk for 1 or 2 minutes. During the walk phase of the routine, take your pulse to see if your target heart rate is where it should be. Over a period of weeks, build up to periods of about 10 to 15 minutes.

Jogging

The term jogging suggests slow and comfortable running. But *how slowly* do you move when you jog? And at what speed should your locomotion be con-

---

THINGS TO REMEMBER WHEN JOGGING OR RUNNING FOR CARDIORESPIRATORY FITNESS

1. Build up to longer distances gradually. Jogging and running are weight-bearing activities and may therefore provide greater vulnerability to more debilitating injuries than nonweight bearing activities such as cycling or swimming.
2. Limit the frequency of your jog or run to 3 or 4 days per week and no more than 30 minutes per workout if you are a beginning exerciser. In this way you'll reduce the likelihood of foot, leg, and knee injury. Use discretion when increasing distance.
3. Try to maintain a steady pace that you can hold for the duration of your jog or run.
4. Systematically and slowly stretch back, foot, and leg muscles before you begin.
5. After your jog or run, walk a few yards. Try not to sit or lie down immediately after completion. You'll adjust to the decreased cardiovascular demands more comfortably. Also, remember to include a reverse stretching routine in your cooldown (see Chapter 3 for a more complete discussion of the cooldown).
6. Plan to take brief stops for sips of water along your route, particularly if your distance is substantial, and the temperature or humidity is high.

---

sidered running? Some sources maintain that a pace slower than 8 minutes per mile is jogging. Others insist that the cutoff speed is 9 minutes per mile. It really makes little difference—decide for yourself. Some of you may feel you are running when you are moving at a 10-minute per mile pace; others may refer to an 8-minute, 30-second pace as a jog. Don't get caught up in unnecessary hair splitting. The factor of speed is far less important in establishing cardiorespiratory endurance than frequency and distance. (You may wish to have another look at Chapter 3, where we discussed your body's response to training.)

Jogging is a terrific aerobic training activity, and we've sung its praises frequently throughout this book. It can be done almost anywhere. Grassy fields provide soft surfaces that are less tiring to leg muscles and bones than asphalt or concrete surfaces. But be careful of stones and holes dug by animals when you are jogging in grass. And the same meadow through which you jog during the summer months can be an exciting and lovely place for physical activity when it is covered with snow in the winter. However, be wary of ice; it's probably the one solid surface that is not conducive to jogging.

Forest trails and parks are also nice places to jog. Your options are broad. That's one of the really nice things about jogging. Pack your jogging gear when you travel. Chances are good that you'll find a suitable place to jog wherever you may be.

Aerobic exercise means uninterrupted activity. However, if you need to stop and drink water, stretch, or rest, particularly during long jogs, don't be hesitant to do so. A brief pause will probably permit you to jog farther and will therefore be beneficial in the long run.

Running

Many of the considerations already noted about jogging also pertain to running. In fact, as we've already suggested, the differences between the two in terms of aerobic fitness are not very important to most people. However, there are some meaningful distinctions. If your exercise or training interests are with competition, then increasingly longer distances and greater speeds become important factors. If you want to run fast, you must acknowledge this goal when designing your training program. (You read about special training programs for speed and endurance in Chapter 3.)

If you run at a fairly high speed, the duration of your run will be compromised. You'll cover a shorter distance the faster you run. Remember, to be considered an aerobic activity, the exercise should be continuous for at least 5 minutes. If you run too fast, you'll be forced to stop before the activity lasts this long.

Other Good Activities

Swimming, rope skipping (Chapter 14 contains descriptions of how these activities should be done and incorporated into a training program), cross-country skiing, and rowing (canoeing, kayaking) are very fine aerobic activities. With the exception of skiing, they may be considered nonweight-bearing exercises, which suggests a lower probability of injury. But all carry an obvious liability. They require special equipment, environments, or weather conditions. In some environments, outdoor cycling may be done year round. This may also be true of skiing, paddling, rowing, and swimming. Therefore, if you declare one of these to be your preferred aerobic exercise, you may very well be in for periods of inactivity when you travel, or if the physical environment changes dramatically wherever you are.

One way to solve this problem is to rely upon the carryover effect we discussed earlier. When you are unable to launch your canoe because it couldn't be taken with you on the plane or bus trip to visit Aunt Helen and Uncle Max, take along your running shoes and shorts. You'll do very well aerobically as long as your large muscles are working in a rhythmic and sustained fashion for a minimal period of time.

SPECIAL FACTORS—PREREQUISITES—CAUTIONS

Assessment

Earlier in this chapter we used the term *beginning exerciser*. There's nothing mysterious about this designation. If you've never done any form of cardiorespiratory exercise, then clearly you are a beginner. But what is your status if you've done *some* exercise during the past year? Are you still a beginner if you've trained fairly heavily for months, laid off due to injury, and are now ready to resume activity? These types of questions imply a need for screening and assessment procedures to indicate your level of readiness for aerobic exercise. Certain of these evaluations should be done under medical auspices. They are discussed in Chapter 4 and include measurement of blood pressure, listening to heart sounds, stress testing, and electrocardiogram. There are, however, some valuable tests which you may administer to yourself, also included in Chapter 4. Remember, your present state of preparedness for cardiovascular training should play a big role in the construction of your exercise program.

In Chapter 4 you were also introduced to the 1.5-Mile Run Test, constructed by Kenneth Cooper. You should be able to conduct this cardiorespiratory endurance test yourself. Follow the procedures carefully and determine your cardiorespiratory fitness category by consulting the table provided. If your score falls with the *very poor*, *poor*, or even *fair* fitness categories, your preparedness for aerobic training is low. You are a beginning exerciser, and your decisions about exercise duration and intensity should be made accordingly.

Age

Another factor that frequently (but not always) influences the construction of cardiorespiratory training programs is age. As we emphasized in Chapter 7, structural and physiological changes occur during aging. Change may be either beneficial or inhibitory at different ages. When children approaching puberty experience gradual increase in muscular strength, we consider this to be developmental and positive. Muscular strength, maximal oxygen intake, and reaction time to sound or light stimuli are examples of human functions that tend to deteriorate significantly in middle age.

Fortunately, these changes, which correlate with decreases in certain kinds of physical performance, are usually not dramatic. Therefore, unless it is measured very finely (for example, in parts of a second), as would be the case in high-track level or swimming competition, some performance decrements may not even be noticeable. However, aerobic exercise may have to be modified somewhat in middle-aged and elderly persons. The volume of blood pumped by the heart in a single stroke tends to be less in the elderly than in youth. Also, the maximal heart rate is lower in the elderly.

These factors have implications for aerobic training. They suggest that age is associated with a comparatively lower cardiorespiratory capacity. But recognition of this simply implies the need to organize the aerobic fitness program with insight and discretion. It doesn't mean that middle-aged and elderly persons cannot or should not participate in activities which stress the cardiorespiratory mechanisms.

Smoking

The essential aspect of any aerobic fitness program is continued and steady demand upon the heart and lungs. Tobacco smoking results in a decreased ability of the cardiorespiratory mechanisms to respond to this demand. The nicotine in cigarette smoke causes blood vessels to constrict, thus inhibiting blood flow. It also causes a rise in resting heart rate (an added and undesirable burden for the heart). Carbon monoxide in cigarette smoke combines with hemoglobin in the blood. As we pointed out in Chapter 2, hemoglobin is an oxygen-carrying agent. The more it combines with carbon monoxide, the less room it has for oxygen. Consequently, oxygen transportation is diminished in smokers. In addition, cigarette smoke causes a narrowing of the small airways in the lungs and thereby interferes with air movement.

The incidence of lung and heart disease is high among smokers. Tobacco is therefore an established risk factor in cardiorespiratory disease. You would do well to avoid its use, particularly if you are eager to improve your aerobic fitness. Fortunately, the ill effects of smoking have been shown for the most part to be reversible—with emphysema (or deterioration of air sacs) a noticeable exception. So if you give up the practice, you may expect improvement in heart and lung function.

The Use of Alcohol

There is some controversy about the effects on physical performance of alcohol taken in the form of beverages such as spirits, beer, and wine. Although it has been established that alcoholic beverages contain a good deal of calories, their vitamin and mineral content is usually low. Therefore alcoholic drinks are not good foods.

Since alcohol depresses the central nervous system, its use prior to performing motor skills that require a high degree of fine neuromuscular accuracy and control is not recommended. On the other hand, moderate intake of alcohol has been shown in some studies to elevate HDL. Earlier in this chapter, we discussed the desirability of a high ratio of HDL to LDL. Remember, a low ratio is linked by research findings to cardiovascular disease.

Despite this information, we are hesitant to recommend the long-term use of alcohol. Since alcohol is absorbed directly from the stomach, it doesn't have to pass through the intestines before it can make its way into the bloodstream. It is therefore quickly metabolized, and its effect upon the nervous system is very rapid. The addictive capacity of alcohol and its potential for causing long-term damage to brain and liver cells should give you cause to consider its regular use very carefully.

Current Fads

Bookstores, drugstores, and supermarkets are laden with sport, fitness, and exercise magazines. There's a specialty magazine for every sport ranging from archery to volleyball. The latest training techniques, equipment, and competitive strategies are creatively presented. Each issue's cover is typically colorful and enticing.

With all this high-powered promotion, it is often difficult to distinguish between the valid training devices that are the result of solid research and testing, and the gimmick machinery about which unproved claims are made. Both kinds of advertisements appear in the popular magazines. There are devices that supposedly elevate cardiorespiratory fitness while you do nothing more than sit on a chair or lie on your back. Other ads recommend wearing specially constructed garments. Heat, dietary supplements, and electrical contraptions are all described as being able to enhance your aerobic fitness.

In this chapter we attempt to establish basic principles for improving cardiorespiratory endurance and provide information about how the cardiorespiratory system works. At this point in your reading, you should understand that aerobic fitness means that the heart and lungs must be able to satisfy the requirement of oxygen for a particular physical activity. When these organs and related systems meet the demand, you are aerobically fit. Activity programs that progressively tax the heart and lungs by increasing the demand load will ultimately produce higher levels of cardiorespiratory fitness. Try to remember these principles of aerobic training and do not be misled by advertisements which suggest training shortcuts. Cardiorespiratory training by definition is taxing and rigorous.

Today, impressively large numbers of Americans are regularly involved in aerobic activities such as running, swimming, and skiing. Evidence of this boom is provided by the manufacturers of sports equipment. Aerobic exercise studios that feature nonstop dancing and/or calisthenics done to music are proliferating nationwide. It is true that our country is in the embrace of a fitness craze. But not all fads are counterproductive, unhealthy, or bad. This one seems to have a positive consequence. Obviously, a profit motive often underlies the encouragement to jog, cycle, or swim coming from manufacturers of sporting goods. But if large numbers of Americans are actually benefiting aerobically from the current popularity of exercise, this is wonderful. Perhaps in time our infatuation with jogging or cycling will diminish in favor of some other exercise form. All well and good, as long as the replacements follow fundamental principles of cardiorespiratory training.

MAINTAINING CARDIORESPIRATORY FITNESS THROUGHOUT LIFE

Intensity, *duration*, and *frequency* are the essential considerations for cardiorespiratory fitness. You have learned about their vital roles in planning your aerobic fitness program. Although cardiorespiratory capacities change due to aging, and exercise programs may therefore require modification, aerobic fitness should be a lifelong goal. Cardiorespiratory well-being is the most critical of all the capacities we discuss in this book. It should not be something that you pursue only when you have time or only when friends are exercising. A realistic, personal training program should be planned and

---

GUIDELINES FOR YOUR CARDIORESPIRATORY FITNESS PROGRAM

1. Cadiorespiratory, cardiovascular, or aerobic endurance refer to persistence in continuing an activity. This involves the ability of the lungs to provide oxygen to the blood, and to the ability of the heart, blood vessels, and blood to transport it to the tissues of the body.
2. Maximum oxygen intake (Max VO_2) is probably the best indicator of cardiovascular and respiratory fitness level. A specially equipped laboratory and trained technicians are required for this value to be determined. *Target heart rate* is therefore an appropriate value to calculate in order to learn how hard you should work during exercise to build heart-lung endurance. The Cooper 1.5-Mile Run Test will provide an estimation of your aerobic fitness category.
3. Select an activity that is rhythmical, performed continuously, and cardiorespiratorily demanding. Be realistic in terms of required equipment, facilities, and weather. Select a back-up activity for occasions when you are unable to participate in your primary exercise. Remember the carryover training potential of aerobic exercise. The best results are provided by training with activities that are specific to your performance goals. Select an activity that you find to be at least moderately enjoyable.
4. Take the time to warm up thoroughly before beginning your training session. Systematically stretch all major muscle groups to be used in the training activity.
5. Don't be misled by advertised claims for rapid and easily acquired improvement in cardiorespiratory status. You will need to train for about 6 to 10 weeks before you can notice substantial improvement in aerobic performance.

---

constructed and implemented regularly. You now have the information to do this.

At this point in your reading, you have learned how the cardiorespiratory system functions; how to assess your cardiorespiratory status; and what activities are best to include in an aerobic training program. In other chapters you have read about cautions to be followed when performing these activities. You have also read about psychological factors that relate to motivation for participating in these activities for extended periods of time. We ended this chapter with a set of guidelines for constructing and maintaining your personal cardiorespiratory fitness program.

SUMMARY

1. Disorders resulting in impairment to arteries delivering blood to the heart muscle itself are known as coronary heart diseases.
2. Risk factors for cardiovascular disease include cholesterol levels, smoking, obesity, age, gender, heredity, and beta/alpha lipoprotein ratio.

3. The terms cardiorespiratory endurance, cardiovascular endurance, or aerobic endurance all refer to the same thing: persistence in continuing an activity.

4. Cardiorespiratory endurance refers to the ability of the lungs to provide oxygen to the blood and to the circulatory system's ability to transport it to the tissues of the body.

5. An aerobic activity is any activity that is rhythmic and sustained for at least 25 to 35 minutes as well as repetitive and rigorous in that it increases heart rate necessary for developing cardiorespiratory fitness.

6. In choosing a cardiorespiratory fitness training program the participant should remember to construct the program relative to his or her state of preparedness.

7. Intensity, duration and frequency are the essential considerations for cardiorespiratory fitness.

8. A cardiorespiratory training program should be planned, constructed, and implemented regularly.

REFERENCES

ACSM Guidelines. *Guidelines for Exercise Testing and Prescription* 3rd ed. Philadelphia: Lea and Febiger, 1986.

BALKE, B. "Prescribing Physical Activity." In A. J. Ryan and F. Allman (eds.), *Sports Medicine*. New York: Academic Press, 1974.

FOX, E. L. *Sports Physiology*. Philadelphia: W. B. Saunders, 1979.

HAYNES, S. G., S. LEVINE, N. SCOTCH, M. FEINLEIB, AND W. B. KANNEL. "The Relationship of Psychosocial Factors to Coronary Heart Disease in the Framingham Study: I. Methods and Risks Factors." *American Journal of Epidemiology* 107 (1978): 362–83.

LEON, A. S. "Age and Other Predictors of Coronary Heart Disease." *Medicine and Science in Sports and Exercise* 19 (1987): 159–67.

McDOUGALL, J. M., T. M. DEMBROSKI, J. E. DIMSDALE, AND T. HACHETT. "Components of Type A, Hostility, and Anger in: Further Relationship to Angiographic Findings." *Health Psychology* 4 (1985): 137–52.

11

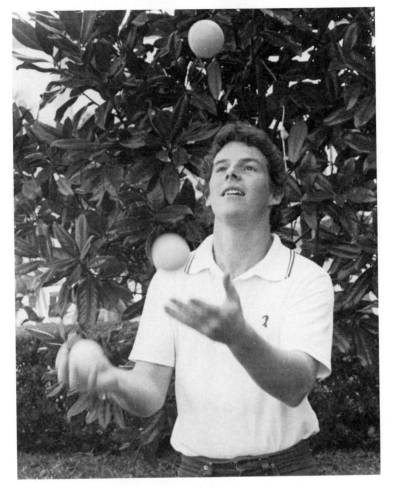

Nutrition
and
Weight Control

Do you care about being too fat? Should you care? How serious a problem is being too fat? Can you do something about the amount of fat you store in your body? These are the kinds of questions we deal with in this chapter. We'll talk about the consequences of being overweight and overfat. We'll examine some of the more important physical and psychological correlates of these conditions, and look at basic principles of weight loss that supposedly underlie many of the currently available weight loss programs. In addition, we'll discuss weight loss and physical activity.

Don't expect to lose weight merely by turning the pages in this chapter; do anticipate acquiring a solid understanding of the mechanics of fat storage and relevant concepts of nutrition.

FAT AND PHYSICAL APPEARANCE

High on our list of personal concerns is physical appearance. Perhaps the word "obsession" more accurately describes this intense interest in the way we look.

It is through descriptions of physical characteristics that we often portray those we know to others. Imagine that a friend has asked you to comment upon a person unknown to him or her—a blind date, if you will. Chances are you would say something about the person's temperament: "He or she is nice or sweet"; then you would probably say something about his or her vocation or status in school; ultimately you would move on to provide detailed information about appearance. You would very likely invest a good deal of time and effort in this part of your response. We seem to place a great deal of importance on how we look as well as on the appearances of those with whom we are linked socially or romantically. Parents are often fearful that their children will embarrass them by looking dirty or unkempt. Somehow we have learned that health and well-being are reflected in our outward appearance. We strive to look well, and those who don't are considered in most circles to be strange.

The way we look is, in very large measure, a function of our body's size and shape. The amount of fat stored beneath the skin (subcutaneous fat) is a determinant of body shape, and thus an important contributor to appearance. If we care about how we look, then we probably care about our fatness. Your physical fitness profile assessment included a determination of your body fat. A faster, yet less accurate, way of determining if you have too much body fat is to use the pinch test. Place your right index finger on your left upper arm just below the point where the arm meets the left shoulder. This area is roughly the location of your deltoid muscle. Pinch the skin here between your thumb and index finger. If you can pinch more than a half inch, you are probably too fat.

It is difficult to trace the origins of our national disdain for fat, but it is certainly well entrenched in our conscious awareness. Perhaps it was our Puritan forefathers who provided this legacy. Their influence upon contemporary values may still be felt, particularly in certain aspects of our culture. They venerated hard work, emphasized a utilitarian philosophy, and abhorred frivolity and excess of any kind. They avoided luxury, and almost everything they did (except worship) was done sparingly. But the condition of overweight poignantly suggests excess. A luxurious collection of fat is usually built up by eating more than is necessary.

Other factors may also contribute to overweight: a sedentary life-style in which very little or no physical exercise is done; metabolic imbalance (thyroid dysfunction), and certain hereditary influences (number of fat cells and effectiveness of cellular enzymatic systems). But overeating is, more often than not, a prime agent in overweight.

Perhaps our current national appreciation of slim waists, trim fannies, and well-toned muscles was bequeathed to us by the ancient Greeks. Through their lifelike statues, engravings, and reliefs they have transmitted across many centuries their love of the human form—or what we would call today the "body beautiful." Ancient Greek civilization has shaped and influenced many of our contemporary values, ideas, and concepts about government, community, and society. It may well be that its emphasis on esthetics underlies our current affinity for slimness and our fascination with physical appearance. But whatever the roots of our obsession may be, we now live in a society that views fatness with disdain. And we are encouraged to take action against fatness, since it is a social as well as a physical liability.

THE OVERWEIGHT SOCIETY

Pick up any newspaper or magazine. Thumb through it and look for advertisements or articles that deal with weight loss. Very shortly you are likely to have quite an assortment of food supplements, appetite depressants, powders, elixirs, capsules, and pills—all touted as aids in weight reduction. Often, "before" and "after" photographs accompany the testimonials of individuals alleging losses of 20, 30, 40 or more pounds of unwanted fat. Photos depicting smiling men and women, virtually swimming in trousers and dresses many sizes too large, add drama to their extraordinary testimony. Their smiles offer credibility to their claims: "Try this treatment," they say. "It has enabled me to lose weight, and see how attractive I am now." Mechanical devices, wraps, belts, and other contraptions are advertised as having miraculous spot-reducing capabilities. Not only is weight loss promised, but the reader is assured that the thigh, bust, or waistline can be made to relinquish the undesired stores of body fat.

But deposits of stored body fat cannot be made to melt away from specific locations. The sites from which stored fat is depleted are highly specific to individuals and cannot be generally predicted. Regular and rigorous physical exercise that emphasizes specific muscle groups may increase tonus and reduce skin looseness, and the result may be a tightening or firmness in certain areas of the body.

Any community of moderate size is likely to have a variety of centers or clinics that cater to dieters. These services, often owned and operated on a franchise basis, emphasize any number of therapeutic approaches. Hypnosis, physical exercise, group counseling, and acupuncture are but a few examples. All approaches have their supporters, and each and every one claims great success.

Look in the Yellow Pages of the telephone directory under "reducing," "diet," or "weight loss." You will be surprised at the number of services listed. The availability of so many opportunities for assistance in weight loss and the variety of treatments can only be viewed as evidence of our national weight consciousness. And in the face of all this focus on overweight and weight loss, one might think that all Americans are slim.

Now examine Table 11.1. The information is striking—almost overwhelming. Probably one in about every 20 Americans may be considered obese.

Table 11.1
Percent of U.S. Population Deviating from Desirable Weight

Age	Men		Women	
	10-19 Percent	20 Percent of More	10-19 Percent	20 Percent or More
20–74	18.1	14.0	12.6	23.8
20–24	11.1	7.4	9.8	9.6
25–34	16.7	13.6	8.1	17.1
35–44	22.1	17.0	12.3	24.3
45–54	19.9	15.8	15.1	27.8
55–64	18.9	15.1	15.5	34.7
65–74	19.1	13.4	17.5	31.5

Source: G. Bray, ed., *Obesity in America,* NIH publication No. 80-359 (1980).

(*Obesity* is a condition wherein an individual's body weight exceeds desirable weight by 25 percent or more.) Although we are eating less than we did 100 years ago, we are unquestionably fatter. Why? Most likely because modern technological advances have resulted in reduced physical work and reduced energy expenditure. Comparatively speaking, we may very well be burning less fuel. Though we may be eating diminished amounts of food, we are probably using much less of it than we did 100 years ago.

However, despite its prevalence in our society, is overweight really a serious or meaningful problem? Bear in mind that not all deviations from medical norms constitute serious health liabilities. Male baldness, for example, is not life threatening. But shall we therefore conclude that overweight, although widespread, is not at all related to any of the leading causes of death? Absolutely not. Overweight has been indicted by medical researchers as a correlate or causal factor in all the conditions listed in Table 1.1.

Physical Liabilities of Overweight

Although innumerable physiological interactions are affected by storage of superfluous fat, perhaps the most important effects are associated with the circulatory and respiratory systems.

Excess body weight causes the heart and vascular system (blood vessels) to work harder. Adipose tissue must be nourished like any other tissue in the body, and the cardiovascular system provides the nourishment (blood). When the overweight person walks or moves, large muscles of the thighs and legs, for example, must contract against a comparatively greater load. Moreover, this load or resistance has no functional value. Bones and teeth add weight to the body; but they are vital to our well-being. Excess fat serves no useful purpose—that's why it's called excess.

Imagine going for a stroll with a 15-, 20-, or 30-pound pack on your back. Figure 11.1 shows some of the negative consequences of having to accommodate the additional load. To be sure that you appreciate the extent of the burden of overweight, let's use one more analogy.

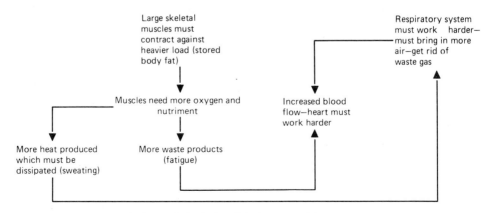

FIGURE 11.1   The added cost of physical work in the overweight

Think of a few additional suitcases tossed on the roof rack of an already heavily loaded, old, subcompact car. As the vehicle attempts to climb a steep grade, engine efficiency decreases. If any of the auto's systems are very weak, the added luggage will cause them to experience overload. This may cause breakdown in the most vulnerable parts. If the transmission is marginally functional, it may fail entirely on the steep grade. If the suspension system is weak, it may fracture under the unaccustomed load.

Exertion due to heavy physical exercise such as running to catch a bus or psychological stress due to receiving news of a death in the family, may elicit more traumatic reaction in the obese than in the nonobese. Physiological systems in the obese may barely be able to cope with the loads imposed by excessive body weight. Additional stress may be critical or even fatal. Many biomechanical and endocrinological functions may be out of kilter in the overweight, affecting essential metabolic processes. Bizarre mechanical stresses may be placed on the skeletal structure, causing postural defects and orthopedic problems. There are other discomforts as well. Heat loss may be inefficient, and heavy sweating may be frequent. Irritation due to the rubbing of thighs or friction caused by ill-fitting clothing may cause skin problems.

An additional and very serious liability of obesity is a greatly enhanced surgical risk. Surgeons are hesitant to operate upon obese patients for fear of "complications" as well as the necessity of slicing through the layers of fat that cover the internal organs to which they seek access.

In a nutshell, if you are overweight, it is unlikely that you can achieve an optimal level of readiness for the type of physical activity required by your vocational or avocational commitments. One popular way of defining physical fitness is in terms of preparedness for the demands of your day. If you deliver the mail, then fitness involves the ability to walk for hours; if you conduct a symphony, you must be able to stand for long periods of time while moving your arms vigorously; if you lay bricks for a living, you must be able to bend, squat, lift, and carry throughout the day. If you are an elementary school child, you must be able to sit comfortably on request, walk, run, crawl, climb, push, and scuffle—if you want to be reasonably content and accepted by your peers.

Obesity or overweightness makes all of these activities difficult to execute. On a superficial level (at least), you cannot claim a reasonably high degree of physical fitness and be overfat. So, have we answered the questions "Should you care about being too fat?" and "How serious a problem is being too fat?" Now, what are your conclusions?

The Social Stigma

Today, thin is in. But this was not always the case. Look at portraits of prominent European personalities of the seventeenth and eighteenth centuries. Notice the corpulence of the men—their large protruding bellies and the folds of skin beneath their chins. In those times, significant storage of body fat was considered a sign of prosperity. It was the unfortunate and the poor who were thin. Observe the portraits of the supposedly wealthy and attractive women. Notice the female nudes, who were obviously selected as models because of their physical beauty. They are almost shockingly wide of hip and ample of buttock, for such were the attributes of physically attractive females of the day. In fact, in certain areas of the world today, such an appearance is deemed very desirable in women. But not so in American society!

Virility, success, and strength were associated with male corpulence in many societies of yesteryear. Today, we hold entirely different ideas about overweight and obesity. In addition to the health and physical performance liabilities associated with these conditions, social stigma is involved.

Researchers tell us that Americans tend to behave in prejudiced ways toward individuals whose physical forms deviate from normative models. Overweight persons are frequently discriminated against when they apply for jobs, promotions, and admission to some colleges and universities. At less than fully conscious levels of awareness, we tend to discriminate against those in our society who are overfat. We don't like fat individuals. Surveys reveal that very fat persons are not usually among the top executives in leading companies.

Furthermore, most of the popular flattering stereotypes about overfat persons are invalid and have never been substantiated through sound research. Supposedly, fat persons are jolly, good dancers, and friendly and have good senses of humor. These attributes are probably distributed among fat persons to the same extent as they are in those of proper weight. They may represent an ill-founded attempt on behalf of nonobese persons to be kind and generous to the obese, for whom they may feel sympathy.

Body Image

Psychologists are confident that the way we feel about our physical selves affects our self-esteem and has an important effect on our overall behavior. *Body image* is the term used to refer to the view we have of our physical selves. Those with positive and strong body images usually have wholesome and positive attitudes about other aspects of the self. The concept of wellness, as we speak of it in this book, is very much dependent upon how we think about and value ourselves. It is very important for us to like ourselves and to think about ourselves in positive terms.

Although grooming (makeup, hair style), skin texture and color, and teeth contribute in important ways to our physical appearance, three factors in particular deserve special mention:

1. The dimensions (length and breadth) of the skeletal framework.
2. The distribution and development of the muscle mass resting upon the skeleton and the amount and location of adipose tissue throughout the body.
3. The clothing that covers the skeleton.

We are able to control the last two factors; the first is a function of genetic forces (for better or for worse). Their individual influences on wellness are enormous, and in combination they practically account for the whole physical image we project.

We should be able to regulate what and how much we eat. Some people relinquish this control. Others are unwilling to invest the effort necessary to deal with this responsibility. To a very large extent, wellness depends on nutrition. The proper control of body weight is a function of nutritional knowledge, habits, and decisions. We have practically uninterrupted opportunities to make highly personal decisions about nutritional matters—perhaps more opportunity than in most other areas of health and wellness.

Here we will review basic principles of weight loss and gain and discuss nutrients and nutritional needs, truths and fallacies. Again, we emphasize that a sound knowledge of nutrition is the cornerstone on which we base our physical appearance, health, and well-being.

THE NUTRIENTS

All foods consist of *nutrients*, which are necessary for the maintenance of life itself. When we are able to satisfy our nutritional needs easily, more time and energy are available for recreational activities. Imagine how little time would be available for sports, reading, and socializing with friends, if we had to forage or hunt for food. Even gathering wild fruits and plants would consume countless numbers of hours within a typical week.

In comparison to other societies in the world, the United States has in recent years benefited from an abundance of food to the extent that it has been able to offer surplus quantities to other nations. Modern technology and science have made hunting and foraging obsolete except for recreational purposes. We have been freed from the awesome responsibilities of providing food through the sweat of our brows and blast of our musket. But the time and energy made available to us as a result of our incredible advancements in science and technology have created other kinds of problems. One set of problems is of paramount concern to us in this chapter: too little exercise and too much food.

Food is something we think of and deal with regularly throughout the day. Since our stomachs are emptied of their contents about five to seven hours after ingestion of food, at about this time our brains receive messages from the stomach which remind us that it is time to eat. When we perceive these signals, which really involve complex neurochemical interactions, we begin to contemplate our next meal. "What's for dinner, Mom?" is an example of such contemplation; "Where shall we meet for lunch?" is another. So confident are we of the regularity of the hunger stimulus that we establish appointments for dining with friends or business acquaintances days and even weeks in advance.

However, some of us are aware of stimuli that visit our consciousness frequently throughout the day, at intervals that do not correspond with the five- to seven-hour stomach emptying cycle. It seems that various mood states may stimulate a desire to eat. At times, some of us are motivated to eat again as a consequence of viewing a picture of food, even though we have very recently taken a large meal. *Appetite* is the term applied to the factors that stimulate interest in eating, but that are more psychologically than physiologically oriented.

Food Intake Versus Needs

As a rule of thumb, when we eat more calories (a *calorie* is a unit of energy contained in food) than the cells in our bodies need for their function, they are stored in the body as fat. We are able to determine the approximate number of calories needed daily according to our height, weight, body build, age, and typical level and kind of daily activities. Table 11.2 provides such information, which may be used as a rough guide for determining daily requirements.

You may wonder how the caloric values for foods are calculated. For example, how can the number of calories contained in an apple or a slice of bread be determined? Known quantities of food are actually burned in a device called a *bomb calorimeter*. The heat (energy) released is trapped, measured (heat is easy to measure), and expressed in terms of calories. A *calorie* is the amount of heat needed to raise 1 gram of water 1 degree Centigrade.

The federal government publishes a detailed listing called *Composition of Foods, Raw, Processed and Prepared*. This is a good resource to consult for an accurate determination of the caloric value of food you eat. It is available in any school library and is the definitive reference used by physicians, diet book authors, and serious-minded weight losers.

To use this book, you need to know the quantity of food eaten. Therefore, the food you eat must be weighed carefully. This requires a special effort, but the result is an accurate assessment of you daily caloric intake. Many of us who swear that we eat very little would be very surprised to discover that our actual daily caloric intake is quite substantial.

Table 11.2
Number of Calories Needed Daily According
to Age and Sex

Age (years)	Calories per Pound per Day	
	Males	Females
10-12	32	29
12-14	24	23
14-18	23	21
18-22	19	19
25 and over	17	15

Basic Nutrients: Fats, Proteins, Carbohydrates, Vitamins, Minerals, Water

We commonly use words such as banana, chocolate, lettuce, pineapple juice, and egg to refer to the food we are eating, preparing, or thinking about. These are everyday or lay terms and have widespread acceptance. But the chemist and nutritionist have a special vocabulary for the components of the foods we eat.

With some exceptions, foods consist of the following nutrients: fats, proteins, carbohydrates, vitamins, minerals, and water (water has no calories). These are present to varying degrees in different foods and are differentiated by their chemical makeup. For example, potato has more carbohydrate than a comparable quantity of celery, carrot more vitamin A and C than green beans, and whole milk (no butterfat removed) more fat than shrimp. A *molecule* (atoms are arranged in groups known as molecules) of carbohydrate contains more of the carbon atom than a molecule of protein.

Although the components of various foods differ, there is considerable overlap in many foods. Foods, therefore, vary in terms of their nutritional value. It is important for us to know which foods contain high or low amounts of these chemical ingredients so that we can organize meals that contain all the essential food components. Sufficient quantities of all nutrients should be included in our daily diets.

A diet that contains the recommended daily allowance (RDA) of essential food nutrients is said to be *balanced*. Although many factors influence our decisions about what we eat, a quest for a balanced diet should always underlie our meal planning and food selection.

Eating Enough of the Right Foods

It is not particularly difficult to satisfy daily carbohydrate, fat, protein, vitamin, mineral, and water requirements in the typical American diet. But even today, malnutrition exists in our country, much to our collective shame and disappointment.

An individual who does not receive adequate supplies of essential food nutrients is said to be malnourished, despite the number of calories ingested daily. All food nutrients are vital to the well-being of the organism, and deficiencies in any of them may result in serious disease. Many of the common foods we eat, such as bread and milk, are *fortified* with essential vitamins and minerals in order that we be assured of recommended daily allowance (RDA) of these.

How can we determine the degree to which a food satisfies our daily minimal requirement for a food nutrient. It is rather easy if the food is packaged or bottled and sold commercially. Law requires that the necessary information be printed on the carton, package, or container. Quite clearly, then, consumers have the responsibility and wherewithal to protect their health and mediate their wellness. Choices abound; you have only to make educated and prudent decisions about what you eat.

Consult Table 11.3 (pp. 222-23) to determine your RDA for the basic food nutrients. Note that the table uses the gram as a basic unit of measurement. The *gram* is a value in the metric system of weight and measurement. One ounce equals 28 grams.

How many grams of carbohydrate, fat, protein, vitamins, and minerals do you require? Have you easily satisfied your RDA for each food nutrient? You probably have. If you haven't, what adjustments will you consider making?

Most of us eat foods that are abundantly or even excessively rich in simple carbohydrates or monosaccharides. Americans typically consume less protein than carbohydrates. This may be due to the comparatively low cost of foods high in carbohydrate (bread, potato, rice) and the higher cost of foods high in protein (beef, fish, poultry, eggs). However, the amount of protein consumed is generally in excess of what we need. Foods popularly known as *staples* are high in carbohydrates and are the basic supporters of dietary needs throughout the world. Protein is an essential food nutrient, but the value of supplemental dietary protein has not been established.

According to a report entitled *Dietary Guidelines for Healthy American Adults* published in 1986 by the American Heart Association, we should reduce our consumption of refined or processed sugars (monosaccharides) by 45 percent or to about 10 percent of our total caloric intake. It is additionally suggested that oligosaccharides and polysaccharides should be increased in the American diet by 17 percent to make a total caloric intake percentage of 45 percent. Thus, for an active athletic individual, a daily nutritional diet should consist of 10–15 percent protein, 25–30 percent fat, and 55–60 percent carbohydrates.

You can approximate your recommended caloric intake by multiplying your ideal body weight (determined by percent body fat measurements) by 18 if you are a moderately active female, and by 20.5 if you are a moderately active male. The sum will provide the amount of calories needed per day to maintain your current body weight.

Vitamins

Although vitamins do not contain energy, they are necessary for good health. They are usually present in adequate amounts in the typical American diet. Eating large quantities of vitamins will not improve your health or enable you to perform exercise in a superior fashion unless a vitamin deficiency has been diagnosed. In fact, large doses of certain vitamins, such as A or D, may be quite harmful.

Vitamin C is found in citrus fruits, tomatoes, cabbage, potatoes, broccoli, and peppers. It plays important roles in forming the tissues of which tendons and ligaments are made, and in protecting against infection. There are a number of B vitamins, and their roles vary from helping to break down carbohydrates, fats, and proteins, to production of red blood cells, to helping to prevent nervous irritability. Most of the B vitamins are found in yeast, liver, leafy vegetables, and wheat germ.

Table 11.3

Recommended Daily Allowance for Food Nutrients

	Age (years)	Weight (lb.)	Height (in.)	Protein (g)	Fat-Soluble Vitamins		
					Vita-min A (µg R.E.)	Vita-min D (µg)	Vita-min E (mg α T.E.)
Infants	0.0-0.5	13	24	kg x 2.2	420	10	3
	0.5-1.0	20	28	kg x 2.0	400	10	4
Children	1-3	29	35	23	400	10	5
	4-6	44	44	30	500	10	6
	7-10	62	52	34	700	10	7
Males	11-14	99	62	45	1000	10	8
	15-18	145	69	56	1000	10	10
	19-22	154	70	56	1000	7.5	10
	23-50	154	70	56	1000	5	10
	51+	154	70	56	1000	5	10
Females	11-14	101	62	46	800	10	8
	15-18	120	64	46	800	10	8
	19-22	120	64	44	800	7.5	8
	23-50	120	64	44	800	5	8
	51+	120	64	44	800	5	8
Pregnant				+30	+200	+5	+2
Lactating				+20	+400	+5	+3

Source: Food and Nutrition Board, *Recommended Dietary Allowances,* 9th ed. Washington, D.C. National Academy of Sciences (1979).

Night blindness and growth problems are associated with vitamin A deficiency. Milk and dairy products and yellow vegetables are good sources of vitamin A. Butter, eggs, milk, and fish oils contain substantial amounts of vitamin D, which is essential for proper bone and tooth development. A deficiency in vitamin E is associated with destruction of red blood cells. It is widely distributed in yellow vegetables, vegetable oils, and wheat germ. Blood clotting is related to vitamin K, which is found in spinach, eggs, liver, and cabbage.

Triglycerides and Cholesterol

Some of the body's fat is stored and some of it is free (appears in the blood). Stored body fat insulates and is vital to maintaining body temperature. It also protects tissues and organs. Some fats are said to be *unsaturated* (derived from plants and tend to be liquid), whereas others tend to be hard (come from animal sources) and are *saturated*. Fat circulating in the blood is an important source of energy for muscular contraction, particularly when muscle glycogen (stored in the muscles) is depleted.

Water-Soluble Vitamins							Minerals					
Vita- min C (mg)	Thia- min (mg)	Ribo- flavin (mg)	Niacin (mg N.E.)	Vita- min B_6 (mg)	Fola- cin (µg)	Vita- min B_{12} (µg)	Cal- cium (mg)	Phos- phorus (mg)	Mag- ne- sium (mg)	Iron (mg)	Zinc (mg)	Iodine (mg)
35	0.3	0.4	6	0.3	30	0.5	360	240	50	10	3	40
35	0.5	0.6	8	0.6	45	1.5	540	360	70	15	5	50
45	0.7	0.8	9	0.9	100	2.0	800	800	150	15	10	70
45	0.9	1.0	11	1.3	200	2.5	800	800	200	10	10	90
45	1.2	1.4	16	1.6	300	3.0	800	800	250	10	10	120
50	1.4	1.6	18	1.8	400	3.0	1200	1200	350	18	15	150
60	1.4	1.7	18	2.0	400	3.0	1200	1200	400	18	15	150
60	1.5	1.7	19	2.2	400	3.0	800	800	350	10	15	150
60	1.4	1.6	18	2.2	400	3.0	800	800	350	10	15	150
60	1.2	1.4	16	2.2	400	3.0	800	800	350	10	15	150
50	1.1	1.3	15	1.8	400	3.0	1200	1200	300	18	15	150
60	1.1	1.3	14	2.0	400	3.0	1200	1200	300	18	15	150
60	1.1	1.3	14	2.0	400	3.0	800	800	300	18	15	150
60	1.0	1.2	13	2.0	400	3.0	800	800	300	18	15	150
60	1.0	1.2	13	2.0	400	3.0	800	800	300	10	15	150
+20	+0.4	+0.3	+2	+0.6	+400	+1.0	+400	+400	+150		+5	+25
+40	+0.5	+0.5	+5	+0.5	+100	+1.0	+400	+400	+150		+10	+50

Cholesterol is a triglyceride or form of fat that has been the focus of much study during the past 25 years. Although it serves many necessary functions, cholesterol has been linked with cardiovascular disease. Therefore we shall briefly discuss it here.

Animal fats that we eat raise the blood triglyceride and cholesterol level. Liver, red meats, egg yolk, butter, and kidney are examples of foods that are high in cholesterol. However, the amount of cholesterol you have in your blood is not due exclusively to dietary factors. Some cholesterol is manufactured by the body itself.

Low-density lipoproteins may deposit their cholesterol in the walls of the coronary arteries which harden into *plaques*. (This is not true of high-density lipids.) Over the years these plaques cause a narrowing of the blood vessel's diameter and the arteries become hard and unelastic (arteriosclerosis). The result is a reduced flow of blood and consequently reduced oxygen supply to the heart muscle. Since it is unlikely that you can regulate blood cholesterol that the body synthesizes, it seems prudent to control volitionally the amount of foods you eat that are high in cholesterol. Your physician can send a sample of your blood to a laboratory where analyses will reveal the amount of triglycerides and low density cholesterol. The relation between dietary cholesterol and arteriosclerosis is an example of how your wellness is dependent upon what you eat.

Fiber

Dietary fiber is carbohydrate from cereal grains, vegetables and fruits that is indigestible. It therefore becomes a residue (referred to as roughage) that stimulates proper digestive function. Since it is not broken down by the body's chemicals, it remains in the lower intestine and retains water that in turn is helpful in bowel movement. For these reasons, fiber is an important dietary consideration.

Salt

Sufficient salt in the body is necessary for the cells to function properly, especially during muscular work. Physical performance will be impaired if salt loss is high. If your body is not well prepared for physical activity, that is, if you are not well trained, you may be inclined to drink a good deal of water during or after exercise. This might result in a decrease of salt concentration. On the other hand, if you drink little or not at all during exercise, your body's salt concentration is likely to increase due to water loss caused by increased sweating. Therefore, exercise can influence salt balance. As a rule, salt tablets which were once prescribed for athletes training in hot weather *should not be used*. Their impact upon proper salt-water balance can be too dramatic.

Sugar

Sugar provides empty calories in that it contains no protein, vitamins, or minerals. But since it has lots of calories, it provides energy. However, it would be wise when seeking sweet tasting foods or supplemental energy sources to consider foods such as fruits and vegetables that also provide vital nutrients. There is much sugar hidden in many of the prepared foods we eat, so it is highly likely that you are already ingesting substantial amounts of sugar. It is not true that large doses of sugar or honey or other forms of carbohydrates taken immediately prior to exercise will necessarily enhance performance. For this type of effect to occur, the physical activity must extend beyond an hour, such as in marathon running.

Diet and Performance

After considering the contents of the preceding sections of this chapter you should be able to appreciate the critical connection between nutrition and performance.

It is through the diet that your body is nourished. Moreover, the food you eat provides the energy that your muscles require to work. You have no control over the natural color of your hair, eyes, or the length of your nose or long bones. But, fortunately, you can regulate your diet. You are in charge of the quantity and quality of what you eat. If you are involved in a regular program of physical exercise that increases your energy requirements, you should give careful and particular attention to what you eat.

The mechanisms that regulate appetite and hunger in humans were developed millions of years ago when our species was very physically active. These mechanisms have not changed very much, but for the most part, our activity patterns have. Today, many individuals living in our society eat too much and are insufficiently physically active. It's up to you to balance the eating activity equation.

Special Nutritional Needs

Many circumstances create special nutritional needs during certain periods in our lives.

Childhood and adolescence are developmental periods in which a considerable amount of physical growth occurs. New tissue and larger organs require additional amounts of nutrients, particularly protein. Adolescents are notoriously prone to fads, including those that relate to diet. They are therefore apt to get into nutritional trouble, since a balanced diet is especially important in this age range.

Skeletal size and amount of muscle mass are determined genetically. Dietary habits, which determine how much and what kind of nutrients will be available to growing cells, enable bones, muscles, and other types of tissue to reach their genetic potential. Iron loss can be a problem in teenage boys on inadequate diets. Women in their teens can also lose a larger than average amount of iron due to menstruation. Iron supplements to the diet are appropriate in both cases.

Individuals who are very active physically burn a lot of calories. Children and adolescents who participate regularly in sport, exercise, and training usually need and request large amounts of food. Parents are sometimes amazed at how trim their children remain despite their enormous appetites. Keeping teenage tummies full can be a formidable challenge. But there are important considerations to make when facing this challenge. For example, proteins and fats are digested more slowly than sugar. Therefore snacks high in sugar and low in protein are undesirable because they stop hunger for only brief periods of time.

Pregnancy is another time in life when special nutritional requirements may be necessary, particularly for protein. The quality and quantity of foods eaten by the pregnant woman not only satisfy *her* nutritional needs, but also those of the developing fetus. This is also true for mothers who are nursing.

The pregnant woman's body weight should be carefully monitored under a physician's direction. Some women tend to gain a lot of weight during the later stages of pregnancy without taking in additional calories. This may be due to a shift in life-style that includes less physical activity. Diets that are low in carbohydrates and salt and include ample amounts of fruits and vegetables are recommended.

Beyond the early twenties, there is a tendency for adults to gain weight. In most cases, the increase is due to accumulation of stored body fat. Fifty-five percent of American men between the ages 50 and 59 are at least 20 percent overweight. The figure for women of this age is 46 percent. But as LaPlace (1980) says,

> It is important to realize that weight need not increase as people get older. Individuals are usually at their ideal or best weight in their mid-twenties. When they are in their mid-sixties, they should still be at this ideal weight. Although the phenomenon of increasing weight with increasing years is common enough to make it seem "natural," it is neither inevitable nor desirable; older people should be no fatter than younger people.

To maintain body weight, elderly men and women will probably have to eat fewer calories. Muscle mass and bone density decrease during this period of life, and therefore even though the scale may reveal no change in overall body weight, the likelihood of an increase in body fat is high.

WEIGHT REGULATION

Approximately 3,500 calories above and beyond the number required to fuel daily activity is needed to account for 1 pound of stored body fat. On the other hand, caloric intake must be reduced by approximately 3,300 calories in order for 1 pound of stored body fat to be *metabolized* (burned) or lost. (See Figure 11.2.) So more calories are needed to add a pound of fat than to lose a pound.

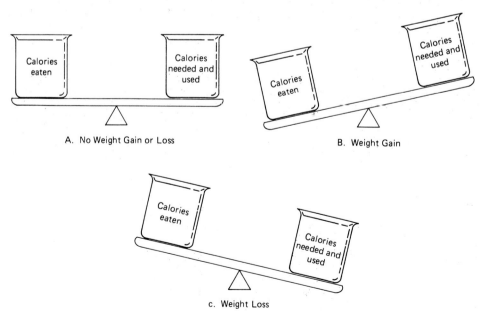

A. No Weight Gain or Loss

B. Weight Gain

c. Weight Loss

FIGURE 11.2   The thermodynamic seesaw

But there is a frequently overlooked aspect of this basic accounting system. In his book, *The High Energy Factor* (1983), Dr. B. Gutin of Teachers College, Columbia University, notes that a "cumulative effect" can exert a hidden but significant influence on weight loss and weight gain.

Dr. Gutin is saying that the balance of incoming (food eaten) and outgoing (energy spent on activity) calories need not be thought of as occurring within any single day. Therefore, a deficit or excess of calories may be accumulated over periods of time. You need not burn up 3,300 calories in one day to lose 1 pound of fat. If you are not in a rush to lose weight, the loss may be accomplished by increasing caloric expenditure while maintaining an unaltered intake of calories. According to Dr. Gutin, the way to do this is through exercise. We'll have more to say about the role of exercise in weight regulation later.

Putting on Weight

Be sure you understand the concept of caloric balance before we proceed. To be on the safe side, let's review a few principles of weight loss and gain.

Assuming that the person in question is physiologically sound, if the number of calories needed to sustain life functions such as walking, studying, reading, and even sleeping is equal to the number of calories available to the body, then no loss or gain of weight will occur. A condition of equilibrium is achieved. Body weight, or more accurately stored body fat, should theoretically remain unchanged. Think of a playground seesaw which is put in equilibrium by two cartons resting on each end of the board. As the contents of one carton are reduced, the balance shifts and the board no longer assumes a horizontal position. Body weight is thus lost or gained according to this model.

Unfortunately, this simple in-out principle doesn't apply exactly as described to all people. Some people may be frustrated in their attempts to lose weight. They may have inherited a large number of fat cells, in the same way that the number of muscle cells or female egg cells are determined by heredity. This means that embedded within their fat-storing tissue is a large number of cells waiting to be filled by unused energy, which is converted to fat. Medical tests sometimes reveal atypical metabolic activity and complicated endocrinological dysfunction in these people. Obese persons, ironically, may be considered to be very efficient processors of food. There is evidence that their systems may utilize food very efficiently (slowly), thereby yielding unneeded calories that are stored as fat. This is like the frugal individual who spends money very cautiously and has some left over to deposit in a savings account.

Psychological Factors

Perhaps it is time to pause and reflect upon an assumption you may very well have been making up to this point. That is, all individuals are motivated to reach and maintain an optimal body weight. Psychologists who probe our hidden motivations through testing and analysis techniques tell us that this is not necessarily true. Some persons are pleased with their over or underweight condition despite the warnings of physicians, height-weight charts, friends,

PSYCHOLOGICAL FACTORS IN WEIGHT REGULATION

There's more to weight gain and loss than calorie counting. Social, emotional, environmental, and vocational factors are important. They dramatically influence dietary practices and choices.

Before beginning a weight regulation program, ask yourself the following questions: your answers may reveal information about why you tend to eat too much too litte:

1. Do I have friends who care about me and about whom I care?
2. Do I participate in joyful or meaningful social activities? How often?
3. Am I sad or angry often? Am I frequently jealous of others?
4. Do I like where I live—my community, my home, my room?
5. Does my job please me? Am I happy in school?

and relatives. They simply reject opinion and advice from others, irrespective of its source or authoritativeness.

Such people may have achieved wellness in spite of their unhealthy weight. On the other hand, their denial may be expressing not only a complacency about their physical appearance, but also a dislike of self or even a wish to experience personal harm. Such dynamics are usually difficult to fathom and require the intervention of trained and competent professionals.

Often much psychological turmoil accompanies obesity. Whether overeating, and ultimately obesity, *result* from the psychic turbulence or whether obesity *causes* or contributes to the development of psychological problems is a difficult and moot question. We consider such issues here because they suggest, quite appropriately, that weight regulation is not always as simple as it appears.

Even those who wish to alter their body weight and appearance to a meaningful extent may discover that the psychological and physiological demands of therapeutic programs are too formidable. Decisions about body weight regulation and physical appearance are highly personal and should be made after considerable thought and reflection. By all means listen to the reactions and advice of others who care about you and integrate their assessments and suggestions into your deliberations. But ultimately, whether or not you lose weight is your decision.

Individual decision making about health matters is a critical element of the *wellness* concept emphasized in this book. Family members, friends, colleagues, and associates who badger an apparently overweight person to lose weight may not only be imprudent and unfair; their efforts may be counterproductive. Certainly, you know from personal experience how irritating it is to hear criticisms of your own behavior and decisions again and again, even though you suspect that the remarks and judgments from others have some truth to them. Some individuals elect to remain overweight or even obese.

Their adjustment to this condition is satisfactory. They function well socially and are not unhappy about their condition.

Intellectual and emotional readiness is needed for success in weight control. As we've noted previously, the basis for marked over- or underweight may very well be psychological in nature (see the accompanying box). *Anorexia nervosa* (a condition in which the ingestion of food is both physically and intellectually repugnant) as well as *obesity* (grossly excessive storage of body fat) are believed to have psychological bases that require attention before changes in the physical condition can be made.

Professionals who counsel the overweight are virtually unanimous in their expressions of confidence about helping clients *lose* weight. But they are usually far less assured about predicting that clients will *maintain* their losses. This may very well be due to the therapeutic program's inability to strike at the problem's core—the *motives* that account for excessive caloric consumption. If these remain unaddressed, there is little hope for a long-term weight loss maintenance. The crucial element in any program that sets out to change caloric consumption is a change in *life-style*. If basic nutritional insights and practices are not altered, any favorable outcomes will be temporary.

Weight Reduction Programs

If it were realistic to count and sort all books published in the last 20 years dealing with health topics, we would very likely find that most of them would be diet books. We tend to be more uneasy about overweight than we are about many other health problems. Apparently our concern has assumed dramatic proportions. As suggested earlier, this is perhaps due to the close relationship between body weight and physical appearance—that is, how we appear to others.

Suppose we are suffering from diabetes. Could we not camouflage this condition successfully? If we had to, because of job-related reasons, could we not keep such a condition a secret? Certainly we could. It is, however, difficult to hide acute overweight. We tend to be terribly conscious of how we look, and since most of us strive to somehow neutralize our unattractive features, at one time or another many of us have been, will be, or know someone who is on a diet.

A veritable cornucopia of weight loss programs is at your disposal. Which one is best? Which are safe? Which programs yield quick results? Answers to these questions need to take into account your particular characteristics. For example, how old are you? How much weight do you want to lose? Do you have any medical problems? Have you previously tried to lose weight? If so, were you successful? What kind of work do you do? Are you married? Answers to these questions should be considered when choosing a weight loss program in addition to general principles about weight loss and weight loss programs.

In addition to the broad principles outlined in the box, you should be wary of fad diets and contraptions or products promoted as yielding immediate and significant loss of fat. An average weight loss of between 2 and 4 pounds per

---

GUIDELINES FOR SELECTING A WEIGHT REDUCTION PROGRAM

1. There is no safe and healthy way to lose fat quickly.
2. Long-range weight control should be a paramount objective of any program.
3. Development of a new or changed life-style (which goes beyond an adjustment of daily caloric intake) should be emphasized.
4. With the exception of severe obesity, regular exercise can be an effective part of weight reduction therapy and should complement other approaches whenever possible.

---

week is safe and realistic. On occasion, some of the weight loss may be attributed to fluid (water) loss rather than to fat.

Further, individuals who are prone to coronary disease should be cautious about high-protein diets, which usually involve high fat intake. The elimination of dietary carbohydrate usually means a severe reduction in vitamin and mineral intake, and you should therefore supplement such a diet with these elements. Any diet that involves caloric reduction will probably result in weight loss. But the aim of any program should be to lose weight *safely*.

Consider taking appetite depressants or other drugs *only* after consulting with a physician. Do not be influenced by claims for dramatic results. Always look for the rational basis that should underlie the success promised by the program. Ask yourself, "Why should this approach work for *me*?" Generate additional questions based on the guidelines given here. Do not make a commitment to a particular regimen until you are confident that all your questions have been answered. Do not let convenience determine your choice. Appendix B presents a summary and evaluation of some widely publicized diets.

Although you may not be in the market for a weight-reducing program at the moment, imagine that you are. Which of the diets in Appendix B do you think would be best for you? How would you go about seeking additional information about a program you felt might be appropriate for your needs?

The Question of Behavior Change

Are there times during the day when you are likely to overeat or eat inadequately? You may have noticed that you tend to eat more than you should when in the presence of certain friends or acquaintances, or that you are never hungry before or after a particular class or activity. Perhaps your "eating behavior" is in need of change. In Chapter 6 we deal with ways to control all kinds of behavior. Perhaps you will be able to apply some of the behavior modification techniques described to your eating routines. You may even learn how to condition yourself to behave in ways that can be helpful when dieting. Reread Chapter 6 with an eye toward your eating behavior.

THE ROLE OF EXERCISE

"I'm out of shape—I've put on a few pounds and I need some exercise." This lament is heard often from college students, business executives, and many middle-aged men and women. Typically, a twofold revelation is being made by those who admit to such conditions:

1. The individual is unhappy with his or her body shape.
2. The individual is acknowledging the role of exercise in weight control.

The Set Point Theory

Exercise may be the only logical way of constructing a weight loss program consistent with a theory that is currently receiving a good measure of support from researchers. It is called the *set point theory* and it suggests that each of us has a biochemically determined range within which our body weight tends to hover. According to the theory, body weight can be nudged out of this "natural" range by dieting. But it is very difficult to do so unless a scrupulous vigil is constantly maintained. Set point theorists argue that exercise may significantly alter the set point so that the boundaries for the so-called natural range are lowered. This, of course, entails regular exercise or training.

Physical activity has widespread acceptance as an important element in weight loss. Laypersons who operate on personal experiential and intuitive levels, as well as scientists and physicians who have the benefit of formal training in such matters, are in agreement that some form of physical activity is beneficial to wellness in general and to weight control programs in particular. So, at this point we need a review of important issues relating to exercise that have specific relevance to weight control.

Selecting the Appropriate Exercise

Although you may recognize the value of exercise, you may need assistance in selecting the appropriate kinds and amounts that will help you regulate your weight optimally. We want you to make healthful and safe decisions about the physical activity program you select.

Not all forms of exercise result in equal amounts of expended energy. These differences are shown in Appendix B. For example, a 170-pound person will use 3.7 calories per minute while horseback riding but 11.7 calories per minute while playing squash.

You should consider some additional factors beyond calorie utilization per minute when deciding whether or not to incorporate an activity into your program. An important question to raise is, "How long can I sustain the activity?" Sprinting will result in 27.3 calories per minute being expended by a 170-pound person. But how long can this activity be endured? In contrast, slow jogging yields 12.1 calories per minute. However, it can be sustained for a much longer period of time than sprinting. The net caloric expenditure for jog-

POINTS TO REMEMBER ABOUT WEIGHT CONTROL

Using up Stored Fat in Ordinary Ways

Exercise uses extra calories. The energy cost of moving large muscles must be met by metabolizing or burning additional fuel. If you do no take in extra quantities of food, then stored body fat will be used as fuel. Approximately 3,300 calories must be metabolized to account for 1 pound of stored body fat. This need not be done all at once. As long as 3,300 calories are used eventually, then 1 pound of fat will be lost. The calories may be expended during the course of a day, week, month, or year. If incoming calories (food) are kept constant and made to equal the number that the body needs to carry out its typical and basic functions (without exercise), the addition of an exercise program to the daily list of activities will result in use of stored energy—fat.

The exercise need not take place in a gymnasium or on a track. You can increase your need for energy by walking up a flight of stairs daily, rather than taking the elevator; or parking your car an extra block away from your destination to experience the extra walk. If walking up one flight of stairs carries an energy cost of 100 calories, then such a climb once a day for 5 days will account for 500 calories, or one-seventh of a pound of fat. If stairs are climbed for 7 weeks (assuming a typical work or school week of 5 days), a pound of body fat should be lost without a change of diet. Approximately 8 pounds could theoretically be lost this way in less than a year. For a more rapid loss, a second flight of climbed stairs could be incorporated into your routine. Or stair climbing and walking an extra block from the parked car could be combined.

This cumulative effect of exercise on weight loss does not require eating less and is therefore relatively "painless," although obviously not an efficient way for very obese persons to lose a lot of weight.

Exercise and Metabolism

Not only are metabolic activities elevated during fairly vigorous rhythmic exercise, but they remain elevated for a considerable amount of time after exercise. When exercise begins, not all muscle cells receive all the oxygen they require, even under aerobic conditions. Therefore, even after a physiological balance occurs during activity and adequate energy is provided to fuel the activities of the body's cells, a deficit remains. So you must repay the oxygen your cells needed and used during the beginning of exercise when it was not available aerobically. We call this *oxygen debt*. It is repaid with heavy breathing, which continues for a while during a period of elevated metabolism after exercise. So, you are using calories even after you have stopped exercising.

Exercise and Appetite

Contrary to popular belief, strenuous exercise has been shown to depress appetite slightly rather than stimulate it, so you probably will *not* be hungry after vigorous physical activity.

Exercise and a Positive Outlook

Increased use of your body may stimulate you to feel better about your body and consequently about yourself. Exercise can be very enjoyable—something to look forward to. It may be done in the company of others; it may be done to music. It can be a time for creative thinking if the exercise is of the rhythmic kind and does not involve competition. Above all, it can provide the feeling that you are doing something *for* yourself rather than depriving yourself of something you like (food).

ging would therefore exceed a minute or two of sprinting, probably the maximum duration for most sprints.

Recreational rowing, jogging, swimming, cycling, and cross country activities, which were recommended for cardiorespiratory endurance training (Chapter 10), are also good exercises for weight reduction. They can be performed for progressively longer periods of time as your aerobic fitness increases. Moreover, they typically require relatively low levels of skill in comparison to activities such as racket sports, wrestling, basketball, handball, and fencing, which yield fairly high amounts of expended energy. Ironically, if your skill level in cross country skiing or rowing is low, your performance will be *inefficient* or wasteful of energy. This means that you will be using more calories than if you performed skillfully. Thus, in terms of weight loss, poorly performed activities could better satisfy your goals. However, factors like safety and a desire to improve your skill levels should counterbalance a purely energy-oriented approach to selecting an activity. You should also consider social aspects, cost, and enjoyment, since it will be necessary to stick with your program for a significantly long period of time.

As we've noted previously, swimming is an excellent activity for people who are overweight or for whom weight-bearing activities are not good (people with arthritis or skeletal problems).

Your exercise program should be conducted in combination with a carefully planned diet. Remember, in order to reduce fatness not only must you increase energy expenditure, you must also moderately reduce energy intake.

CONCLUSION

In this chapter we have discussed the various elements found in food (fats, carbohydrates, proteins). Requirements for each of these were considered, as were special nutritional needs occurring at certain periods of life.

Weight regulation was discussed from the standpoint of theory as well as practical approaches. Last, we reviewed the important role of exercise in weight control.

SUMMARY

1. Overweight has been indicated by medical researchers as a correlate or causal factor in most of the leading diseases of our time.
2. Although innumerable physiological interactions are affected by storage of superfluous body fat, perhaps the most important effects are associated with the circulatory and respiratory systems.
3. Body image is the term used to refer to the vision we have of our physical selves. Those with positive and strong body images usually have wholesome and positive attitudes about other aspects of the self.
4. All foods consist of nutrients which are necessary for the maintenance of life itself.
5. A calorie is the amount of heat needed to raise one gram of water one degree centigrade.
6. Foods consist of the following nutrients: fats, proteins, carbohydrates, vitamins, minerals, and water.
7. An individual who does not receive adequate supplies of essential food nutrients is said to be malnourished, despite the number of calories ingested daily.
8. All food nutrients are vital to the well-being of the organism, and deficiencies in any of them may result in serious disease.
9. Eating large quantities of vitamins will not improve your health or enable you to perform exercise in a superior fashion.
10. Exercise programs should be conducted in combination with a carefully planned diet.

REFERENCES

AMERICAN HEART ASSOCIATION. *Dietary Guidelines for Healthy American Adults*. Dallas, TX: AHA, 1986.

BRAY, G. (ed.). *Obesity in America*. National Institutes of Health Publication No. 80-359, 1980.

DINTIMAN, G., AND J. GREENBERG. *Health through Discovery*, 2nd ed. Reading, MA: Addison-Wesley, 1983.

FOOD AND NUTRITION BOARD, National Academy of Sciences—National Research Council. *Recommended Dietary Allowances*, 9th ed. Washington, DC: National Academy of Sciences, 1979.

GUTIN, B. *The High Energy Factor*. New York: Random House, 1983.

LAPLACE, J. *Health*. Englewood Cliffs, NJ: Prentice-Hall, 1980.

12

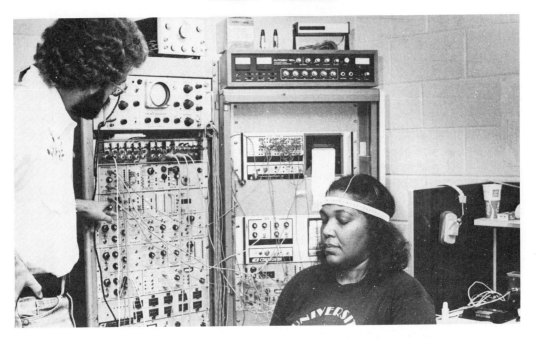

Stress Management
and
Physical Fitness

In his book *Comprehensive Stress Management*, one of your authors describes personal involvement with stress (Greenberg, 1986, p. 3-4):

> It was a pleasant spring day—about seventy degrees, with the sun shining and a slight breeze. It was the kind of day I would have enjoyed celebrating by playing tennis, jogging, and helping my son learn how to ride his bicycle. . . . Instead, I was on the shoulder of a country road in upstate New York with my hands on my knees, vomiting. . . . At the time, I was an assistant professor. . . . I had become quite successful in each of three areas the university established as criteria for promotion and tenure: teaching, research and other publications, and university and community service.
>
> To meet the community service standards of acceptance for promotion and tenure, I made myself available as a guest speaker to community groups. I soon found that I was able to motivate groups of people through speeches or workshops on numerous topics, both directly and tangentially related to my area of expertise—health education. I spoke to the local Kiwanis Club on the topic "Drug Education Techniques" and to the Green Acres Cooperative Nursery School parents and teachers on "Drug Education for Young Children." I was asked to present the senior class speech at Medaille College on "Sex Education," and wound up conducting workshops for local public school districts on such concerns as "Why Health Education," "Values and Teaching," "Group Process," and "Peer Training Programs for Cigarette-Smoking Education." Things started jelling and I expanded my local presentations to state and national ones, presenting papers at various state and national meetings.
>
> My life changed rapidly and repeatedly. I came to Buffalo as an assistant professor and was promoted twice, leaving as a full professor with tenure and administrative responsibility for the graduate program in

health education . . . I had published over forty articles in professional journals, and my second book was soon to come off the presses. During my tenure . . . I appeared on radio and television programs, and was the subject of numerous newspaper articles. I bought my first house, fathered my first two children, and won my first tennis tournament: In short, I became a success.

So why the vomiting? Well, I was experiencing too much change in too short a period of time. I wondered if I was as good as others thought I was or if I was just lucky. I worried about embarrassing myself in front of other people and became extremely anxious when due to speak in front of a large group—so anxious that on a nice spring day, about seventy degrees, with the sun shining and a slight breeze, as I was on my way to address a group of teachers, school administrators, and parents in Wheatfield, New York, I became sick to my stomach.

What I didn't know then, but know now, is that I was experiencing stress—too much stress. I also didn't know what to do. Everything seemed to be going very well; there seemed to be no reason to become anxious or ill. Well, I think I understand it all now and want to explain it to you. I want to help you learn about stress and how to manage it so that your life will be better, and you will be healthier.

One way to manage stress is through exercise. We will discuss this idea in more detail later in this chapter. Now, though, let's set the basis for that discussion by learning about stress, stressors, and stress management.

STRESS: SOME DEFINITIONS

In spite of there being several definitions of stress offered by the experts, it is necessary for us to agree upon one so we know what we're studying. Even before that, however, we need to define *stressor* and *stress reactivity*. A *stressor* is a stimulus with the potential of triggering the fight-or-flight response. This response was first described by Walter Cannon in his classic *The Wisdom of the Body* (1932) and was later verified by the father of stress research, Hans Selye (1956). To understand the fight-or-flight response, let's imagine you are walking through a dark alley at night. The streets are quiet and no one else is visible. As you're halfway through the alley, you see someone enter it from the other side and begin walking toward you. Your heart begins beating rapidly, you start perspiring, your breathing becomes shallow and rapid, and your muscles are tensed. What you may not know is that your blood pressure rises, your body retains sodium, your pupils and bronchial tubes dilate, your liver releases glucose, and you have an increase in free fatty acids in your blood. All this is part of the fight-or-flight response. The intention is to prepare your body so it may fight the threat or run away from it. Your body is prepared to do something physical. Another name for the fight-or-flight response is *stress reactivity*. So a stressor is a threat of some kind that has the potential of eliciting stress reactivity.

Stress can now be defined: It is the combination of a stressor and stress reactivity. Each by itself is only a part of what we call stress. As we shall soon see, this conceptualization has implications for the management of stress.

Common Stressors

Stressors come in many forms. Some are biological, such as toxins, heat, or cold. Others are psychological, such as threats to self-esteem or depression. Still others are sociological, such as unemployment or the death of a loved one. And there are philosophical stressors, such as how best to use time and deciding on a purpose in life.

We all encounter stressors; situations, people, or things to which we must adapt and which have the potential of triggering a stress reaction. You may have stressors associated with your schooling: getting good grades, exams, having your teachers think well of you. You may have stressors associated with your work: too much to do in a given time, not really understanding what you are to do, having one person expecting you to do something different from another person. You may have stressors associated with your family: still being treated as a child when you are an adult, arguing often, lack of trust. Or you may have stressors associated with your social life: making friends, telephoning for dates, deciding on your level of sexual activity. In addition to these, your own traits might serve as stressors: You may be shy, jealous, or easily angered. Your weight may be a stressor. So may your lack of physical fitness or low level of sport skills.

A word of caution: These stressors do not necessarily mean you are stressed. They only have the *potential* for triggering stress reactivity. They need not do so; and we will later show you how you can prevent them from doing so.

Stress Reactivity

When a stressor results in the fight-or-flight response, several things happen. One of these is an increase in your heart rate. To demonstrate this effect, turn to Figure 12.1 and follow the instructions.

Another component of stress reactivity is increased muscle tension. As you begin to read this, FREEZE. Don't move at all. Now pay attention to your body. In particular, pay attention to your muscle tension. If you think you could drop your shoulders, that means your muscles are unnecessarily raising them. If your forearm muscles can be relaxed, you're unnecessarily tensing them. If your body is seated in a position where you are "on edge," maybe you really are on edge. Is your forehead muscle too tense? Can your stomach, buttocks, thigh, or calf muscles be relaxed?

When your muscles are unnecessarily tensed as though you are about to do something physical when you really aren't, that is called *bracing*. Bracing is a part of stress reactivity and, we shall soon see, can lead to illness.

Other components of stress reactivity include rapid and shallow breathing, opening of bronchial tubes (air passages to and from the lungs), increased

While seated in a comfortable position, determine how fast your heart beats at rest using one of the following methods. (Use a watch that has a second hand.)
1. Place the first two fingers (pointer and middle finger) of one hand on the underside of your other wrist, on the thumb side. Feel for your pulse and count the number of pulses for thirty seconds. (See the drawing.)
2. Place the first two fingers of one hand on your lower neck, just above the collar bone; move your fingers toward your shoulder until you find your pulse. Count the pulses for thirty seconds.
3. Place the first two fingers of one hand in front of your ear near your sideburn, moving your fingers until you find your pulse. Count the pulses for thirty seconds. Multiply your thirty-second pulse count by two to determine how many times your heart beats each minute while at rest.

Now close your eyes and think of either someone you really dislike or some situation you experienced that really frightened you. If you are recalling a person, think of how that person looks, smells, and what he or she does to incur your dislike. Really feel the dislike, don't just think about it. If you recall a frightening situation, try to place yourself back in that situation. Sense the fright, be scared, vividly recall the situation in all its detail. Think of the person or situation for one minute and then count your pulse rate for thirty seconds, as you did earlier. Multiply the rate by two and compare your first total with the second.

Most people find that their heart rate increases when experiencing the stressful memory. This increase occurs despite a lack of any physical activity; just thoughts increase heart rate. This fact demonstrates two things: the nature of stressors and the nature of stress reactivity. The stressor is a stimulus with the potential of eliciting a stress reaction (physiological arousal).

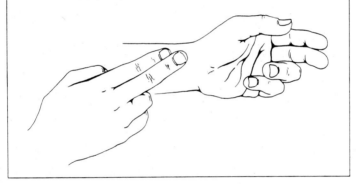

FIGURE 12.1   Stress and stress reactivity

Source: Jerrold S. Greenberg, *Comprehensive Stress Management* (Dubuque, IA: Wm. C. Brown, 1986), p. 11.

blood pressure, opening of the arteries to the heart, widening of the pupils of the eyes, secretion of hydrochloric acid in the stomach, increased perspiration, and a decrease in the effectiveness of the immunological system because of fewer T lymphocytes to fight allergens and bacteria. In addition, the blood vessels to the skin of the arms and legs constrict, resulting in the fingers and toes getting cold and people being described as being "white as a ghost."

Stress Psychophysiology

The reason the body changes in response to a stressor as it does is called *stress psychophysiology*; as the term implies, both the mind and the body are involved. Think for a moment of an arcade with computer games. These arcades are like our bodies, the computer games like our brains, and their programming like our minds. As arcades project a cacophony of noise and a rainbow of colors and lights, so do our bodies (so to speak) when we experience stress. As a computer collects and processes data, so do our brains. As these data are processed, depending on the programming of the computer, so does the interpretation we give to stress-related data depend on the perception of our minds. For example, we have to give a speech to a large audience. The brain takes the situation objectively (me the speaker, 200 people in the audience), while the mind interprets that data (this is a threat since I could make a fool of myself and be thought of as incompetent). The body reacts to this threat by speeding up its heart rate, making itself perspire, increasing its blood pressure, and so on.

Stress psychophysiology is complicated and extensive. We will just summarize this response here so you can develop an appreciation for the effect of stress within the body and better understand the need to manage it (see Figure 12.2).

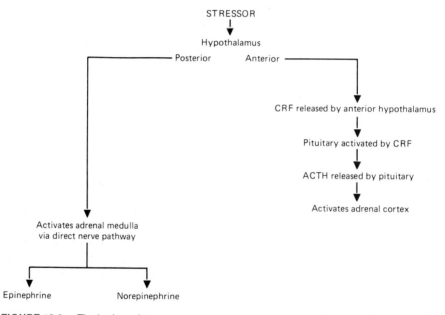

FIGURE 12.2   The brain and stress

When stressors are encountered, the brain is notified via messages passed along nerves. When the hypothalamus of the brain is told a stressor exists, it activates the endocrine system two ways: (1) From the posterior portion of the hypothalamus, a message is sent along nerves directly to the adrenal medulla; (2) from the anterior portion of the hypothalamus, corticotrophin-releasing factor (CRF) is released (see Figure 12.3). The direct nerve message results in the adrenal medulla secreting the hormone epinephrine (adrenalin) and norepinephrine (noradrenalin). CRF causes the pituitary gland to release

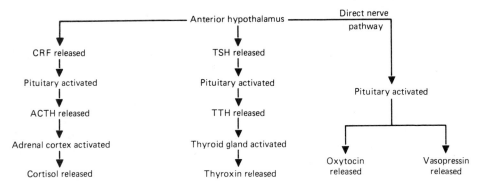

FIGURE 12.3   Stress and the anterior hypothalamus

adrenocorticotrophin hormone (ACTH), which in turn results in the adrenal cortex secreting the hormone cortisol. In addition, the thyroid gland is instructed to secrete the hormone thyroxin, and the pituitary gland secretes the hormones oxytocin and vasopressin. While all this is occurring, other messages passed along nerves instruct various body organs to become activated. It is because of all this activity that the body undergoes the stress reactivity changes noted earlier.

Stress, Illness, and Disease

When you were walking through the dark alley, stress reactivity was beneficial. If you were attacked by the person walking toward you, you would be grateful for your body's preparedness to fight or run away. However, if that person just walked peacefully by you, your body would have been prepared to do something physical, and yet no physical action was needed. It is on such occasions that stress reactivity becomes a threat to your health. If the fight-or-flight response occurs often, is prolonged, or goes unabated, it can lead to illness and disease (see the box, "Stress and You"). The reason this is so relates to the changes that take place within the body at these times. It stands to reason that if your blood pressure is raised often, if free fatty acids are frequently roaming about in your blood, and if hydrochloric acid is often secreted in large amounts into your stomach, you will eventually become ill.

Illnesses and diseases associated with stress are labeled *psychosomatic*. This does not mean that these diseases are "just in your mind"; they actually exist. However, the mind is involved by preparing the body to become ill. This relationship of mind and body can be illustrated with allergies.

Assume you are allergic to pollen. What this means is that you have a threshold level of pollen—an amount below that level will not affect you, but at or above that level, you have an allergic reaction. Another way of describing this threshold is to say that the immunological system is effective in controlling a certain amount of pollen in the body. At any amount above that, the system loses its effectiveness. We have already said that when one is stressed the immunological system is less effective (fewer T lymphocytes). Consequently, when you experience stress it takes less pollen to set off an allergic reaction than when you are not experiencing stress. The mind, perceiving a threat, has changed the body (fewer T lymphocytes) so that it becomes ill (an allergic reaction).

A number of illnesses and diseases are suspected of being stress related. The mechanisms leading stress to cause or exacerbate these conditions are described elsewhere (see Greenberg, 1986). Here we list only the illnesses and diseases and note that the relationship of stress to some of these conditions is more controversial than to some of the others. Stress has been implicated in hypertension, stroke, coronary heart disease, ulcers, migraine headaches, tension headaches, cancer, allergies, asthma, hay fever, rheumatoid arthritis, backache, and diabetes mellitus. The controversial relationships concern hypertension, ulcers, and cancer.

The causes of hypertension are not well known. Some people seem genetically predisposed to it; others may come to it through obesity, salt-laden diets, or cigarette smoking. However, since we know the stress response includes elevated blood pressure, health scientists believe someone with a stressful life style will have a chronic elevation of blood pressure and therefore be hypertensive. Ulcers, a cut in the lining of a part of the digestive system, is suspected of resulting from the increase presence of hydrochloric acid that is a part of the stress response. However, many people who are highly stressed never develop ulcers, and therefore this relationship is also far from proved. Last, cancer is really several diseases with several different causes. Some cancers are caused by chemicals we ingest in our foods, some by environmental toxins we inhale, and some by viruses with which we come in contact. However, the fact that our immunological systems are less effective during stress and that researchers have identified certain life events and personality traits cancer victims seem to have in common (Pelletier, 1977) leads experts to believe stress is involved. But this relationship, too, is far from clear.

A MODEL OF STRESS

Imagine that you are a college senior and that all you need to do is pass a physical fitness class to graduate this semester. Imagine further that you fail this class! You might say to yourself: "This is terrible. I won't be able to start work. I must be a real dummy. What will all my friends and relatives think?" This example illustrates two stages of a model of stress we would like you to consider. Once you understand this model, you will be able to intervene and prevent stress from leading to illness and disease.

The model begins with a life situation. Failing the course is the life situation that has the potential of triggering stress reactivity. In other words, failing the course is the stressor. However, the operative word here is *potential*. In the example, you perceived failing the course as distressing. This *perception* will lead to various *emotions*—for example, insecurity, embarrassment, anger, disappointment. Those emotions will lead to a stress *reaction*—for example, high blood pressure, muscle tension, decreased T lymphocytes—which

STRESS AND YOU

In the space provided, indicate how often each of the following effects happens to you either when you are experiencing stress, or following exposure to a significant stressor. Respond to each item with a number between 0 and 5, using the scale that follows (Allen and Hyde, 1980, pp. 101-5).

0=never
1=once or twice a year
2=every few months

3=every few weeks
4=once or more each week
5=daily

Cardiovascular Symptoms
_____ Heart pounding
_____ Heart racing or beating erratically
_____ Cold, sweaty hands
_____ Headaches (throbbing pain)
_____ *Subtotal*

Respiratory Symptoms
_____ Rapid, erratic, or shallow breathing
_____ Shortness of breath
_____ Asthma attack
_____ Difficulty in speaking because of poor breathing control
_____ *Subtotal*

Gastrointestinal Symptoms
_____ Upset stomach, nausea, or vomiting
_____ Constipation
_____ Diarrhea
_____ Sharp abdominal pains
_____ *Subtotal*

Muscular Symptoms
_____ Headaches (steady pain)
_____ Back or shoulder pains
_____ Muscle tremors or hands shaking
_____ Arthritis
_____ *Subtotal*

Skin Symptoms

_____ Acne
_____ Dandruff
_____ Perspiration
_____ Excessive dryness of skin or hair
_____ *Subtotal*

Immunity Symptoms

_____ Allergy flare-up
_____ Catching colds
_____ Catching the flu
_____ Skin rash
_____ *Subtotal*

Metabolic Symptoms

_____ Increased appetite
_____ Increased craving for tobacco or sweets
_____ Thoughts racing or difficulty sleeping
_____ Feelings of crawling anxiety or nervousness
_____ *Subtotal*
_____ Overall symptomatic total (add all seven subtotals)

What Does Your Score Mean?

0 to 35   =   Moderate physical stress symptoms
              A score in this range indicates a low level of physical stress mani-
              festations, hence a minimal overall probability of encounter with
              psychosomatic disease in the near future.

36 to 75 =   Average physical stress symptoms
              Most people experience physical stress symptoms within this range.
              It is representative of an increased predisposition to psychosomatic
              disease, but not an immediate threat to physical health.

76 to 140 =   Excessive physical stress symptoms
              If your score falls in this range, you are experiencing a serious
              number and frequency of stress symptoms. It is a clear indication
              that you may be headed toward the experience of one or more
              psychosomatic disease states sometime in the future. You should
              take deliberate action to reduce your level of stress.

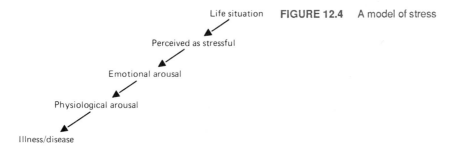

FIGURE 12.4   A model of stress

if chronic, prolonged, or unabated, can lead to *illness* or *disease*. This is the stress model (see Figure 12.4).

Now let's use the same example, but this time you perceive failing the course as not so distressing. You might say to yourself, "It's not good that I failed this course, but I still have my health and people who love me. They'll help me get through this." If we imagine that a road goes through the town of Life Situation, Perceived as Stressful, Emotional Arousal, Physiological Arousal, and Illness/Disease (our model), we can also imagine roadblocks along this road. Changing your perception of life situations is such a roadblock: It blocks the stressor from proceeding down the road to illness or disease. This is stress management—controlling or eliminating the negative effects of stress.

STRESS MANAGEMENT

We conceptualize *stress management* as reponses to each level of the stress model. We need to manage each and every level, since no technique is totally effective, and some filtering to the next level invariably occurs. We will now consider how to intervene to lessen our chances of becoming ill from the stress we experience.

Intervention: Setting Up Roadblocks

We've said that stress management is the setting up of roadblocks at different points in the stress model. The higher up on the model we can set up our roadblock, the better off we are. So, if you can prevent a life situation (stressor) from occurring in the first place, that would be preferable to waiting to intervene at some other level. Perceiving the life situations that do occur as less distressing can be an important next step.

If we can learn to relax and to exercise some control over our emotions so we diminish our anxiety to stressors, that is preferable to waiting to intervene at some level lower down on the model. And if we can exercise away built-up stress waste products—for example, increased serum cholesterol, raised heart and respiratory rates, and muscle tension—that is preferable to waiting to intervene after illness or disease occurs.

Many books on stress management are available (Girdano and Everly, 1986; Friedman and Rosenman, 1974; Friedman and Ulmer, 1984), so here we will briefly describe some ways to set up stress roadblocks.

Life Situation Interventions

One of the best ways to prevent stressful life situations from occurring is to keep a diary of your stressors and your reactions to them. We have presented a format for that diary in Figure 12.5. The diary would include:

1. Stressors for that day
   a. Routine stressors (experienced often)
   b. Unique stressors (seldom encountered)
2. Reactions to *each* stressor encountered
   a. Physical reactions (perspiration, increased pulse rate, muscle tension)
   b. Psychological reactions (fear, anxiety, confusion)
3. Means of coping with *each* stressor
4. Better means of coping
5. Relaxation techniques tried that day
6. Effectiveness of these techniques
7. Ailments during that day
   a. Physical (headache, stomach discomfort, backache)
   b. Psychological (anxiety attack, feelings of insecurity, sense of being rushed)

When three weeks are up, read your diary in one sitting and ask yourself the following questions:
1. What stressors do you frequently experience?
2. Do you need to, or want to, continue experiencing these stressors?
3. If you do not, which routine stressors can you eliminate? How?
4. How does your body typically react to stressors?
5. How does your psyche typically react to stressors?
6. Can your body's or mind's reactions to stress teach you ways to identify stress early in its progression so as to make it less harmful?
7. Are there any coping techniques that you use more than others?
8. Do these techniques work for you or against you?
9. Are there any coping techniques that you believe would be helpful, but that you don't use often enough?
10. How can you get yourself to use these coping techniques more often?
11. Are any particular relaxation techniques more effective for you than others?
12. Are you experiencing difficulty in employing a relaxation technique? No time? No place? No quiet?
13. How can you better organize your life to obtain periods of relaxation?

Stressor	Reactions		Means of coping	Means of coping better
	Physical	Psychological		
1. Routine				
a.				
b.				
2. Unique				
a.				
b.				

3 Relaxation techniques tried	Effectiveness of techniques
1.	
2.	
3.	

Ailments

Physical   Psychological

FIGURE 12.5   The stress diary

Source: Jerrold S. Greenberg, *Comprehensive Stress Management* (Dubuque, IA: Wm. C. Brown, 1986), pp. 67–68.

14. Are there any physical ailments that you usually experience either preceding or following stressful events?
15. Are there any psychological ailments that you usually experience either preceding or following stressful events?
16. Are there ways to prevent either physiological or psychological ailments from being associated with your stress?

You can learn a lot about what causes you stress by keeping this diary, as well as what to eliminate to make your life less stressful. You can also learn a lot about how you try to cope with stress, whether you are successful at these efforts, and how you might cope better.

Perception Interventions

One way of perceiving life situations as less distressing is to use *selective awareness.* Selective awareness is consciously choosing what to be aware of in a situation. For example, rather than focusing on the displeasure of standing on a line at the checkout counter, you could choose to focus on the pleasure of

LIFE CAN BE A CELEBRATION

Life can be a celebration if you take the time to celebrate.

Whenever I think of the importance of perception in general, and selective awareness in particular, I recall one day in 1980 that seemed to be heading downhill in a hurry. Before noon I had received a telephone call notifying me that some consulting work I was attempting to organize wasn't coming together, a letter stating that a grant proposal I had submitted would not be funded, and a manuscript I had submitted was rejected. As you might imagine, I was down in the dumps. I was feeling very sorry for myself, forgetting all the other consultations I had successfully completed, the other research studies I had funded, and the other manuscripts I'd written and had published. Now I can say (the fog was too thick at the time) that I chose to be selectively aware of the defeats of that day rather than focus upon past and anticipated future successes.

Well, a proper perspective was soon achieved with just two phone calls. First I received a call from a colleague at a university at which I had previously taught. He told me about two former deans under whom we had worked. It seems that the married daughter of one of them awoke in the middle of the night and, not being able to sleep, arose from bed to get something in another room. Her husband, who was still sleeping when she arose, heard noises in the house, reached for his gun, and thinking her to be a burglar, shot his wife in the head. As I write this she is still in a coma. My heart went out to Harry when I heard about his daughter's ordeal (and, consequently, his).

The second story my colleague told me during that phone call described the recent accident another dean of ours had while pruning a tree. To get the top of the tree pruned, he extended a ladder and proceeded to climb it. When he found part of the tree out of his reach, he leaned and stretched toward that part, tipping the ladder, falling, and landing on a tree stump. Since he was still in the hospital, I called him to offer whatever feeble support I could. When I reached him, he described the accident and his severe injuries (to this day he experiences pain daily) and the physical therapy he would need. But he said two things that I'll always remember. He said it took 20 minutes for the ambulance to arrive, during which time he was afraid to move since he had landed on his back and feared a spinal injury. When he was placed on the stretcher, though, he wiggled his toes and fingers, and the knowledge that he was able to do that made him cry. The other thing he said was how great the hospital staff treated him, how competent the ambulance drivers were, and how lucky he was to be alive and to be able to move. I called him with the intention of cheering him up, and it turned out that he cheered me up.

After those telephone calls, my consulting, grant proposal, and manuscript did not seem very important. I had my health, a lovely family, and a job I really enjoyed. The rest of my day would, I decided, be appreciated. I would focus on the positive.

Source: Jerrold S. Greenberg, *Comprehensive Stress Management* (Dubuque, IA: Wm. C. Brown, 1986), pp. 109–10.

being able to do nothing when your day is usually so hectic. The value of selecting what to be aware of is illustrated in the accompanying box.

In your life, you might want to choose something good to focus upon rather than something upsetting. For example, while exercising you can focus upon the good you're doing for your health and the calories you are using, rather than the discomfort you are experiencing. Or, when speaking in front of a group of people, you can keep in mind the opportunity you have to present your ideas, rather than the fear of saying something foolish. It's all up to you.

Relaxation Techniques

Many relaxation techniques can help you react less emotionally to stressors and lead you to a physiological state opposite of fight-or-flight. These include meditation, autogenic training, yoga, progressive relaxation, biofeedback training, and other activities that require you to focus on something other than your stressors. We will not discuss these here, but you should know of their existence and the availability of literature describing these techniques (Greenberg, 1986; Girdano and Everly, 1986; Benson, 1975; Davis, McKay, and Eshelman, 1980).

Time Management

A whole set of interventions that needs its own category so as to emphasize its importance is called time management. Time spent is time gone forever. In spite of what we often profess, we cannot save time. Time moves continually and it is used—one way or another. If we waste time, there is no bank where we can withdraw time we previously saved to replace the time wasted. The techniques described in this section will not save you time, but will instead free some of your time from other things. The result should be plenty of time to plan and participate in a regular exercise program—as well as have time for some other activities which you have been neglecting.

- **Assessing How You Spend Time.** As a first step in managing time better, you might want to analyze how you spend your time now. To do this, divide your day into 15 minute segments. Then, record what you are doing every 15 minutes. Afterward, review this time diary and total the time spent on each activity throughout the day. For example, you might find you spent 3 hours watching television, 15 minutes exercising, 1 hour reading, and 2 hours shopping. Next, evaluate the use of your time. You might decide you spent too much time watching television and too little time exercising. Based on this evaluation, adjust how you spend your time; but be specific. For example, "I will watch only 1 hour of television and will exercise one hour."
- **Setting Goals.** The most important thing you can do to manage time is to set goals: daily, weekly, monthly, yearly, and long range. If you don't have a clear sense of where you are headed, you will not be able to plan how to get there. Your use of time should be organized to maximize the chances of achieving your goals.
- **Prioritizing.** Once you have your goals defined, you need to prioritize them and your activities. Not all of your goals will be equally important. To help prioritize your goals and your activities designed to achieve these goals, develop A, B, C lists. On the A list are those activities which *must* get done. For example, if an assignment is due next week and you haven't

as yet begun the library research necessary to complete that assignment, getting to the library goes on the A list. On the B list are those activities you'd like to do today and need to be done. However, if they don't get done today, it wouldn't be terrible. For example, if you haven't spoken to a close friend and have been meaning to telephone, you might put that on your B list. Your intent is to call today, but if you don't get around to it, you can always call tomorrow or the next day. On the C list are those activities you'd like to do if you get done all your A and B list activities. If the C list activities never get done, that would be just fine. In addition, make a list of things *not to do*. For example, if you tend to waste your time watching television, you might want to include that on your not-to-do list.

- *Scheduling.* Once you've prioritized your activities, you can then schedule them into your day. Don't forget to also schedule some time for relaxation and some time for exercise since those are two good stress management techniques.

- *Saying No.* Because of guilt, concern for what others might think of us, or a real desire to engage in that activity, we have a hard time saying "no." The A, B, C lists and the schedule of activities will help identify how much time remains for other activities and make saying no easier.

- *Delegating.* When possible, get others to do those things which need to be done but which do not need your personal attention. Conversely, avoid taking on chores which others try to delegate to you. This does not mean to get others to help you but don't help other people. It means not to hesitate to seek help when you are short on time and overloaded. Help others only when they really need it and you have time available.

- *Limiting Interruptions.* Don't make your schedule so tight that there is no room for interruptions. On the other hand, try to keep these interruptions to a minimum. There are several ways to accomplish that. You cannot accept phone calls between certain hours. Ask your roommate or secretary to take messages and call back later. Do the same with visitors. Ask visitors to return at a more convenient time, or you should schedule a visit with them for later. If you are serious about making better use of your time, you will need to adopt some of these tactics of limiting interruptions.

By using these time management techniques, you can free up time for almost anything you want. Certainly, a lack of time should no longer be an excuse for not engaging in a physical fitness program. We all have the time, we just choose to use it differently. Recognizing that, you can decide to use your time more consistent with your best interests if you choose to. It's really up to you.

THE ROLE OF EXERCISE IN MANAGING STRESS

Now that you have an understanding of stress and how to manage it, we can consider the role of exercise as an intervention. Exercise is a unique intervention, since it can be plugged in at many levels on the stress model. It is a life situation intervention when you give up stressful habits (for example, cigarette smoking) because they interfere with your exercising. When you make friends through participating in a training program, you may also be using exercise as a life situation intervention, since your loneliness and social isolation may be remedied.

Exercise can be a perception intervention as well. We have previously described how the brain produces endorphins during exercise, and the euphoric, analgesic affects of these endorphins. This is one example of the ability of exercise to effect our perceptions. In addition, exercise can be a relaxation technique. While exercising, we focus on what we are doing and away from our problems and stressors.

In this section we discuss the role of exercise in managing stress by considering tension, progressive relaxation, the use of stress by-products, psychological relief, and selective awareness.

Tension

Tension is muscular contraction resulting from stress. We saw earlier in this chapter how some of our muscles are tensed more than necessary and longer than necessary. This tension can lead to headaches or neck or back pain. Regular exercisers tend to be more attuned to their bodies and therefore more apt to recognize when they are muscularly tense. Once aware of this tension, they are better able to control those muscles and relax them. Another way of stating this is that regular exercisers are better able to recognize physical manifestations of stress and to remedy inappropriate physiological responses to stressors.

Progressive Relaxation

One relaxation technique uses familiarity with the body as the basis for controlling stress and tension. It is called *progressive relaxation* (Jacobson, 1938). Progressive relaxation requires you to tense a muscle group for 10 seconds, all the while paying attention to the sensations created. Then you relax that muscle, paying attention to that sensation. The idea is to learn what muscular tension feels like so you will be more likely to recognize it when you are experiencing it; and to be familiar with muscular relaxation so that when you are tense, you can relax those muscles. It is called "progressive" because you progress from one muscle group to another throughout the body. Figure 12.6

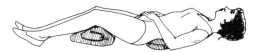

FIGURE 12.6   Reclining position for progressive relaxation exercise

Source: Jenny Steinmetz, et al., *Managing Stress Before It Manages You* (Palo Alto, CA: Bull, 1980), pp. 20–27.

shows the body position for progressive relaxation. Here is an example of how to do progressive relaxation (Steinmetz et al., 1980, pp. 20-27):

RELAXATION OF THE ARMS (4 OR 5 MINUTES)

- Settle back as comfortably as you can and let yourself relax to the best of your ability.
- Now, as you relax, clench your right fist.
- Clench it tighter and tighter, and study the tension as you do so.
- Keep it clenched and feel the tension in your right fist, hand and forearm.
- Now relax . . .
- Let the fingers of your right hand become loose . . .
- Observe the contrast in your feelings.
- Now, let yourself go and try to become more relaxed all over.
- Once more, clench your right fist really tight.
- Hold it, and notice the tension again.
- Now, let go, relax, let your fingers straighten out . . .
- Notice the difference once more.
- Now repeat that with your left fist.
- Clench your left fist while the rest of your body relaxes.
- Clench that fist tighter and feel the tension.
- And now relax . . . Again, enjoy the contrast.
- Repeat that once more, clench the left fist, tight and tense.
- Now do the opposite of tension—relax and feel the difference . . .
- Continue relaxing like that for awhile.
- Clench both fists tighter and tighter, both fists tense, forearms tense.
- Study the sensations . . . and relax . . .
- Straighten out your fingers and feel that relaxation . . .
- Continue relaxing your hands and forearms more and more.
- Now bend your elbows and tense your biceps.
- Tense them harder and study the tension feeling.
- All right, straighten out your arms . . .
- Let them relax and feel the difference again . . .
- Let the relaxation develop.
- Once more, tense your biceps.
- Hold the tension and observe it carefully.
- Straighten the arms and relax . . .
- Relax to the best of your ability . . .
- Each time pay close attention to your feelings when you tense up and when you relax . . .
- Now straighten your arms, straighten them so that you feel most tension in the triceps muscles along the back of your arms.
- Stretch your arms and feel the tension.
- And now relax . . .

- Get your arms back into a comfortable position . . .
- Let the relaxation proceed on its own . . .
- The arms should feel comfortably heavy as your allow them to relax.
- Straighten the arms once more so that you feel the tension in the triceps muscles.
- Feel that tension . . . and relax.
- Now let's concentrate on pure relaxation in the arms without any tension . . . Get your arms comfortable and let them relax further and further.
- Continue relaxing your arms even further . . .
- Even when your arms seem fully relaxed, try to go that extra bit further...
- Try to achieve deeper and deeper levels of relaxation.

RELAXATION OF THE FACE, NECK, SHOULDERS, AND UPPER BACK (4 OR 5 MINUTES)

- Let all your muscles go loose and heavy.
- Just settle back quietly and comfortably.
- Wrinkle up your forehead now, wrinkle it tighter.
- And now stop wrinkling up your forehead.
- Relax and smooth it out . . .
- Picture the entire forehead and scalp becoming smoother, as the relaxation increases . . .
- Now frown and crease your brow and study the tension.
- Let go of the tension again . . .
- Smooth out the forehead once more.
- Now, close your eyes.
- Keep your eyes closed, gently, comfortably, and notice the relaxation.
- Now clench your jaws, push your teeth together.
- Study the tension throughout the jaws.
- Relax your jaws now . . .
- Let your lips part slightly . . .
- Appreciate the relaxation.
- Now press your tongue hard against the roof of your mouth.
- Look for the tension.
- All right, let your tongue return to a comfortable and relaxed position.
- Now purse your lips, press your lips together tighter and tighter.
- Relax the lips . . .
- Notice the contrast between tension and relaxation . . .
- Feel the relaxation all over your face, all over your forehead, and scalp, eyes, jaws, lips, tongue, and throat . . .
- The relaxation progresses further and further.
- Now attend to your neck muscles.
- Press your head back as far as it can go and feel the tension in the neck.
- Roll it to the right and feel the tension shift . . .

- Now roll it to the left.
- Straighten your head and bring it forward.
- Press your chin against your chest.
- Let your head return to a comfortable position and study the relaxation...
- Let the relaxation develop.
- Shrug your shoulders right up.
- Hold the tension.
- Drop your shoulders and feel the relaxation . . .
- Neck and shoulders relaxed.
- Shrug your shoulders again and then move them around.
- Bring your shoulders up and forward and back.
- Feel the tension in your shoulders and in your upper back.
- Drop your shoulders once more and relax . . .
- Let the relaxation spread deep into the shoulders right into your back muscles.
- Relax your neck and throat, and your jaws and other facial areas, as the pure relaxation takes over and grows deeper . . . deeper . . . even deeper.

RELAXATION OF THE CHEST, STOMACH, AND LOWER BACK (4 OR 5 MINUTES)

- Relax your entire body to the best of your ability.
- Feel that comfortable heaviness that accompanies relaxation.
- Breathe easily and freely in and out . . .
- Notice how the relaxation increases as you exhale . . .
- As your breathe out, just feel that relaxation.
- Now breathe right in and fill your lungs.
- Inhale deeply and hold your breath.
- Study the tension.
- Now exhale, let the walls of your chest grow loose, and push the air out automatically . . .
- Continue relaxing and breathe freely and gently . . .
- Feel the relaxation and enjoy it.
- With the rest of your body as relaxed as possible, fill your lungs again.
- Breathe in deeply and hold it again.
- Now breathe out and appreciate the relief, just breathe normally . . .
- Continue relaxing your chest and let the relaxation spread to your back, shoulders, neck and arms . . .
- Merely let go and enjoy the relaxation.
- Now let's pay attention to your abdominal muscles, your stomach area.
- Tighten your stomach muscles, make your abdomen hard.
- Notice the tension.
- And relax, let the muscles loosen and notice the contrast.
- Once more, press and tighten your stomach muscles.

- Hold the tension and study it.
- And relax, notice the general well-being that comes with relaxing your stomach.
- Now draw your stomach in.
- Pull the muscles right in and feel the tension this way.
- Now relax again . . . Let your stomach out . . .
- Continue breathing normally and easily and feel the gentle massaging action all over your chest and stomach.
- Now pull your stomach in again and hold the tension.
- Once more pull in and feel the tension.
- Now relax your stomach fully . . .
- Let the tension dissolve as the relaxation grows deeper.
- Each time you breathe out, notice the rhythmic relaxation both in your lungs and in your stomach . . .
- Notice how your chest and your stomach relax more and more . . .
- Try to let go of all contractions anywhere in your body.
- Now direct your attention to your lower back.
- Arch up your back, make your lower back quite hollow, and feel the tension along your spine.
- Now settle down comfortably again, relaxing the lower back.
- Just arch your back up and feel the tension as you do so.
- Try to keep the rest of your body as relaxed as possible.
- Try to localize the tension throughout your lower back area.
- Relax once more, relaxing further and further . . .
- Relax your lower back, relax your upper back, spread the relaxation to your stomach, chest, shoulders, arms and facial area . . .
- These parts are relaxing further and further and further and even deeper.

RELAXATION OF THE HIPS, THIGHS, AND CALVES (4 OR 5 MINUTES)

- Let go of all tensions and relax.
- Now flex your buttocks and thighs.
- Flex your thighs by pressing down your heels as hard as you can.
- Relax and notice the difference.
- Straighten your knees and flex your thigh muscles again.
- Hold the tension.
- Relax your hips and thighs . . .
- Allow the relaxation to proceed on its own.
- Press your feet and toes downward, away from your face, so that your calf muscles become tense.
- Study that tension.
- Relax your feet and calves.

- This time, bend your feet toward your face so that you feel tension along your shins.
- Bring your toes right up.
- Relax again . . . Keep relaxing for awhile . . .
- Now let yourself relax further all over . . .
- Relax your feet, ankles, calves and shins, knees, thighs, buttocks and hips...
- Feel the heaviness of your lower body as you relax still further.
- Now spread the relaxation to your stomach, waist and lower back.
- Let go more and more deeply . . .
- Make sure no tension has crept into your throat.
- Relax your neck and your jaws and all your facial muscles.
- Keep relaxing your whole body like that for awhile . . .
- Let yourself relax.
- Now you can become twice as relaxed as you are merely by taking in a really deep breath and slowly exhaling, with your eyes closed, so that you become less aware of objects and movements around you, and thus prevent any surface tensions from developing.
- Breathe in deeply and feel yourself becoming heavier.
- Take in a long, deep breath and exhale very slowly . . .
- Feel how heavy and relaxed you have become.
- In a state of perfect relaxation, you should feel unwilling to move a single muscle in your body.
- Think about the effort that would be required to raise your right arm.
- As you think about that, see if you can notice any tension that might have crept into your shoulders and arm.
- Now you decide not to lift the arm, but to continue relaxing . . .
- Observe the relief and the disappearance of the tension.
- Just carry on, relaxing like that . . . Continue relaxing . . .
- When you wish to get up, count backward from four to one.
- You should now feel fine and refreshed, wide awake and calm.

Using Stress By-products

We have previously described the body's response to stress as preparing the body to do something physical. Using the body's preparedness by actually doing something physical relieves the stress. That is why some people throw dishes when they are stressed and angry. That is why some people beat up other people. That is why we have so much child and spouse abuse. It *feels good*! But there *are* more socially acceptable ways to use these stress by-products. For example, beating up a mattress or pillow is very effective in relieving stress. As you've probably guessed by now, so is exercise. Exercise is doing something physical and therefore uses the stress by-products in the manner in which they were intended to be used. That is why many of us feel better after exercising; and feel less stressed.

Beating up a mattress or pillow is effective in relieving stress. The pounding will feel good because it uses the stress by-products, and it does not hurt your hands or another person. You could also take a long piece of foam rubber and use it to pound a wall. The wall will stay intact, and so will your loved ones. Running around the block as fast as you can will use the stress by-products and do wonders for your disposition. Dribbling a basketball up and down the court mimicking several fast breaks, or serving 30 tennis balls as hard as you can, or biking as fast as you can for as long as you can, or swimming several laps at breakneck speed, as well as other tiring exercises can also relieve stress. Remember, throwing a baseball at a fence or wall beats throwing a book at the person you live with.

Psychological Relief

Exercise results in production of endorphins which, in turn, make us feel better. Our pain is lessened by the analgesic effect of endorphins. As a result, long-distance runners can tolerate the pain in a race and injured players can continue playing in spite of what, under other conditions, would be incapacitating pain. Further, endorphins have a euphoric effect that allows us to feel better about ourselves and our lives, and to be less distressed.

One important psychological benefit of exercise is an improvement in self-esteem. Exercise provides a sense of accomplishment while it improves our health and our body's ability to function. The result of all this is that we feel better about ourselves. When we hold ourselves in high regard, we are less apt to be made ill or to feel badly from a stressor. Exercise, therefore, can provide psychological relief and help us manage stress.

Selective Awareness

We have already discussed our ability to choose what to focus upon—the positive or negative in any situation. This selective awareness can be obtained through exercise. In *The Inner Game of Tennis* (1974), Tim Galway discusses this concept. Galway says that the mind often interferes with the body and prevents the body from doing what it can naturally do. For example, you're playing tennis and the ball is hit to your backhand. The backhand is a natural swing, but the mind says: "Oh, oh. Here it comes to my weak shot. I hope I make it. Boy is this a tough one. I always net this shot." As a result, your muscles get tense and you don't swing fluidly. The consequence is a backhand hit into the net—a self-fulfilling prophecy. To prevent this from happening, Galway suggests trying to read the label on the ball as it travels toward you or to focus on the ball's rotation. The idea is to focus on something other than your fear of backhands.

In a sense, exercise itself can be the focus of selective awareness. If you concentrate on your exercise—its effect on your body, what it feels like, your technique—you will not be able to concentrate on your stressors. Remember, you are in charge of what *you* will be aware of. You can focus on your stressors or focus on your exercising. The choice is yours.

CONCLUSION

One of us used to play tennis with a fellow named Dick. Although a fairly skilled player, Dick would always lose. His problem was that he tried to "cream" every shot, and did—except that the ball more often than not landed off the court. When it was suggested that Dick hit the ball easier but place it better, he objected vehemently: "That ball is my wife, my boss, and everyone else I get angry with. No way am I going to hit that sucker any easier." Although Dick lost, he won. Tennis allowed him to achieve greater wellness by relieving stress and tension in a socially acceptable way.

Exercise has tremendous potential for enhancing wellness. Kenneth Cooper, the founder of the aerobic fitness movement, has recognized this in one of his books, *The Aerobics Program for Total Well-Being* (1983), when he speaks of the physical-mental-spiritual balance of regular exercise. One way exercise helps us to achieve wellness is to put us more in control of ourselves and our lives.

You cannot achieve high-level wellness if you are not in control of you. A person who is manipulated by his or her environment or by people in it by definition is not well. Regular exercise helps you to be more in control of you by conditioning both your mind and your body so you are able to take control when necessary. You will have the cardiorespiratory endurance, muscular strength and endurance, flexibility, and confidence in your abilities to meet life's challenges (stressors) by exercising control over them, if you have trained to achieve these capacities. When you feel prepared, your mind will not interfere with your body doing what it needs to do during stressful moments. With a history of meeting these challenges successfully, each subsequent challenge seems less threatening and more manageable. And it is: Once you have the tools and know you can use them skillfully, what once seemed insurmountable seems easy.

With the management of stress also comes a spiritual enhancement. The ability to focus on exercising leads to a greater likelihood that we will experience oneness with our environment. We also will be better able to focus upon the mental aspects of our exercise activity, given that our stress is under control.

In all these ways, the use of exercise to manage stress has a significant influence on wellness. Stress management is possible; and exercise is a major weapon in the control process.

SUMMARY

1. A stressor is a stimulus with the potential of triggering the fight-or-flight response. Another name for the fight-or-flight response is stress reactivity. Stress is the combination of a stressor and stress reactivity.
2. Stressors can be biological (such as toxins or heat), psychological (such as threats to self-esteems), sociological (such as unemployment), or philosophical (such as deciding on a purpose in life).

3. Stress reactivity includes an increase in heart rate and muscle tension, rapid and shallow breathing, opening of the bronchial tubes, increased blood pressure, opening of the arteries to the heart, widening of the pupils, secretion of hydrochloric acid in the stomach, increased perspiration, and a decrease in the effectiveness of the immunological system.

4. Some body organs and systems involved in responding to stress are the brain; the pituitary, endocrine, and thyroid glands; the gastrointestinal, muscular, cardiorespiratory, and the immunological systems, and the skin.

5. Stress can result in several psychosomatic illnesses such as hypertension, stroke, coronary heart disease, ulcers, migraine headaches, tension headaches, cancer, allergies, asthma, hay fever, rheumatoid arthritis, backache, and diabetes mellitus.

6. One model of stress begins with a life situation that is perceived as distressing. That leads to emotional arousal, which in turn leads to physiological arousal. If the stress remains chronic, and prolonged, or goes unabated it can lead to illness and disease.

7. Stress interventions can occur at the life situation, perception, emotional arousal, or physiological arousal levels.

8. Examples of relaxation techniques that can be used to respond to stress are meditation, autogenic training, yoga, progressive relaxation, biofeedback training, and other activities that require focusing on something other than one's stressors.

9. Time management techniques include assessing how time is now spent, setting goals, prioritizing, scheduling, saying "no," delegating, and limiting interruptions.

10. Exercise is a stress intervention that responds to many different levels on the stress model. Exercise can help alleviate muscular tension, help one more readily identify physical signs of stress, use the body's preparedness to do something physical (the fight-or-flight response), and produce endorphins that make one feel better.

REFERENCES

ALLEN, R. J., AND D. HYDE. *Investigations in Stress Control.* Minneapolis, MN: Burgess, 1980.

BENSON, H. *The Relaxation Response.* New York: Avon, 1975.

CANNON, W. B. *The Wisdom of the Body.* New York: W. W. Norton, 1932.

COOPER, K. *The Aerobics Program for Total Well-Being.* New York: M. Evans, 1983.

DAVIS, M., M. MCKAY AND E. R. ESHELMAN. *The Relaxation and Stress Reduction Workbook.* Richmond, CA: New Harbinger, 1980.

FRIEDMAN, M., AND R. H. ROSENMAN. *Type A Behavior and Your Heart.* New York: Alfred A. Knopf, 1974.

FRIEDMAN, M., AND D. ULMER. *Treating Type A Behavior and Your Heart*. New York: Alfred A. Knopf, 1984.

GALWAY, W. T. *The Inner Game of Tennis*. New York: Random House, 1974.

GIRDANO, D., AND G. EVERLY. *Controlling Stress and Tension*. Englewood Cliffs, NJ: Prentice-Hall, 1986.

GREENBERG, J. S. *Comprehensive Stress Management*. Dubuque, IA: Wm. C. Brown, 1986.

JACOBSON, E. *Progressive Relaxation*. Chicago: University of Chicago Press, 1938.

MOSS, G. E. *Illness, Immunity and Social Interaction*. New York: John Wiley, 1973.

PELLETIER, K. R. *Mind as Healer, Mind as Slayer*. New York: Dell, 1977.

SELYE, H. *The Stress of Life*. New York: McGraw-Hill, 1956.

STEINMETZ, J., ET AL. *Managing Stress Before It Manages You*. Palo Alto, CA: Bull, 1980.

13

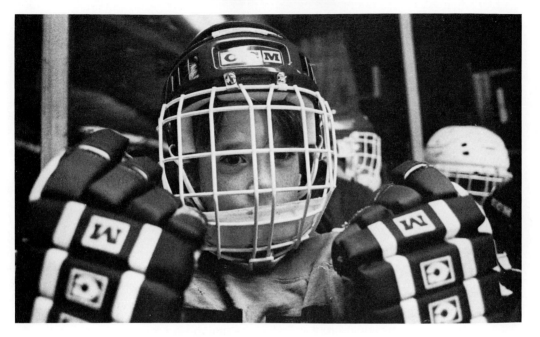

Common
Fitness Injuries

It has been a long, enjoyable autumn with unusually good tennis weather. To be out on the tennis court wearing a short-sleeved shirt late in October in Buffalo, New York, was a pleasant surprise. But it wasn't the only surprise! As I ran to my left to attempt to hit a ball that Wilt Chamberlain would not have reached, I felt myself being hit by a baseball just behind my ankle. Since the baseball field adjacent to the tennis court was inhabited by children just as delighted with the weather as I was, this was not surprising. The surprise came when I turned to look for my assailants, and no one was there. Furthermore, there was no baseball: I had an ankle injury instead. I knew how serious the injury was when I had to forfeit the match—a practice I considered in the same category as turning over top secret information to a foreign spy. My injury turned out to be a ruptured Achilles tendon which required surgery, immobilization (a cast to the knee) for 7 weeks, and a period of rehabilitation.

We can all suffer accidents at some time or another, but many athletic injuries are preventable, and many can be made less serious with the application of a little knowledge and common sense. The injury just described, for example, might have been avoided if I had stretched my Achilles tendon prior to playing tennis. In this chapter we discuss some of the more common injuries, how to prevent them, and what to do about them when they do occur. We begin with prevention, which is the better way to handle injury.

PREVENTING INJURY

If you can minimize your chances of injury, and you can, you are far better off than trying to treat injuries once they occur. The situation is like the town that found too many of its citizens falling off a cliff into the valley below. Some of the townspeople lobbied for allocating money in the next year's budget so that an ambulance could be purchased, parked in the valley, and be on the alert to treat the injured. Others, however, argued for a fence to be built at the top of the cliff to prevent people from falling into the valley in the first place. In this section we will discuss how to build a fence, in a manner of speaking, to prevent injuries from physical activity.

Principles of Prevention

To prevent fitness-related injury, several principles are helpful:

1. Don't do too much too soon.
2. Train, don't strain.
3. Hard days, easy days.
4. Know your body.
5. Warm up and cool down.

Don't Do Too Much Too Soon.   Exercising regularly is like dieting. The best way to do it is a little at a time over a long period of time. In fact, it should be a change in your life-style rather than a temporary adaptation. A diet that stops will shortly lead to the return of fat; an exercise program that ceases will shortly lead to a loss of physical and psychosocial benefits. Dieting and exercising, to be effective, must become a part of your regular routine forever. This seems like common sense, and yet each of us has seen an over-weight person threatening his or her life by jogging in a rubberized or cotton sweatshirt on a hot day. Ask them what they are doing, and they'll reply they are exercising to lose weight. Come back in a few weeks, and these people will have long since ceased exercising. The frustration accompanying their failure to "keep it up" has probably led to their overeating once again.

Beyond failing to lose weight, however, trying to do too much too soon can lead to injuries. Weight should be lost gradually, cardiorespiratory endurance developed slowly and muscular strength and endurance build up over several months. Building flexibility illustrates this prevention principle very well. Too often people stretch by bouncing into the stretch, rather than stretching slow-ly and only as far as is comfortable. The "bouncers" are going to touch their toes no matter what and too often that "no matter what" is an injury to some connective tissue. With a regular flexibility program, injury can be prevented and the toes become accessible.

If you are beginning a running program, start by walking and then run-ning short distances at a slow pace. If you are beginning an aerobic dance program, keep the sessions short at first. And, if you are weight training, begin with manageable weight and gradually increase the weight you lift or the repetitions you do.

Train, Don't Strain.   Training should be a gradual and an enjoyable process. The old principle "no pain, no gain" has long since been discarded. If you have pain, you are overdoing it. That doesn't only mean pain *during* exer-cising, but your feelings *afterward* as well. You shouldn't be walking around the next day feeling stiff or fatigued; if you are, you are training incorrectly and are likely to be injured.

Hard Days, Easy Days.   Your muscles need to recover from a heavy workout since (Mirkin and Hoffman, 1978, p. 31): (1) Muscle fiber is damaged by hard exercise and, like any other tissue in the body, requires healing time proportionate to the amount of injury. (2) Muscle fuel, called glycogen, is used up. It takes the body 10 hours to 10 days to replenish it. (3) Potassium, a mineral released from the muscle cell to control heat, is also depleted. It takes up to 48 hours to restore the supply.

To allow the body to heal itself, you should exercise hard on one day and either easily on the next day, or not at all. For example, if you run a long distance on a Saturday, run a short distance on Sunday or take the day off.

Know Your Body.   Be aware of how your body usually feels so you can recognize when it doesn't feel right. For example, if you usually feel energetic and today you feel weak and tired, then you may have overtrained. If you experience any of the following signs of overtraining, cut down on your fitness program or you may wind up with an "overuse" injury:

1. Soreness in muscles or joints
2. Heaviness in arms or legs
3. Inability to relax
4. Persistent tiredness
5. Loss of appetite
6. Loss of weight
7. Constipation or diarrhea
8. Repeated injury

Table 13.1 offers advice regarding health warnings that can occur during or as a result of exercise.

Table 13.1
Warnings and What to Do About Them

	Symptom	Cause	Remedy
Stop — See a physician before resuming	1. Abnormal heart action, for example, —pulse becoming irregular —fluttering, jumping, or palpitations in chest or throat —sudden burst of rapid heartbeats —sudden very slow pulse when a moment before it had been on target. (immediate or delayed)	Extrasystoles (extra heartbeats), dropped heartbeats, or disorders of cardiac rhythm. This may or may not be dangerous and should be checked out by physician.	Consult physician before resuming exercise program. He or she may provide medication to temporarily eliminate the problem and allow you to safely resume your exercise program, or you may have a completely harmless kind of cardiac rhythm disorder.

Symptom	Cause	Remedy
2. Pain or pressure in the center of the chest or the arm or throat precipitated by exercise or following exercise. (immediate or delayed)	Possible heart pain	Consult physician before resuming exercise program.
3. Dizziness, lightheaded-ness, sudden incoordina-tion, confusion, cold sweat, glassy stare, pallor, blueness or fainting. (im-mediate)	Insufficient blood to the brain.	Do not try to cool down. Stop exercise and lie down with feet elevated, or put head down between legs until symptoms pass. Later consult physician before next exercise session.
4. Persistent rapid heart action near the target level even 5-10 minutes after the exercise was stopped. (immediate)	Exercise is probably too vigorous.	Keep heart rate at lower end of target zone or below. Increase the vigor of exercise more slowly. If these measures do not control the excessively high recovery heart rate, consult physician.
5. Flare up of arthritic condition or gout which usually occurs in hips, knees, ankles, or big toe (weight bearing joints). (immediate or delayed)	Trauma to joints which are particularly vulnerable.	If you are familiar with how to quiet these flareups of your old joint condition, use your usual remedies. Rest up and do not resume your exercise program until the condition subsides. Then resume the exercise at a lower level with protective footwear on softer surfaces, or select other exercises which will put less strain on the impaired joints; for example, swimming will be better for people with arthritis of the hips since it can be done mostly with the arms. If this is new arthritis, or if there is no response to usual remedies, see physician.
6. Nausea or vomiting after exercise. (immediate)	Not enough oxygen to the intestine. You are either exercising too vigorously or cooling down too quickly.	Exercise less vigorously and be sure to take a more gradual and longer cooldown.
7. Extreme breathlessness lasting more than 10 minutes after stopping exercise. (immediate)	Exercise is too taxing to your cardiovascular sys-tem or lungs.	Stay at the lower end of your target range. If symptoms persist, do even less than target level. Be sure that while you are exercising you are not too breathless to talk to a companion.

Remedies which may be self-administered*

*Treat initially yourself but see physician if condition persists.

Can be remedied without medical consultation

Symptom	Cause	Remedy
8. Prolonged fatigue even 24 hours later. (delayed)	Exercise is too vigorous.	Stay at lower end of target range or below. Increase level more gradually.
9. Shin splints (pain on the front or sides of lower leg). (delayed)	Inflammation of the fascia connecting the leg bones, or muscle tears where muscles of the lower leg connect to the bones.	Use shoes with thicker soles. Work out on turf which is easier on your legs.
10. Insomnia which was not present prior to the exercise program. (delayed)	Exercise is too vigorous.	Stay at lower end of target range or below. Increase intensity of exercise gradually.
11. Pain in the calf muscles which occurs on heavy exercise but not at rest. (immediate)	May be due to muscle cramps due to lack of use of these muscles, or exercising on hard surfaces. May also be due to poor circulation to the legs (called claudication).	Use shoes with thicker soles, cool down adequately. Muscle cramps should clear up after a few sessions. If "muscle cramps" do not subside, circulation is probably faulty. Try another type of exercise; e.g. bicycling instead of jogging in order to use different muscles.
12. Side stitch (sticking under the ribs while exercising). (immediate)	Diaphragm spasm. The diaphragm is the large muscle which separates the chest from the abdomen.	Lean forward while sitting, attempting to push the abdominal organs up against the diaphragm.
13. Charley horse or muscle-bound feeling. (immediate or delayed)	Muscles are deconditioned and unaccustomed to exercise.	Take hot bath and usual headache remedy. Next exercise should be less strenuous.

Source: Lenore R. Zohman, *Beyond Diet . . . Exercise Your Way to Fitness and Heart Health.* Best Foods, 1979, pp. 24-25.

Warm Up and Cool Down.   Every workout should begin with a warmup to prepare the body. Every workout should end with a cooldown to help the body recover. Eliminating these parts of your exercise session is flirting with danger. The warmup is designed to increase the general body temperature and deep muscle temperature as well as to stretch the ligaments and other tissues to increase flexibility (Klafs and Arnheim, 1981, p. 98). The increased flexibility will prevent muscle tears, muscle soreness and strained ligaments (Ellis and Yavorsky, 1986). The cooldown assists the pumping of the blood from your extremities back to your heart.

Special Precautions

In addition to the practices already described, there are other precautions you can take to prevent athletic injuries.

Training in Hot Weather.   When the temperature or humidity are high, special precautions should be taken. Wear loose-fitting, lightweight clothing when training in the heat. Try to train early in the morning or in the evening when the temperature is at its lowest. Drink plenty of fluids before, during, and after the exercise. Salt tablets, often used during exercise in hot weather to replace salt eliminated through perspiration, should not be used. Salt tablets may actually lead to high blood pressure, clots, or heat exhaustion.

An important addition to your exercise outfit in hot (especially sunny) weather is a hat. It will protect you from the heat, and if you pour water on it, can cool your head. If your vision becomes blurred, your mouth becomes parched, you feel dizzy or nauseous, or you have difficulty thinking rationally, you may be suffering from heat stroke. Stop exercising *immediately*, get into the shade or a cool room, find a drink, and immerse yourself in cool water.

Training in Cold Weather.   The temperature isn't the only thing to worry about in the winter. You must also be concerned with the wind chill factor. The combination of temperature and wind velocity creates a lower temperature to your skin than the actual air temperature. Table 13.2 (p. 286) shows how cold the air feels for various combinations of temperature and wind velocity.

When exercising in cold weather, dress appropriately. The best way to do that is to dress in layers of clothing which will trap air between them, warm the air, and thus keep you warm. Make sure to protect parts of your body that receive relatively little blood and consequently little warmth: fingers, toes, ears, nose.

Do not exercise in the cold unless you have trained for it. If you live in Florida and, just your luck, you choose the worst day of winter to visit friends in Montana, don't exercise outdoors that day. Or if you do, exercise for only a short period of time.

Hypothermia, a drop of one or more degrees Fahrenheit of core body temperature as a result of cold, is a real danger when exercising in severe cold. If you experience any of the signs of hypothermia—slurred speech, lack of coordination, or mental confusion—get indoors immediately. Another danger of cold weather training is *frostbite*, the destruction of body tissue by freezing. The signs of frostbite include burning and stinging skin, numbness, redness, and poor coordination. As with hypothermia, if you experience any of the signs of frostbite, get indoors immediately.

Nutritional Needs.   During exercise, body tissue is broken down. Nutrients aid in the repair of this tissue. One way to help prevent injury is to eat a nutritionally sound diet so tissue can be repaired before it is once again

Table 13.2
Wind Chill Factor Chart

Wind Speed (mph)	Local Temperature (°F)										
	32	23	14	5	−4	−13	−22	−31	−40	−49	−58

	Equivalent Temperature (°F)										
	Little danger for properly clothed persons*			Considerable danger*		Very great danger*					
Calm	32	23	14	5	−4	−13	−22	−31	−40	−49	−58
5	29	20	10	1	−9	−18	−28	−37	−47	−56	−65
10	18	7	−4	−15	−26	−37	−48	−59	−70	−81	−92
15	13	−1	−13	−25	−37	−49	−61	−73	−85	−97	−109
20	7	−6	−19	−32	−44	−57	−70	−83	−96	−109	−121
25	3	−10	−24	−37	−50	−64	−77	−90	−104	−117	−130
30	1	−13	−27	−41	−54	−68	−82	−97	−109	−123	−137
35	−1	−15	−29	−43	−57	−71	−85	−99	−113	−127	−142
40	−3	−17	−31	−45	−59	−74	−87	−102	−116	−131	−145
45	−3	−18	−32	−46	−61	−75	−89	−104	−118	−132	−147
50	−4	−18	−33	−47	−62	−76	−91	−105	−120	−134	−148

* Danger from freezing of exposed flesh

Source: Courtesy U.S. Army Antarctic Research Laboratory, Chart 20-12.

physically stressed. Even in terms of preventing injury, you need to be concerned with what you eat.

Competing.　The positive side of competition is that it can motivate you to achieve your potential. One of its negative aspects, however, is its potential for contributing to injury. We say *potential*, because it need not; that's up to you. We heard of a golfer so competitive that, in the middle of a poor scoring round, he tossed his clubs and cart off a small bridge into a creek and walked away. Some time later he returned, rolled up his trouser legs, waded into the creek until he reached his clubs, unzipped a compartment, reached in and removed his pack of cigarettes, and left, never to see his golf clubs again.

It's that kind of competition that motivates parents to show their children how athletic they once were, a situation sure to result in an injured parent. It's that kind of competition that leads to hamstring muscle pulls during the annual picnic. And it's that kind of competition that results in a black eye from an argument during a pick-up basketball game.

When you find yourself in a competitive situation and seek to prevent injury, consider how important a victory really is, and what price you're willing to pay for it. In most instances, such clear-headed thinking will serve to rein you in so that you compete within your limitations. You'll enjoy and profit from the competition more (even if you don't win) than you would have if you had competed irresponsibly and injured yourself.

Have the Proper Equipment.   A mountain climber would never find him or herself on a mountain without the proper equipment. That would be worse than foolish; it would be suicidal. You should not engage in any physical activity without the proper equipment. Don't box without a mouth guard, and don't jog without good running shoes. Don't play football without a helmet, and don't play racketball without a protective eye guard. Don't bike without bicycle clips on your trousers, and don't jump rope on a cement floor. If you exercise with the proper equipment and use the proper facilities, your chances of injury will be greatly reduced (Richie, Kelso, Bellucci, 1985).

Structural Analysis

If your body is not structured so that you are balanced, you will put undue stress on its parts. Such stress can result in injury. No one's body is perfectly symmetrical. Many people know that when they buy a long-sleeved shirt, one sleeve will appear longer than the other; in actuality, it is one arm that is longer than the other (usually the dominant arm). Such imbalances do not usually cause problems. However, other structural abnormalities can lead to injury.

For example, one leg that is just a quarter of an inch shorter than the other can result in pelvic tilt, which means greater stress on the hip joint on the longer leg side. This pelvic tilt can also result in pinched nerves and lower back aches. Take a moment to test your body for unequal leg lengths, using the following procedure:

1. Have a partner measure the distance from the floor to the top of each side of your pelvis as you stand straight with your heels together. The distances should be equal.
2. Seated with your toes pointed forward and your heels together, place a carpenter's leveler on your knees. If the bubble is not in the middle, there is an unequal distance between the floor and your knee, so your problem lies below the knee.

Foot abnormalities are another cause of fitness-related injuries. These can range from *pronated feet* (ankles rolling inward) to *high-arched feet*. Excessive pronation causes strain on the ankle, knee, and hip joints, resulting in an increased tendency toward hamstring muscle pulls, shin splints, strains, and bone spurs (Vinger and Hoerner, 1981, p. 262). High-arched feet result in a diminished "shock absorber effect," with the result often being stress fractures and painful knees and hips. Some people are *bowlegged* and susceptible to lower back pain. If when standing straight, with your heels together, you can place two fingers between your knees, you are bowlegged. Some people's knees bend inward. This is called being *knock-kneed* and may lead to knee problems. If when standing straight you have trouble putting your heels together, you are knock-kneed.

Spinal malalignments may also lead to injury. Scoliosis (sideways curvature of the spine) and lordosis (a forward curvature of the spine) are two such examples. Hip, back, and neck problems are more likely in people with these conditions.

CARE OF COMMON INJURIES

In spite of what we do to prevent injuries, it seems that they are inevitable. We can decrease the probability of acquiring an injury or its severity when it does occur, but sooner or later all active people will be injured. When all sports are considered, the most frequently injured body parts are these (Muckle, 1982, p. 8):

knee	24%	ankle	10%	head	2%
hip	16%	thigh	9%	foot	2%
shin	14%	groin	5%	chest	1%
elbow	13%	wrist	4%		

In this section, for some of the common injuries we will describe what to do once you are injured.

Self-care

There are many injuries you can care for yourself. A little heat, a little cold, a little tape, a little rest, a little change in routine, or a little adjustment in equipment is often all that is needed. A good medical care book (for example, Vickery and Fries, 1976), or sports medicine book (for example, Mirkin and Hoffman, 1978) can be an invaluable aid. So can experts in your community (for example, a professor, athletic trainer, physician, or podiatrist).

When to See a Professional

A first and major consideration once an injury occurs is whether to treat it yourself or to seek the help of a professional. Although there are no absolute guidelines regarding this question—each injury and each person is slightly different from each other injury and each other person—Mirkin and Hoffman (1978, pp. 93–94) suggest you consult professionals for:

1. All traumatic joint injuries.
2. Any injury accompanied by severe pain.
3. Any pain in a joint or bone that persists for more than two weeks.
4. Any injury that doesn't heal in three weeks.
5. Any injury that concerns you enough that you'd feel more comfortable having it checked.

6. Any infection in or under the skin manifested by pus, red streaks, swollen lymph nodes, or fever.

To Exercise or Not to Exercise?

Here's where we often get ourselves into trouble. Whether an injury requires rest or whether you can exercise without doing any further damage is a difficult question to answer. Some people argue that if an injury pains you while resting, don't exercise. Others believe you can exercise as long as when you do, the injury feels no worse. Here too there are no strict guidelines. We do know one thing: even if the injury limits your physical activity, often you can still be physically active. If your ankle is sprained, you might be able to swim using just your upper body and arms; if your tennis elbow is acting up, you might be able to jog. Certainly some injuries require total rest, but don't assume that in every case. When in doubt about whether to continue or to cease exercising, it might be wise to consult a professional.

COMMON KINDS OF INJURIES

Injuries to Muscles

Muscles are located throughout your body. They are connected to your bones by tendons and when they contract, muscles are responsible for your ability to move any body part. Sometimes muscles are injured as a result of physical activity. The most common injuries are muscle pulls (strains) and muscle cramps.

Muscle Pulls.   A muscle pull is a stretch, tear, or rip in the muscle and is properly known as a muscle *strain*. Muscle pulls may be a result of insufficient warmup, imbalance in muscle strength, poor flexibility, mineral imbalance caused by a great deal of sweating or faulty diet, or overtraining.

When a muscle pull occurs, a sharp pain will be felt, and any further movement of that part of the body will hurt. When touched, that muscle will hurt, and there may be some spasms visible (rapid contractions).

To treat a muscle pull, apply ice immediately (never directly on the skin, but through a towel or ice pack), compress the muscles with an elastic bandage, and elevate the body part. This treatment will limit the amount of swelling and speed recovery. Some experts suggest replacing the ice with heat after 24 to 48 hours to increase the blood supply to the muscle, and consequently nutrients to and transportation of fluids from the area. Others recommend ice throughout.

Physical activity involving that area of the body can usually begin anywhere from two days to two weeks and should be governed by the pain—start slowly and stop if you experience pain.

Muscle Cramps.   A muscle cramp is an involuntary sustained contraction of the muscle that may be caused by a mineral deficiency (salt, potassium, magnesium, or calcium), an injury to the muscle, or an insufficient supply of blood to the area to remove built-up waste products (lactic acid). One common form of muscle cramp is a *stitch*; a sharp pain, usually on the sides of the upper abdomen. It is believed that this is a cramping of the diaphragm, which controls breathing.

Stitches can be prevented by not eating just before exercising (Reilly, 1981, p. 81). Once they happen, exercise should stop. Place the palm of your hand over the stitch, and exhale several breaths. When the pain stops, you can resume exercising. For other muscle cramps, rest and a more minerally nutritious diet (more fruit and vegetables) is the best treatment.

Injuries to Connective Tissue

Tendons connect muscle to bone. *Ligaments* connect bone to bone to limit movement in the *joint* (where two bones meet and range of motion is possible; see Figure 13.1). *Cartilage* surrounds the ends of the bones at the joint to prevent bones from rubbing against one another. All these are connective tissues, and all can be injured in physical activity. Common injuries are tendonitis, Achilles tendon rupture, shin splints, sprained ankle, water on the knee, plantar fascia strain, and tennis elbow.

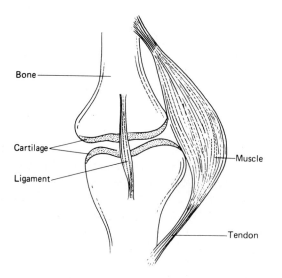

FIGURE 13.1   Tissue at a joint

Bone

Cartilage

Ligament

Muscle

Tendon

Tendonitis.   Tendonitis is an inflammation of a tendon that results in swelling and pain. The pain of tendonitis is worse when *not* exercising, since the muscle to which the tendon is attached is not stretched and creates a greater pull on the tendon.

Since exercise actually relieves the pain of tendonitis, the tendency is to continue exercising, with the result often being a worsening of the condition.

Tendonitis, most common in the Achilles tendon (just above the heel), requires rest, with stretching of the muscle to which the tendon is attached only when the pains subsides. Applying ice to the tendon after exercise to decrease the inflammation is also recommended.

Achilles Tendon Rupture.   Occasionally the pull on the tendon will be so great or the condition of the tendon so deteriorated that it will actually rupture. As with tendonitis, the most likely tendon to rupture is the Achilles tendon. If the rupture is complete, surgery is usually required; if it is not complete, immobilization in a cast for several weeks may be all that is necessary (Williams, 1980, pp. 117–118).

Shin Splints.   The term *shin splints* is used to refer to several conditions, but generally means pain in the shin region of the leg. There is usually an inflammation of the tendon or muscle in that area (Allen, 1979, p. 59). The exact causes of shin splints are not known, but an educated guess involves "faulty posture alignment, falling arches, muscle fatigue, overuse stress, body chemical imbalance, or a lack of proper reciprocal muscle coordination between the anterior and posterior aspects of the leg" (Klafs and Arnheim, 1981, p. 38).

To treat shin splints, some experts recommend taking two aspirins and applying ice to the region prior to exercising or gradual stretching before and after exercising. Heat applied at other than times of exercise has also been recommended. Taping of the shin may also provide some relief.

Sprained Ankle.   Sprained ankle, a common fitness-related injury, results from a twisting of the ankle. Usually this injury involves a partial tear of the ligament. Treatment involves applying ice, wrapping with tape or an elastic bandage, and elevating the ankle to decrease swelling. Activity can be resumed when the pain subsides.

Water on the Knee.   Medically known as *bursitis*, water on the knee usually results from trauma to the knee. When the knee is hit, the bursa (a fluid membrane that facilitates joint movement) may become inflamed, and an excess of fluid may develop. Treatment includes removal of fluid by syringe, local injection of corticoids, protection against being bumped, and wrapping of the knee with an elastic bandage. In addition, aspirin and warm compresses to reduce the inflammation have been recommended.

Plantar Fascia Strain.   Planter fascitis or plantar fascia strain involves inflammation of the plantar fascia, resulting in pain in the heel. The fascia cover all the tissues in the body (muscles, ligaments, organs). The plantar fascia covers the plantar ligament in the bottom of the foot, and the inflammation usually occurs where the ligament attaches to the heel bone (see Figure 13.2). Plantar fascia strains are easy to identify because they create pain when running or walking, especially when the person has not warmed up. Getting out of bed in the morning and walking will create pain in the heel.

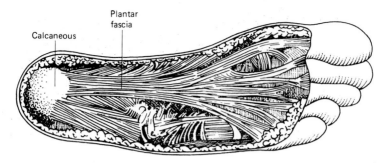

FIGURE 13.2   Plantar fascia strain

Treatment involves protecting the painful area by using a plastic heel cup or some "cushiony" material such as felt. Injection of cortisone in the area may be helpful, as may stretching the Achilles tendon, since a tight Achilles tendon often contributes to this injury.

Tennis Elbow.   This condition is common in tennis players (therefore its name), but can result from any twisting of the elbow joint. Baseball pitchers throwing curve balls and tennis players using topspins are prone to this injury.

Tennis elbow (medically known as *lateral epicondylitis*) is inflammation and/or tears in the muscle attachment just above the elbow joint (at the large upper arm bone called the humerus). The elbow joint is painful and hurts, especially when touched or accidentally bumped. In tennis players, this condition may be caused by "too large or too small a racket grip, racket strings either too tight or too loose or an improper stroke, particularly the backhand . . . , playing too much tennis too early in the season or playing significantly more tennis in a day than one normally plays" (Apple and Cantwell, 1979, p. 111).

The recommended treatment for tennis elbow is rest with forearm strengthening exercises once the pain subsides. In some cases, injections of cortisone in the area will provide relief.

Injuries to Bones

The 206 bones in the body are also subject to fitness-related injury. We will discuss the following injuries to bone: bone bruises, fractures, and stress fractures.

Bone Bruises.   A blow to a bone can be quite painful, but often not very serious. Some blood vessels may be ruptured, causing skin discoloration, and some pain may linger. However, application of ice and a few days' rest is usually all that is needed.

Fractures.   Sometimes the blow to the bone, or the stress upon it, is so great that the bone actually breaks. Aside from the pain and damage to structure and mobility, broken bones may cause secondary problems. For example, if not kept immobile, the jagged edges of the broken bone can injure blood vessels, nerves, or other tissues. Further, such secondary damage and any broken skin exposing the body to bacteria can result in infection.

Broken bones call for immediate immobility (with a splint if possible) until a physician can set the bone and immobilize it with a plaster cast. Depending on the nature, severity, and location of the break, traction may be necessary. Healing can take anywhere from 1 to 6 months.

Stress Fractures.   Sometimes called a *fatigue fracture*, a stress fracture is a small crack on the surface of the bone that can be recognized by the pain when it is pressed on *both* from above and from below. Other injuries will usually pain only when pressed from above *or* below, but not both. Stress fractures are difficult to diagnose because even X rays do not always pick them up. Treatment involves resting that area of the body for several weeks to allow the bone to repair itself.

An interesting observation has recently been made regarding stress fractures and women athletes (in particular, runners). Women runners have been found to experience amenorrhea (or cessation of menstruation) in greater numbers than women in general. The cause of this condition is still being investigated, but one result of amenorrhea is a decrease in estrogen produced by the body. Decreased estrogen production results in a weakening of the bones, and that is why postmenopausal women are more susceptible to broken bones. The bottom line to this observation is that stress fractures are being seen in greater numbers in women athletes, and especially in those who have stopped menstruating.

It is recommended that such women increase the amount of calcium in their diets to strengthen their bones. If you find yourself in this situation, drink milk, and eat yogurt, cheese, or other foods high in calcium. Much has been written on amenorrhea and the physically active female, and you should consult that literature if you need more information on the topic (for example, Shangold, 1981).

Injuries to the Skin

Injuries to the skin are usually more bothersome than serious, and yet they can limit physical activity. The skin injuries we will discuss are hematomas, "jock itch," "athlete's foot," blisters, and abrasions.

Hematomas.   A hematoma is a collection of blood pooled in a particular area as a result of a blow to that area. The treatment for a hematoma includes an ice pack applied immediately, a pressure bandage, and keeping the part immobilized and elevated. After several days, heat should be used to encourage absorption of the blood. In some instances, where the pooled blood is extensive or creating pressure on adjacent structures, aspiration by needle may be required. In most instances, however, this is unnecessary.

Jock Itch.   The red, flaky rash that develops on the inner skin of the upper thighs is usually the result of a fungus infection irritated by warm weather, excessive perspiration, or wearing wet underclothes. "Jock itch" can be quite uncomfortable. Several measures can be taken to prevent this condition: drying well after bathing; wearing loose, clean, dry clothing; and the liberal use of talcum powder (Vinger and Hoerner, 1981, p. 195). Once jock itch occurs, an antifungal cream should be applied to kill the fungus. Tolnaftate is the cream recommended by several experts.

Athlete's Foot.   The extreme itching on the soles of the feet and between the toes is known as athlete's foot. Its medical name is *tinea pedis*. Athlete's foot is caused by a fungus that thrives in a warm, moist, dark environment. To prevent this condition in the first place, talcum powder should be applied to the feet twice daily; the feet should be thoroughly dried after

---

INJURY INSIGHTS

List the fitness-related injuries you have incurred within the past year. If you've had more than five such injuries, list the five most serious ones.

1. _____

2. _____

3. _____

4. _____

5. _____

On a separate sheet of paper, answer the following questions for *each* injury listed:

1. What contributed to this injury?
2. How could this injury have been prevented?
3. How were your fitness activities affected by this injury?
4. How did you feel about this injury?
5. How might you have felt better? Worse?
6. How did you treat your injury?
7. How might you have treated it better? Worse?
8. How have *you* changed or how have you changed your environment to prevent this injury from occurring again?
9. What have you learned by answering these questions?

showering; shoes and socks should be kept dry by liberal use of talcum powder; and clean socks should be worn. Once athlete's foot develops, use talcum powder frequently, wear clean socks, and use a fungicide such as Desenex or Tinactin (or a stronger fungicide for more serious infections).

Blisters.   The constant rubbing of soft skin can cause a blister. What is occurring is a separation of the outer layer of skin (the epidermis) from the next layer (the dermis), with fluid accumulating between the layers. To prevent blisters, apply tincture of benzoin followed by talcum powder to protect the skin, or wear something soft between the skin and what it will rub against (for example, two pair of athletic socks on the feet or gloves on the hands).

Once the blister occurs, cut out a donut-shaped bandage to separate the blister from anything it might rub against. Some people recommend puncturing the blister to drain the fluid. However, puncturing introduces the possibility of infection and should be done only to prevent tearing of the blister. When puncturing a blister is necessary, use a sterile needle applied to one edge of the blister and apply a pressure bandage to prevent refilling of fluid. The application of an antiseptic to the blister prior to securing the pressure bandage is recommended.

Abrasions.   When the skin is scraped against a rough surface and the epidermis and dermis are worn away, the result is known as an abrasion. Small blood vessels are usually ruptured, resulting in minor bleeding and the possibility of infection. Abrasions should be treated by cleansing the area with soap and water; applying an antiseptic and a petroleum-based ointment; and covering with a sterile, nonadhering bandage. The bandage should be changed each day.

CONCLUSION: WELLNESS IN SPITE OF INJURY

When you read of all the possible injuries that can result from physical activity, and how common some of them are, you might want a warning label on athletic equipment like that on packs of cigarettes: *Warning—the Surgeon General has determined that exercise is hazardous to your health.* What you should remember, however, is that *lack* of exercise may be more hazardous to your health—and by now you should realize we mean your social, mental, emotional, and spiritual, as well as your physical health. First, the more common fitness injuries tend to be relatively inocuous, especially compared to the potential for ill health from lack of exercise. Second, the more serious fitness injuries are less likely to occur. And, last, most of these injuries can be prevented with a modicum of care and can be treated easily if they should occur.

Exercise has been said to result in a "positive addiction." One runner we know has had two stress fractures directly attributed to her running, and yet she still runs. Why? Well, she's positively addicted. She misses running when she can't do it. She gets irritable and frustrated during those times. Her relationships with people around her suffer. For her, running is healthy in spite of that threat it creates to her *physical health*. She is more *well* running than not running. We're sure you know people like this as well. Perhaps you're one of them.

The sensible way to manage such a situation—at least *we* think it sensible—is to cut down on any activity that causes a threat, add some different types of exercise, and work at preventing potential injury. So the runner now runs less than before, has added swimming and bicycling to her routine, and has begun weight training to strengthen her legs.

What can you do to achieve the benefits of regular exercise while limiting *your* potential for illness. Will you do it? Remember, it's up to you.

Last, we want to emphasize the fact than an injury need not destroy your exercise program. With adaptations consistent with your limitations, you can maintain your program. The knowledge you acquire in this book should help you make such adaptations, and we hope you'll consult experts for further assistance.

SUMMARY

1. To prevent fitness-related injury, follow these principles: don't do too much too soon; train, don't strain; hard days, easy days; know your body; and warm up and cool down.

2. The signs of overtraining are soreness in muscles and joints, heaviness in arms and legs, inability to relax, persistent tiredness, loss of appetite, loss of weight, constipation or diarrhea, and repeated injury.

3. When training in hot weather, try to train early in the morning or in the evening when the temperature is at its lowest. Also drink plenty of fluids, wear a hat, and wear loose-fitting lightweight clothing.

4. When training in cold weather, pay attention to the wind chill factor. Also wear layers of clothing and protect the fingers, toes, ears, and nose.

5. To prevent athletic injuries, don't get carried away with competition, use the proper equipment, and eat well.

6. The most frequently injured body parts are the knee, hip, shin, elbow, and ankle—in that oder.

7. Many fitness-related injuries can be cared for by oneself. However, a professional should be consulted for all traumatic joint injuries, all injuries accompanied by severe pain, any pain in joint or bone that persists for more than 2 weeks, all injuries that don't heal in 3 weeks, and any infection in or under the skin manifested by pus, red streaks, swollen lymph nodes, or fever.

8. Fitness-related injuries can occur to muscles, connective tissue, bone, or skin.

9. Fitness-related injuries to muscles include muscle pulls (strains) and muscle cramps.

10. Fitness-related injuries to connective tissue can affect tendons, ligaments, or cartilage. They include tendonitis, Achilles tendon rupture, shin splints, sprained ankle, water on the knee, plantar fascia strain, and tennis elbow.

11. Fitness-related injuries to bone include bone bruises, fractures, and stress fractures.
12. Fitness-related injuries to skin include hematomas, jock itch, athlete's foot, blisters, and abrasions.

REFERENCES

ALLEN, R. C. "Shin Splints." *The Athletic Journal* 60 (1979): 59.

APPLE, D. F., AND J. D. CANTWELL. *Medicine for Sport.* Chicago: Year Book Medical Publishers, 1979.

ELLIS, J., AND P. YAVORSKY. "Stretching Specifics: The Right Stretch Gets Directly to a Trouble Spot to Prevent Injury." *Runner's World*, July 1986, pp. 40-45.

KLAFS, C. E., AND D. ARNHEIM. *Modern Principles of Athletic Training.* St. Louis: C.V. Mosby, 1981.

MIRKIN, G., AND H. MARSHALL. *The Sportsmedicine Book.* Boston: Little, Brown, 1978.

MUCKLE, D. S. *Injuries in Sport.* Bristol, Eng.: John Wright, 1982.

RICHIE, D. H., S. F. KELSO, AND P. A. BELLUCCI. "Aerobic Dance Injuries: A Retrospective Study of Instructors and Participants." *The Physician and Sportsmedicine* 13 (1985): 130–40.

REILLY, T. (ed.). *Sports Fitness and Sports Injuries.* London: Faber and Faber, 1981.

SHANGOLD, M. "The Woman Runner: Her Body, Her Mind, Her Spirit." *Runner's World* 16 (July 1981): 34.

VICKERY, D. M., AND J. F. FRIES. *Take Care of Yourself.* Reading, MA: Addison-Wesley, 1976.

VINGER, P. F., AND E. F. HOERNER (eds.). *Sports Injuries: The Unthwarted Epidemic.* Littleton, MA: PSG, 1981.

WILLIAMS, J. G. P. *Color Atlas of Injury in Sport.* Chicago: Year Book Medical Publishers, 1980.

14

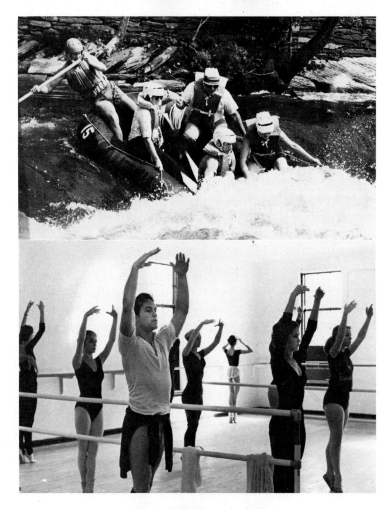

A Word
on Popular Exercises

Now that you know what physical fitness and wellness are, now that you know what health benefits accrue from regular exercise, now that you have determined your fitness profile and have an arsenal of behavioral techniques to begin and maintain a program of regular exercise, we are able to add the accoutrements—the little extras that will maximize the benefits you derive from any particular activities you choose to include in your fitness regimen. Although space and your interests dictate that this discussion be brief and by no means all-inclusive, you should find some useful suggestions for ways of better achieving the health benefits that really mean increased wellness.

In this chapter, we will present some considerations you might want to take into account when deciding to achieve physical fitness and wellness by engaging in particular activities. The activities we present all have the potential for wellness. They include a cardiorespiratory, a muscular, and a flexibility component. In addition, they also have the potential to improve your mental, emotional, social, and spiritual health.

WALKING AND JOGGING

Walking and jogging are excellent ways to keep fit. They improve cardiorespiratory performance (in particular, brisk walking), enhance muscular strength and endurance, and can be a spiritual experience if you pay attention to the birds, the trees, and the clouds. If you walk or jog with a friend, you can also respond to your social health needs.

A Walking-Jogging Program

To start you out on a walking-jogging exercise program, we include the Red, White, and Blue Program suggested by the President's Council on Physical

Fitness (*An Introduction to Physical Fitness,* 1980). Remember to warm up beforehand and to cool down afterward. With exercise programs such as this, flexibility exercises should be an integral part of the warmup and cooldown.

RED WALKING PROGRAM

Week	Daily Activity
1	Walk at a brisk pace for 5 minutes, or for a shorter time if you become uncomfortably tired. Walk slowly or rest for 3 minutes. Again walk briskly for 5 minutes, or until you become uncomfortably tired.
2	Same as week 1, but increase pace as soon as you can walk 5 minutes without soreness or fatigue.
3	Walk at a brisk pace for 8 minutes, or for a shorter time if you become uncomfortably tired. Walk slowly or rest for 3 minutes. Again walk briskly for 8 minutes, or until you become uncomfortably tired.
4	Same as week 3, but increase pace as soon as you can walk 8 minutes without soreness or fatigue.

When you have completed week 4 of the Red program, begin at week 1 of the White program.

WHITE WALKING-JOGGING PROGRAM

Week	Daily Activity
1	Walk at a brisk pace for 10 minutes, or for a shorter time if you become uncomfortably tired. Walk slowly or rest for 3 minutes. Again walk briskly for 10 minutes, or until you become uncomfortably tired.
2	Walk at a brisk pace for 15 minutes, or for a shorter time if you become uncomfortably tired. Walk slowly for 3 minutes.
3	Jog 20 seconds (50 yards). Walk 1 minute (100 yards). Repeat 12 times.
4	Jog 20 seconds (50 yards). Walk 1 minute (100 yards). Repeat 12 times.

When you have completed week 4 of the White program, begin at week 1 of the Blue program.

BLUE JOGGING PROGRAM

Week	Daily Activity
1	Jog 40 sec. (100 yds.) Walk 1 min. (100 yds.) Repeat 9 times.
2	Jog 1 min. (150 yds.) Walk 1 min. (100 yds.) Repeat 8 times.
3	Jog 2 min. (300 yrds.) Walk 1 min. (100 yds.) Repeat 6 times.
4	Jog 4 min. (600 yds.) Walk 1 min. (100 yds.) Repeat 4 times.

5	Jog 6 min. (900 yds.) Walk 1 min. (100 yds.) Repeat 3 times.
6	Jog 8 min. (1200 yds.) Walk 2 min. (200 yds.) Repeat 2 times.
7	Jog 10 min. (1500 yds.) Walk 2 min. (200 yds.) Repeat 2 times.
8	Jog 12 min. (1700 yds.) Walk 2 min. (200 yds.) Repeat 2 times.

Jogging

Running is very popular. Surveys show that more than 17 million adult Ameicans are running regularly and over 50,000 Americans have completed at least one marathon (26 miles, 385 yards). Running is such a good form of exercise because it requires a minimum of equipment (the only expense is a good pair of running shoes); it can be done almost anywhere and anytime; and it does not require a special skill.

What to Wear.   The most important apparel for the runner is a pair of sturdy, properly fitting running shoes. Training shoes with heavy, cushioned soles and arch supports are preferable to flimsy sneakers and racing flats. (Some running magazines annually rate major brands and popular models.)

Weather Will Dictate the Rest of Your Attire.   As a general rule, you will want to wear lighter clothing than temperatures might seem to indicate. Running generates lots of body heat.

Light-colored clothing that reflects the sun's rays is cooler in the summer, and dark clothes are warmer in the winter. When the weather is very cold, it's better to wear several layers of light clothing than one or two heavy layers. The extra layers help trap heat, and it's easy to shed one of them if you become too warm.

You should wear something on your head when it's cold, or when it's hot and sunny. Wool watch caps or ski caps are recommended for winter wear, and some form of tennis or sailor's hat that provides shade and can be soaked in water is good for summer.

If you dress properly, you can run in almost any weather, but it's advisable not to run when it's extremely hot and humid. On such days, plan to run early in the morning or in the evening (President's Council on Physical Fitness, *An Introduction to Running*, 1980).

Warmup and Cooldown.   To minimize the chances of injury or soreness, the following exercises (Figures 14.1-14.5) should be done *before* and *after* running. If you find the exercises difficult to perform, you may want to do them twice when warming up to increase flexibility. Stretch slowly and do not bounce to attain prescribed positions. The text and captions from the adapted illustrations are from a 1980 publication of the President's Council on Physical Fitness and Sports (*An Introduction to Running*).

Running Style.   In most sports we are taught to run for speed and power. In running for fitness, the objectives are different and so is the form.

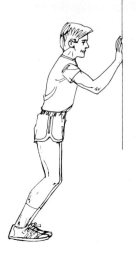

FIGURE 14.1 Achilles tendon and calf stretch

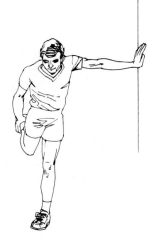

FIGURE 14.2 Thigh stretcher

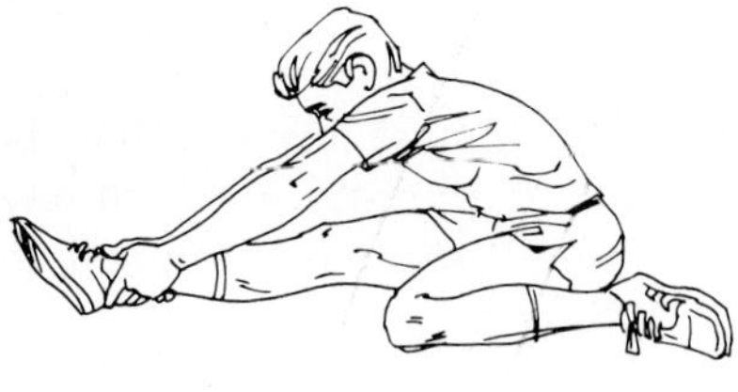

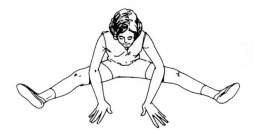

FIGURE 14.3 Hurdler's stretch
(Caution: Do not lean backward)

FIGURE 14.4 Straddle stretch

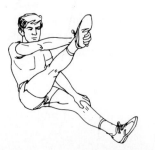

FIGURE 14.5 Leg stretcher

Here are some suggestions to help you develop a comfortable, economical running style.

1. Run in an upright position, avoiding excessive forward lean. Keep your back as straight as you comfortably can and keep your head up. Don't look at your feet.
2. Carry arms slightly away from the body, with elbows bent so that forearms are roughly parallel to the ground. Occasionally shake and relax arms to prevent tightness in shoulders.
3. Land on the heel of the foot and rock forward to drive off the ball of the foot. If this proves difficult, try a more flat-footed style. Running only on the balls of your feet will tire you quickly and make the legs sore.
4. Keep your stride relatively short. Don't force your pace by reaching for extra distance.
5. Breathe deeply with your mouth open.

Beginner's Timetable.   The American Podiatry Association (undated) recommends the following running program:

1–6 WEEKS

* Warm up with walking and stretching movement
* Jog 55 yards, walk 55 yards (four times)
* Jog 110 yards, walk 110 yards (four times)
* Jog 55 yards, walk 55 yards (four times)
* Pace: 110 yards in about 45 seconds

6–12 WEEKS

* Increase jogging and reduce walking
* Pace: 110 yards in 30-37 seconds

12–24 WEEKS

* Jog a 9-minute mile

30+ WEEKS

* The second workout each week, add variety—continuous jogging, or running and walking alternately at a slow varying pace for distances up to two miles.

ROPE JUMPING

When I was 13, my friend Steven and I both fell head over heels in love with 12-year-old, blonde-haired, adorable, vivacious (yes, even at that age) Jill. I'm talking about the heart-pounding, palm-perspiring, any-spare-time-spent-with-her love. Steven and I would do anything for Jill. We even spent hours playing "Who Stole the Cookie from the Cookie Jar?" while our friends played baseball or basketball. That was the summer I learned to jump rope, the whole time made frantic by the thought that this was a "sissy" activity. If my other friends had seen me, I would have died.

Well, I'm no longer crippled by that thought because I have since learned that the sex you were born with need not stop you from engaging in an enjoyable activity, and that rope jumping is an excellent way to develop cardiorespiratory endurance, strength, agility, coordination, and a sense of wellness. Fortunately, many other people have learned a similar lesson, and rope jumping has become very popular. Here are some pointers for jumping rope:

1. Determine the best length for your rope by standing on the center of the rope. The handles should then reach from armpit to armpit.
2. When jumping, keep your upper arms close to your body, with your elbows almost touching your sides. Have your forearms out at right angles, and turn the rope by making small circles with your hands and wrists. Keep your feet, ankles, and knees together.
3. Relax. Don't tense up. Enjoy yourself.
4. Keep your body erect, with your head and eyes up.
5. Start slowly.
6. Land on the balls of your feet, bending your knees slightly.
7. Maintain a steady rhythm.
8. Jump just 1 or 2 inches from the floor.
9. Try jumping to music. Maintain the rhythm of the music.
10. When you get good, improvise. Create new stunts. Have fun.

The American Heart Association (1983) recommends the rope jumping stunts shown in Figure 14.6. Try them out yourself.

---

1. Side Swing
  1. Twirl rope to one side
  2. Repeat on the opposite side
  3. Twirl rope alternately from side to side
Teaching Hints: Keep hand together, keep feet together

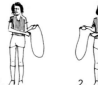

1.   2.   3.

---

2. Basic Bounce (single bounce)
  1. Jump on both feet
  2. Land on balls of feet
Teaching Hints: Keep feet, ankles and knees together.

1.   2.

Figure 14.6   Rope jumping stunts
(Courtesy American Heart Association. Reprinted with permission.)

Figure 14.6 (continued)

3. Double side swing and jump
1. Twirl rope to left side
2. Twirl rope to right side
3. Jump over rope

Teaching Hints: Keep hands together on side swings, keep feet together.

1.   2.   3.

4. Single side swing and jump
1. Twirl rope to left side   3. Twirl rope to right side
2. Jump over rope   4. Jump over rope

Teaching Hints: Keep hands together on side swings, keep feet together.

1.   2.   3.   4.

5. Skier (side to side)
1. Jump left
2. Jump right

Teaching Hints: Feet move laterally 4-6" to each side, keep feet together.

 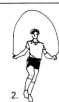

1.   2.

6. Bell (forward and backward)
1. Jump forward
2. Jump backward

Teaching Hints: Feet move 4-6" forward & backward as a bell clapper, keep feet together.

 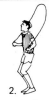

1.   2.

7. Side straddle (spread together)
1. Jump to a straddle position
2. Return to basic bounce

Teaching Hints: Spread feet shoulder width apart.

1.   2.

8. Forward straddle (scissors)
1. Jump to stride position with left foot forward
2. Jump and reverse position of feet

Teaching Hints: Feet 8-12" apart.

1.   2.

9. X motion (straddle, cross)
1. Jump to straddle position
2. Jump to crossed legs

Teaching Hints: Feet shoulder width apart.

1.   2.

Figure 14.6 (continued)

10. Wounded duck (alternate toes/heels together)
  1. Jump, toes & knees touch, heels spread
  2. Jump, heels touch, toes and knees spread
  Teaching Hints: Alternate toes touching and heels touching.

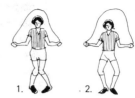

11. Criss cross (cross arms)
  1. Cross arms and jump
  2. Open rope, basic bounce
  Teaching Hints: Cross right arm over left, cross left arm over right.

12. Full turn (one complete circle with rope in front)
  1. Turn body left, with right turn of rope
  2. Side swing right, body turns right
  3. Full turn body makes full turn to right
  4. Jump rope forward
  Teaching Hints: Follow rope, rope and body may turn left.

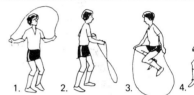

13. Heel to Heel
  1. Jump and touch left heel
  2. Jump and touch right heel
  Teaching Hints: Heel touches are forward.

14. Toe to toe (alternate toe touch)
  1. Hops on left foot, touch right toe
  2. Hops on right foot, touch left toe
  Teaching Hints: Keep body over weighted foot.

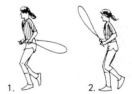

15. Forward 180 (half turn rotating rope from forward
  position to backward jumping position)
  1. Side swing left, half turn of body right
  2. Jump over backward turning rope
  Teaching Hints: Follow rope, rope and body may turn to left.

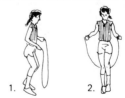

16. Backward 180 (turn keeping rope in front of face)
  1. Jump backward, turning rope
  2. Half turn of body left, facing rope
  3. Jump rope forward
  Teaching Hints: Follow rope, rope and body may turn left.

Figure 14.6 (continued)

17. Heel-toe (alternate heel-toe touch)
1. Hop on left foot, touch right heel forward
2. Hop on left foot again, touch right toe backward
3. Repeat on opposite side
Teaching Hints: Heel-toe as in a polka.

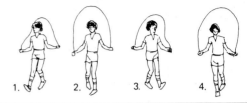

18. Kick swing (alternate kick or swing feet, forward, sideward, backward)
1. Hop on left foot, swing right leg forward
2. Hop on right foot, swing left leg forward
Teaching Hints: Repeat directions sidward and backward.

19. Peek-a-boo (alternate toe touch sideways)
1. Hop on left foot, touch right toe right
2. Hop on right foot, touch left toe left
Teaching Hint: Keep feet close to floor.

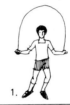

20. Double peek-a-boo (double toe touch sideways)
1. Hop on left foot, touch right toe right about 6''
2. Hop on left foot again, touch right toe right about 12''
Teaching Hints: Keep feet close to floor.

 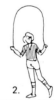

21. 360 (conbine forward 180 and backward 180)
1. Execute numbers 18 and 19 in a continuous sequence
2. Repeat 2 or more times
Teaching Hints: Follow rope.

22. Twist (rotate hips from side to side)
1. Jump and rotate hips right
2. Basic jump
3. Jump and rotate hips left
Teaching Hints: Advanced twise, execute nos. 1 & 3 in a continuous sequence.

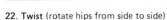
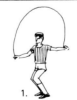 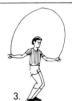

23. Can Can (knee-up-touch kick)
1. Hop on right foot, left knee up
2. Hop on right foot, touch left toe
3. Hop on right foot, kick left leg
4. Basic jump
Teaching Hints: Knee lift and kick are waist high, repeat on opposite leg.

Figure 14.6 (continued)

24. Shuffle (side step and touch)
1. Step sideways to the right, touch left toe beside right foot
2. Step sideward to the left, touch right toe beside left foot
Teacing Hints: Keep feet close together.

1.   2.

25. Side swing criss cross (alternate side turn — cross — side turn — cross)
1. Twirl rope on right side   3. Twirl rope on left side
2. Criss cross (number 11)   4. Criss cross
Teaching Hints: On criss crosses, number 2 right arm crosses over left number 4 left arm crosses over right.

1.   2.   3.   4.

26. Double under (2 rotations of rope with one jump)
1. Whip rope to increase speed
2. Rope passes under feet twice during one jump
Teaching Hints: Jump higher than normal at first.

1.   2.

27. Grapevine
1. Step right on right foot
2. Left foot crosses behind right
3. Step right on right foot
4. Kick the left leg forward right
Teaching Hints: Each step is taken over the rope, repeat to the left, have students say "step, behind, step, kick."

1.   2.   3.   4.

Note: All the above stunts can be performed with the rope turning backward as well as forward.

SWIMMING

As of January 1, 1980, there were 1,927,000 in-ground swimming pools in the United States. Of these, 1,530,000 were residential pools; 207,790 were in hotels, motels, or apartments; 57,275 were in private clubs; 51,315 in public recreation agencies; 31,170 in schools, colleges and universities; and 48,450 miscellaneous, including camps. Since 1965, an average of 88,000 in-ground pools have been built each year. In addition, it is estimated that there are over 2 million pools installed above the ground.

Obviously, swimming is popular. It is also a very good activity for physical fitness. What's more, it enhances physical fitness in a manner that diminishes the chances of injury. The reason is that when submerged up to the neck in water, you experience an apparent loss of 90 percent of your weight (President's Council on Physical Fitness and Sports, 1981, p. 1). If you weigh

130 pounds, when you're in water to your neck, your feet and legs have to support a weight of only 13 pounds. Therefore, you are less apt to cause injury to your legs and feet.

Many people who use swimming for conditioning do lap swimming; that is, they swim back and forth. When lap swimming, you should periodically check your heart rate to determine if you are at your target.

But lap swimming is not appropriate for everyone. Backyard pools usually are not large enough. Most residential pools are no larger than 36 ft. long by 17 ft. wide, with approximately 600 sq. ft. of water surface, ranging from 3 to 8.5 ft. in depth. In a swimming pool of this size, a workout would have to be adjusted considerably from that usually practiced in the typical school, college, or athletic club pool. Otherwise, swimming in the backyard pool becomes largely diving in, gliding across, and climbing out. For the typical person, it would mean only inactive bathing. But swimming pools, regardless of size, have a high potential as exercise facilities. This potential can be realized as individuals learn how to exercise in limited water areas.

The President's Council on Physical Fitness and Sports recommends an exercise program for limited water areas in its booklet *Aqua Dynamics* (1981). The program involves standing water drills (for example alternate toe touching, side straddle hopping, toe bouncing, and jogging in place), pool-side standing drills (such as stretching the arms out, pressing the back flat against the wall, and raising the knees to the chest), gutter-holding drills (such as knees to chest, hop twisting, front and back flutter kicking, and side flutter kicking), bobbing, and treading water. If you have your own pool and feel it is too small for lap swimming, you might want to write to the President's Council on Physical Fitness and Sports, Washington, DC 20201, for the *Aqua Dynamics* booklet. Another good source is Jane Katz's 1986 article, "The W.E.T. Workout."

CAUTIONS FOR POPULAR EXERCISES

Although exercise can lead to physical fitness, health, and wellness, when done incorrectly it can result in just the opposite. In this section we discuss some cautions you should observe when participating in some of the more popular exercises.

Tennis

Tennis is so popular that it deserves a special mention. As with all fitness activities, duration and intensity will determine how much your tennis game contributes to your physical fitness. You can see in Table 14.1 that a doubles game of tennis generally results in less of a workout than does a game of singles. In fact, a doubles match will use up about 330 calories in one hour of play, whereas a game of singles will use up 390 calories per hour.

Table 14.1

Relative Merits of Various Exercises in Inducing Cardiovascular Fitness

Energy Range	Activity	Comment
1.5-2.0 Mets* or 2.0-2.5 cals/min or120-150 cals/hr.	Light housework such as polishing furniture or washing small clothes	Too low in energy level and too intermittent to promote endurance.
	Strolling 1.0 mile/hr	Not sufficiently strenuous to promote endurance unless capacity is very low.
2.0-3.0 Mets or 2.5-4.0 cals/min or 150-240 cals/hr.	Level walking at 2.0 miles/hr	See "Strolling"
	Golf, using power cart	Promotes skill and minimal strength in arm muscles but not sufficiently taxing to promote endurance. Also too intermittent.
3.0-4.0 Mets or 4-5 cals/min or 240-300 cals/hr.	Cleaning windows, mopping floors, or vacuuming	Adequate conditioning exercise if carried out continuously for 20-30 minutes.
	Bowling	Too intermittent and not sufficiently taxing to promote endurance.
	Walking at 3.0 miles/hr.	Adequate dynamic exercise if low capacity.
	Cycling at 6 miles/hr.	As above.
	Golf, pulling cart	Useful for conditioning if reach target rate. May include isometrics depending on cart weight.
4.0-5.0 Mets or 5-6 cals/min or 300-360 cals/hr.	Scrubbing floors	Adequate endurance exercise of carried out in at least 2 minute stints.
	Walking 3.5 miles/hr.	Usually good dynamic aerobic exercise.
	Cycling 8 miles/hr.	As above.
	Table tennis, badminton and volleyball.	Vigorous continuous play can have endurance benefits but intermittent, easy play only promotes skill.
	Golf, carrying clubs	Promotes endurance if reach and maintain target rate, otherwise merely aids strength and skill.
	Tennis, doubles	Not very beneficial unless there is continuous play maintaining target rate—which is unlikely. Will aid skill.
	Many calisthenics and ballet exercises.	Will promote endurance if continuous, rhythmic and repetitive. Those requiring isometric effort such as pushups and situps are probably not beneficial for cardiovascular fitness.

Energy Range	Activity	Comment
5.0-6.0 Mets or 6-7 cals/min or 360-420 cals/hr.	Walking 4 miles/hr.	Dynamic, aerobic and of benefit.
	Cycling 10 miles/hr.	As above.
	Ice or roller skating	As above if done continuously.
6.0-7.0 Mets or 7-8 cals/min or 420-480 cals/hr.	Walking 5 miles/hr.	Dynamic, aerobic and beneficial.
	Cycling 11 mile/hr.	Same.
	Singles tennis	Can provide benefit if played 30 minutes or more by skilled player with an attempt to keep moving.
	Water skiing	Total isometrics; very risky for cardiacs, precardiacs (high risk) or deconditioned normals.
7.0-8.0 Mets or 8-10 cals/min or 480-600 cals/hr.	Jogging 5 miles/hr.	Dynamic, aerobic, endurance building exercise.
	Cycling 12 miles/hr.	As above.
	Downhill skiing	Usually ski runs are too short to significantly promote endurance. Lift may be isometric. Benefits skill predominantly. Combined stress of altitude, cold and exercise may be too great for some cardiacs.
	Paddleball	Not sufficiently continuous but promotes skill. Competition and hot playing areas may be dangerous to cardiacs.
8.0-9.0 Mets or 10-11 cals/min or 600-660 cals/hr.	Running 5.5 miles/hr.	Excellent conditioner.
	Cycling 13 miles/hr.	As above.
	Squash or handball (practice session or warmup)	Usually too intermittent to provide endurance building effect. Promotes skill.
Above 10 Mets or 11 cals/min or 660 cals/hr.	Running 6 miles/hr=10 Mets 7 miles/hr=11.5 8 miles/hr=13.5	Excellent conditioner.
	Competitive handball or squash	Competitive environment in a hot room is dangerous to anyone not in excellent physical condition. Same as singles tennis.

*Met=multiple of the resting energy requirement: for example, 2 Mets require twice the resting energy cost. 3 Mets triple, and so on.

Note: Energy range will vary depending on skill of exerciser, pattern of rest pauses, environmental temperature, and so on. Caloric values depend on body size (more for larger person). Table provides reasonable "relative strenuousness values."

Source: Lenore R. Zohman, *Beyond Diet . . . Exercise Your Way to Fitness and Heart Health* (Best Foods, 1979), pp. 20-21.

The contribution of tennis to wellness, however, is another matter. As we've so often stated in this book, even if your physical health is improved, if the other components of your health suffer you have not improved your health. Playing tennis may improve the efficiency of your heart, but if your attitude and behavior on the court loses you friends, results in your not enjoying youself, or frustrates you, you would be better off not playing at all. In spite of exercising, you are making yourself *less well*. Two answers seem to make the most sense to us: Approach tennis with a different attitude, or select a less competitive exercise to engage in regularly.

When stroking the ball, if you roll over the shot too much (too much top-spin), you can contribute to tennis elbow. Using too much wrist in the shot will lead you to roll over; instead, you should stroke through the ball with your wrist locked. If tennis elbow does develop, you can switch to a lighter racket to aggravate the elbow less. Applying ice after playing will also help.

A warmup that includes stretching is a must. Tennis involves dynamic, quick movements with a great deal of stretching to reach the ball. Therefore, if you are not flexible enough, you may be prone to muscle and connective tissue injury, such as muscle pulls or sprained ligaments.

Racketball, Handball, and Squash

In Chapter 8 we discussed the risk of eye injury from racketball, handball, and squash. To decrease this risk, you need to wear an eye protector made of polycarbonate.

Another risk involved in these sports relates to the environment in which they are played. To exercise in a hot room can be hazardous unless you take certain precautions. You should drink plenty of water before starting to play and intermittently take breaks to replenish the water you lose through perspiration. You should not play longer than you are in condition to play; to overdo it in a hot room can be risky. Know when to stop.

Last, you must be in good physical condition before engaging in these sports. Since they are highly competitive, since they are usually played in a hot environment, and since they involve dynamic (stop and go) and stretching movements, if you are not in good physical condition you may injure yourself. If you *are* in good condition, these sports are excellent activities to help you remain fit.

Aerobic Dance

One of the best fitness activities is dance, especially if you're serious about your training. Look at the bodies of dancers. They are remarkably muscularly developed, incredibly supple, and ready to meet the demands strenuous exercise places on their hearts, circulatory systems, and respiratory systems. Dance is one good way to develop and maintain physical fitness.

The traditional dance programs were tap, ballet, and modern dance. In recent years a different form of dance has swept the country and become a significant part of the fitness movement. This form of dance combines calisthenics and a variety of dance movements, all done to music, and is called *aerobic dance*. The term, coined by Jacki Sorenson (1979), involves choreographed routines that include walking, jumping, hopping, bouncing, kicking, and various arm movements designed to develop cardiorespiratory endurance, flexibility, and muscular strength and endurance. What's more, it's fun. Dancing to music is an enjoyable activity for many people who would not otherwise seek to exercise. And since aerobic dance is often done in groups, the social contact makes it even more enjoyable.

To maximize the fitness benefits of aerobic dance, you should maintain the dancing for approximately 35 to 45 minutes and work out three or four times a week. In addition, you should check periodically to see if you are maintaining your target heart rate. Since many communities offer aerobic dance classes (some may be called Dancercize or Jazzercise) through YM/YWCAs, colleges, and local schools, and even on morning television programs, maintaining a regular dance regimen should not be difficult. The only equipment you will need is a good pair of aerobic dance shoes with good shock absorbency, stability, and outer sole flexibility (Ocker and Rosenbaum, 1986) and clothes to work out in. One caution: Don't dance on a concrete floor, since the constant pounding could result in shin splints. A wooden floor is ideal.

Low-Impact Aerobics

Several factors associated with aerobic dance has led some experts to question the manner in which it is usually conducted. A study by the American Aerobics Association found 80 percent of its teachers and students were getting injured during workouts, and another questionnaire administered to aerobics instructors found 55 percent reported significant injuries (Rosenbaum, 1984). Among the causes of these injuries are bad floors (too hard), bad shoes (too little shock absorbency and stability), and bad routines offered by poorly trained instructors (Schwinn, 1986). With the popularity of aerobics, it is not surprising what is done in its name. Even a "pet aerobics" routine has been developed for that pudgy dog or cat. It is therefore no surprise that many aerobics instructors are poorly trained and teach routines that are inappropriate and injury-producing, using surfaces which result in high-impact injuries.

To respond to these concerns, several developments have occurred. One is the certification of aerobics instructors. Organizations such as the American College of Sports Medicine, the Aerobics and Fitness Association of America, International Dance and Exercise Association, Ken Cooper's Aerobics Way, and the Aerobic Center have all instituted certification for aerobics instructors. Unfortunately, the requirements for certification by these organizations vary greatly. However, some form of certification is probably better than none.

Another attempt at limiting the injuries from aerobics is the development of *low-impact* aerobic routines. Low-impact aerobics features one foot on the ground at all times and the use of light weights. The idea is to cut down on the stress to the body caused by jumping and bouncing while at the same time deriving the muscle toning and cardiorespiratory benefits of high-impact aerobics. These routines have become more and more popular as the risk of injury from high-impact aerobics has become better known. Something called "chair aerobics" has even been developed (Green, 1986). It involves routines done while seated in a chair. However, low impact aerobics is not risk free. Injuries to the upper body caused by the circling and swinging movements with weights are not infrequent (Weldon, 1986). However, many of these injuries can be treated at home and are not serious. With any form of physical activity there is always the chance of injury. However, the benefits to the cardiorespiratory system and the rest of the body—benefits that we have described in this book—are often worth the slight chance of injury.

Bicycling

We have discussed bicycling in Chapter 8, so its presentation here will be brief. However, mention should be made of certain precautions bicyclers should take when incorporating cycling into their exercise routines. First and foremost is to follow the guidelines presented in Chapter 8 regarding selecting equipment which is both safe and effective in enhancing fitness and wellness. That includes the bike itself, a helmet, gloves, pants clips, and any clothes specific to bicycling you choose to wear. When biking, keep your elbows slightly bent, lower your upper body for a streamlined position, don't grip the handle bars too tightly, wear bright clothing so motorists can easily see you, obey traffic laws, always lean into the turn, learn hand signals that indicate which way you are turning, and leave the Walkman radio at home since you should be focused on the road (Vaz, 1986). Following these rules should help to ensure your bicycling is done both safely and in a manner in which you will derive maximum physical fitness benefits.

CONCLUSION: SOME LAST WORDS ON WELLNESS

- To be well, pay attention to your body. If you do, you will know when it is doing fine, and when it needs special care.
- Pay attention to your mind. When choosing an activity to include in your fitness routine, choose one that is enjoyable, one you look forward to doing. Not only will this improve the chances of your continuing that activity, it will also increase your wellness by making you feel good.
- Pay attention to your spirit too. Gain spiritual health from your fitness selections. Feel closer to nature or to a Supreme Being. Feel connected to your past and your future. To do so is to move toward high-level wellness.
- Be aware of the effects of your fitness choices on your mental and social health. Do your choices add to your knowledge? To your learning? Do they improve your relationships or help you establish new ones?
- Remember, improving one component of your health to the neglect of the others is not being well. Wellness is coordinating and integrating your physical fitness activities with the mental, social, emotional, and spiritual parts of your life.

We can think of no better image to leave you with than that of the Special Olympics—althetic competition for the mentally and physically handicapped. These athletes try their best, train long and hard, and feel good about participating and competing. What better example of wellness is there? The learning (mental health) that must precede the competition, the good feelings developed between athletes and their coaches and competitors (social health), the satisfaction derived from trying one's best (emotional health), and the sense of oneness and closeness developed in competition (spiritual health), not to mention the physical fitness level needed to participate in the first place (physical health), evidences the wellness of these competitors. They may not be totally healthy, but they certainly are WELL.

We wish for all of you the same degree of wellness, and we hope this book helps you to achieve it.

SUMMARY

1. Walking and jogging are excellent ways to keep fit. They can improve cardiorespiratory performance, enhance muscular strength and endurance, and can be a spiritual experience if one pays attention to the birds, trees, and clouds. Participating with a friend can also respond to social health needs.

2. Before beginning to walk or jog, warm up; afterward, cool down. Flexibility exercises should be an integral part of the warmup and cooldown.

3. When running for exercise, wear training shoes which have heavy, cushioned soles and arch supports; light-colored clothing; lightweight clothing in the heat and layered clothing in the cold; and something on the head when it's either cold or hot and sunny.

4. The proper running style includes running in an upright position, carrying the arms slightly away from the body with elbows bent so the forearms are parallel to the ground, landing on the heel and rocking forward, keeping the stride relatively short, and breathing deeply with an open mouth.

5. Rope jumping can be an excellent physical fitness exercise. To jump rope properly, determine the best length for the rope, keep the arms close to the body with elbows touching the sides, don't tense up, keep the body erect, start slowly, land on the balls of the feet, and maintain a steady rhythm.

6. Swimming can enhance physical fitness by lap swimming or by participating in exercise in limited water areas. Such exercises may include standing water drills, pool-side standing drills, gutter-holding drills, bobbing, or treading in water.

7. For tennis to enhance wellness as well as physical fitness, the competitive aspect of the game must not be exaggerated. In addition, to prevent tennis elbow, don't roll over the shot too much by using too much wrist. Rather, stroke through the ball with the wrist locked.

8. Racketball, handball, and squash should all be played wearing eye protectors made of polycarbonate. In addition, plenty of water ought to be drunk before starting to play and intermittent breaks should be taken so more water can be ingested.

9. Aerobic dance is a popular fitness activity that can improve cardiorespiratory endurance, and muscular strength and endurance and can help to maintain proper body weight. To maximize the fitness benefits of aerobic dance, the routine ought to be maintained approximately 40 minutes and be done three or four times per week.

10. Low-impact aerobics developed in response to the number of injuries experienced by high-impact aerobic exercisers. Low-impact aerobics features one foot on the ground at all times and the use of light weights.

11. When bicycling as part of a fitness program, use safe and effective equipment, keep the elbows slightly bent, lower the upper body for a streamlined position, don't grip the handlebars too tightly, wear bright clothing, and obey traffic rules.

REFERENCES

AMERICAN HEART ASSOCIATION. *Jump for the Health of It.* Dallas, TX: American Heart Association, 1983.

AMERICAN PODIATRY ASSOCIATION. *Jogging Advice from Your Podiatrist.* Washington, DC: American Podiatry Association, undated.

GREEN, T. "My Favorite Routine: Chair Aerobics." *Shape*, June 1986, 150–53.

KATZ, J. "The W.E.T. Workout: A Swimmers Guide to Water Exercise Techniques." *Shape*, June 1986, 82–88ff.

PRESIDENT'S COUNCIL ON PHYSICAL FITNESS AND SPORTS. *Aqua Dynamics.* Washington, DC: President's Council on Physical Fitness and Sports, 1981.

PRESIDENT'S COUNCIL ON PHYSICAL FITNESS AND SPORTS. *An Introduction to Physical Fitness.* Washington, DC: President's Council on Physical Fitness and Sports, 1980.

PRESIDENT'S COUNCIL ON PHYSICAL FITNESS AND SPORTS. *An Introduction to Running.* Washington, DC: President's Council on Physical Fitness and Sports, 1980.

ROSENBAUM, J. "Aerobics Without Injury." *Medical Self-Care*, Fall 1984, 30–33.

SCHWINN, B. "Burned in Pursuit of the Burn." *Washington Post, Health*, August 14, 1986, 12.

SORENSON, J. *Aerobic Dancing.* New York: Rawson, Wade, 1979.

U.S. CONSUMER PRODUCTS SAFETY COMMISSION. *National Electronic Injury Surveillance System.* Bethesda, MD: National Injury Information Clearinghouse, 1976.

VAZ, K. "Shifting to Two Wheels." *Washington Post, Health*, October 7, 1986, 12–14.

WELDON, G. "The ABC's of Aerobics Injuries." *Shape*, September 1986, 86–90ff.

Appendix A:
Weight Regulation
and Nutrition

WIDELY PUBLICIZED DIETS: AN EVALUATION

Diet	Special Claims	Allowable Foods	Evaluation
Gimmick Diets Pritikin Program	Low-fat and exercise combine to produce weight loss.	Whole grains, vegetables, legumes, fruit; snack on raw vegetables all day and 1 portion from dairy, grain, and fruit groups.	High fiber content causes gas and diarrhea; protein is insufficient; difficult to follow; contains one-quarter normal fat intake; fairly well rounded; devoid of cholesterol, salt, and artificial sweeteners.
Save Your Life Diet	Fiber in foods leads to weight loss which increases by rapid transport of food through the digestive tract	Vegetable group emphasized, and 1 cup of bran added to six foods; meats and eggs deemphasized.	Side effects may include flatulence; frequent defecation; and soft, bulky stools. Too much fiber binds to some trace minerals and may cause them to pass through the system without being absorbed.
Nibbling Diet	Eating smaller portions will result in fewer calories than eating three meals per day and snacking.	Low-carbohydrate, high-protein, and nutritious snacking.	With careful calorie counting, weight loss is likely to occur, but difficult to get a balanced diet, and not easy to follow for long periods of time.
Cellulite Diet	Promises removal of the "fat gone wrong" (so-called fat, water, and toxic wastes).	High in fruits and vegetables, low fat and carbohydrate intake; involves kneading the skin, massage under heat lamps to melt the fat away.	No medical condition known as cellulite exists. The fat being described as cellulite cannot be eliminated by a combination of diet and massage.
Cooper's Fabulous Fructose Diet	"Fructose" (sugar from fruit) is used to help lose weight, maintain constant blood-sugar level, keep up energy, and satisfy the sweet tooth.	High protein intake and 1.0 to 1.5 oz. fructose supplement.	Weight loss may occur from caloric deficit, not from use of a fructose supplement. Fructose does not help you consume fewer calories and contains the same number of calories as sucrose (4 per gram).
Lecithin, Vinegar, Kelp, and B6 Diet	Grapefruit and lecithin burn off fat by regulating metabolic rate.	One teaspoon of vinegar with each meal of normal foods.	No one claim (grapefruit or vinegar) can be supported.

Diet	Special Claims	Allowable Foods	Evaluation
The Body Clock Diet	When you eat is nearly twice as important as the number of calories you consume. Lose by eating "breakfast like a king, lunch like a prince, and dinner like a pauper."	Any type of food can be consumed or any diet adapted to the body clock diet.	There is no convincing evidence that eating the big meals early in the day will cause significant weight loss without very close calorie counting. The somewhat hidden implication that calories don't count is inaccurate.
High-Protein Diets Women Doctor's Diet for Women New You Diet Doctor's Quick Weight Loss Diet Complete Scarsdale Medical Diet Miracle Diet for Fast Weight Loss	"Specific Dynamic Action" (SDA) is the basis for some high-protein diets: extra calories burned through the process of digesting protein.	Lean meats and poultry, fish, seafood, eggs, and low-fat cheese, no calorie counting.	SDA has no basis. Protein calories are no more or less important than carbohydrate calories. Diets are boring; hard to follow; lacking in vitamins, minerals, and fiber; and can increase blood serum cholesterol levels; dangerous for pregnant women and a poor choice for anyone who wants weight loss to be permanent after a change in eating habits. Ketosis can be dangerous to *some people.*
High-Fat Diets Dr. Atkins Super Energy Diet Calories Don't Count Diet	In the absence of carbohydrates, stored fat is mobilized and burned for energy. Fat-mobilizing hormone (FMH) is said to be activated to fuel your body with the fat stores.	Unlimited fatty foods: bacon, meat, mayonnaise, rich cream sauces, etc. No calorie counting and avoidance of fruits, vegetables, sugars, starches, bread, and potatoes.	Carbohydrates are needed to oxidize fat completely. If in short supply, fat cannot be used completely and fatigue occurs. Ketone bodies build up in the blood and are excreted in the urine. The existence of a fat-mobilizing hormone has never been substantiated. The diet neglects the four food groups, is dangerous for pregnant women, and is high in cholesterol. Most weight loss is water, which is temporary.

Diet	Special Claims	Allowable Foods	Evaluation
Low Carbohydrate Diets Diet of a Desperate Housewife The Drinking Man's Diet No Breakfast Diet Dr. Yudkin's Lose Weight, Feel Great Diet The Brand New Carbohydrate Diet	Claims are similar to those for high-protein diets: a state of ketosis provides a condition conducive to fat loss.	Protein in unlimited amounts with few or no carbohydrates permitted.	Most weight loss is water, and temporary fatigue results from insufficient carbohydrate intake. Ketosis is potentially dangerous over prolonged periods of time. These diets fail to provide adequate foods from the basic four food groups and are difficult to follow.
One Food Diets Grapefruit, egg, poultry, melon, banana, steak, beer, fruit, juice, yogurt, rice, etc.	Dieters must concentrate on the food they choose, use a multiple vitamin, and drink plenty of fluid.	Only the one food is permissible.	Impossible to obtain the proper nourishment, even with the vitamin supplement, boring and nearly impossible to follow. Fails to change eating habits, short-term approach. Potentially very dangerous because it it impossible to obtain proper nutrition from the four food groups.
Pill Diets Appetite suppressants: Anorexiants (amphetamines, Dexedrine, Digitilis)	Appetite is depressed; metabolism is increased.	Medication is designed to restrict total caloric intake. Often used in conjunction with specific diets.	Anorexiants curb appetite and increase metabolic rate. Nervousness, depression, and dependence (physical and mental) are some of the possible side effects.
Metabolic medication: Thyroid hormone	Increases metabolic rate and energy output to burn more calories. Promotes breakup of lipids.	Used in conjunction with numerous diets.	No evidence is available to support the breakup of lipids. Additional calories are burned as metabolic rate increases. Thyroid hormone induces a stage of hyperthyroidism and is dangerous to people with heart disease. It also disrupts the entire endocrine system.
Diuretics: Thiazides	Excess body fluid is lost.	Used in conjunction with numerous diets. Additional potassium is needed* to replace that lost through fluid.	Does not increase caloric expenditure. Fluid loss is unrelated to fat and permanent weight loss. Can cause dehydration, nausea, weakness, and drowsiness.

Diet	Special Claims	Allowable Foods	Evaluation
Cathartics (laxatives)	Speeds food through the intestine so nutrients are not absorbed.	Used in conjunction with numerous diets.	May result in bowel difficulty, dehydration, and poor nutrition. Not an effective method of weight loss.
Nonprescription drugs: Sugar candy	Curbs appetite when taken prior to meal.	Used in conjunction with numerous diets.	Only mildly effective. Claims of advertisements are not met.
Benzocaine and methylcellulose	Deadens taste buds to kill hunger and provides a feeling of fullness in stomach.	Used in conjunction with numerous diets.	The amount that can be legally sold is not enough to be effective.
Starvation and Fasting Diets The Zip Diet Lockjaw Zen Macrobiotic Diet Liquid Protein Diet	Diets eliminate practically everything but liquids. Jaws wired shut (lockjaw diet) to aid will power. With no calories from chewable foods, weight loss will occur rapidly.	Liquids and some foods.	Extremely dangerous; lacking in vitamins, minerals, roughage. Anemia is likely. The Liquid Protein Diet may have caused over 60 deaths. Weight loss is dramatic at first, then slows considerably, even though you are consuming practically no calories. Quality of weight loss is poor. Too much loss of lean muscle mass, along with fat loss, keeps you flabby.
Vegetarian Diets Vegetarian	Reduction in animal fats and cholesterol and less likelihood of excess body fat and heart disease.	Only foods of plant origin, including seeds, grains, nuts fruits, and vegetables.	Studies in the United States indicate that vegetarians have heart attacks 10 years later in life than meat eaters. An excellent, healthy way to lose weight and keep it off.
Lacto-vegetarian		Foods of plant origin, plus foods made of milk (yogurt, cheese, and cream).	The diet is safe, providing sufficient protein, iron, calcium, and vitamin B12 can be consumed (an iron and B12 supplement may be needed).
Lacto-ovo-vegetarian		All plant foods, plus dairy products and eggs.	Have your physician confirm that you do not have a peptic ulcer or other inflammation of the digestive tract. On the negative side, the new habits of cooking, purchasing, and eating are not easy to follow at first.

Source: George B. Dintiman and Jerrold S. Greenberg, *Health Through Discovery*. New York: Random House, 1986, pp. 179-182.

CALORIE EXPENDITURE PER MINUTE FOR VARIOUS ACTIVITIES

Body Weight in Pounds

Activity	90	99	108	117	125	134	143	152	161	170	178	187	196	205	213	222	231	240	249	257	266	275
Archery	3.1	3.4	3.7	4.0	4.5	4.6	4.9	5.2	5.5	5.8	6.1	6.4	6.7	7.0	7.3	7.6	7.9	8.2	8.5	8.8	9.1	9.4
Badminton (recreation)	3.4	3.8	4.1	4.4	4.8	5.1	5.4	5.6	6.1	6.4	6.8	7.1	7.4	7.8	8.1	8.3	8.8	9.1	9.4	9.8	10.1	10.4
Badminton (competition)	5.9	6.4	7.0	7.6	8.1	8.7	9.3	9.9	10.4	11.0	11.6	12.1	12.7	13.3	13.9	14.4	15.0	15.6	16.4	16.7	17.3	17.9
Baseball (player)	2.8	3.1	3.4	3.6	3.9	4.2	4.5	4.7	5.0	5.3	5.5	5.8	6.1	6.4	6.6	6.9	7.2	7.5	7.7	8.0	8.3	8.6
Baseball (pitcher)	3.5	3.9	4.3	4.6	5.0	5.3	5.7	6.0	6.4	6.7	7.1	7.4	7.8	8.1	8.5	8.8	9.2	9.5	9.9	10.2	10.6	10.9
Basketball (half-court)	2.5	3.3	3.5	3.8	4.1	4.4	4.7	4.9	5.3	5.6	5.9	6.2	6.4	6.7	7.0	7.3	7.5	7.6	8.2	8.5	8.8	9.0
Basketball (moderate)	4.2	4.6	5.0	5.5	5.9	6.3	6.7	7.1	7.5	7.9	8.3	8.8	9.2	9.6	10.0	10.4	10.8	11.2	11.6	12.1	12.5	12.9
Basketball (competition)	5.9	6.5	7.1	7.7	8.2	8.8	9.4	10.0	10.6	11.1	11.7	12.3	12.9	13.5	14.0	14.6	15.0	15.2	16.3	16.9	17.5	18.4
Bicycling (level) 5.5 mph	3.0	3.3	3.6	3.9	4.2	4.5	4.8	5.1	5.4	5.6	5.9	6.2	6.5	6.8	7.1	7.4	7.7	8.0	8.3	8.6	8.9	9.0
Bicycling (level) 13 mph	6.4	7.1	7.7	8.3	8.9	9.6	10.2	10.8	11.4	12.1	12.7	13.4	14.0	14.6	15.2	15.9	16.5	17.1	17.8	18.4	19.0	19.6
Bowling (nonstop)	4.0	4.4	4.8	5.2	5.6	5.9	6.3	6.7	7.1	7.5	7.9	8.3	8.7	9.1	9.5	9.8	10.2	10.6	11.0	11.4	11.8	12.2
Boxing (sparring)	3.0	3.3	3.6	3.9	4.2	4.5	4.8	5.1	5.4	5.6	5.9	6.2	6.5	6.8	7.1	7.4	7.7	8.0	8.3	8.6	8.9	9.2
Calisthenics	3.0	3.3	3.6	3.9	4.2	4.5	4.8	5.1	5.4	5.6	5.9	6.2	6.5	6.8	7.1	7.4	7.7	8.0	8.3	8.6	8.9	9.2
Canoeing, 2.5 mph	1.8	1.9	2.0	2.2	2.3	2.5	2.7	3.0	3.2	3.4	3.6	3.7	3.9	4.1	4.7	4.4	4.6	4.8	5.0	5.1	5.3	5.5
Canoeing, 4.0 mph	4.2	4.6	5.0	5.5	5.9	6.3	6.7	7.1	7.5	7.9	8.3	8.7	9.2	9.4	10.0	10.5	10.8	11.2	11.6	12.0	12.4	12.9

Body Weight in Pounds

Activity	90	99	108	117	125	134	143	152	161	170	178	187	196	205	213	222	231	240	249	257	266	275
Dance, modern (moderate)	2.5	2.8	3.0	3.2	3.5	3.7	4.0	4.2	4.5	4.7	5.0	5.2	5.4	5.7	5.9	6.2	6.4	6.7	6.9	7.2	7.4	7.6
Dance, modern (vigorous)	3.4	3.7	4.1	4.4	4.7	5.1	5.4	5.7	6.1	6.4	6.7	7.1	7.4	7.7	8.1	8.4	8.7	9.1	9.4	9.7	10.1	10.4
Dance, fox-trot	2.7	2.9	3.2	3.4	3.7	4.0	4.2	4.5	4.7	5.0	5.3	5.5	5.8	6.0	6.3	6.6	6.8	7.1	7.3	7.6	7.9	8.1
Dance, rumba	4.2	4.6	5.0	5.4	5.8	6.2	6.6	7.0	7.4	7.8	8.2	8.6	9.0	9.4	9.8	10.2	10.6	11.0	11.5	11.9	12.3	12.6
Dance, square	4.1	4.5	4.9	5.3	5.7	6.1	6.5	6.9	7.3	7.8	8.1	8.5	8.9	9.3	9.7	10.1	10.5	10.9	11.3	11.7	12.1	12.4
Dance, Waltz	3.1	3.4	3.7	4.0	4.3	4.6	4.9	5.2	5.5	5.8	6.1	6.4	6.7	7.0	7.3	7.6	7.9	8.2	8.5	8.8	9.1	9.4
Fencing (moderate)	3.0	3.3	3.6	3.9	4.2	4.5	4.8	5.1	5.4	5.6	6.0	6.2	6.5	6.8	7.1	7.4	7.7	8.0	8.3	8.6	8.9	9.2
Fencing (vigorous)	6.2	6.8	7.4	8.0	8.6	9.2	9.8	10.4	11.0	11.6	12.2	12.8	13.4	14.0	14.6	15.2	15.8	16.4	17.0	17.6	18.2	18.8
Football (moderate)	3.0	3.3	3.6	4.0	4.2	4.5	4.8	5.1	5.4	5.7	6.0	6.2	6.5	6.8	7.1	7.4	7.7	8.0	8.3	8.6	8.9	9.2
Football (vigorous)	5.0	5.5	6.0	6.4	6.9	7.4	7.9	8.4	8.9	9.4	9.8	10.3	10.8	11.3	11.8	12.3	12.8	13.2	13.7	14.2	14.7	15.2
Golf, two-some	3.3	3.6	3.9	4.2	4.5	4.8	5.2	5.5	5.8	6.1	6.4	6.7	7.1	7.4	7.7	8.0	8.3	8.6	9.0	9.3	9.6	10.0
Golf, four-some	2.4	2.7	2.9	3.2	3.4	3.6	3.9	4.1	4.3	4.6	4.8	5.1	5.3	5.5	5.8	6.0	6.2	6.5	6.7	7.0	7.2	7.4
Handball	5.9	6.4	7.0	7.6	8.1	8.7	9.3	9.9	10.4	11.0	11.6	12.1	12.7	13.3	13.9	14.4	15.0	15.6	16.1	16.7	17.3	17.9
Hiking, 40 lb. pack, 3.0 mph	4.1	4.5	4.9	5.3	5.7	6.1	6.5	6.9	7.3	7.7	8.1	8.5	8.9	9.3	9.7	10.1	10.5	10.9	11.3	11.7	12.1	12.5
Horseback riding (walk)	2.0	2.3	2.4	2.6	2.8	3.0	3.1	3.3	3.5	3.7	3.9	4.1	4.3	4.5	4.7	4.9	5.1	5.3	5.5	5.7	5.8	6.0
Horseback riding (trot)	4.1	4.4	4.8	5.2	5.6	6.0	6.4	6.8	7.2	7.6	8.0	8.4	8.8	9.2	9.6	10.0	10.4	10.8	11.2	11.6	12.0	12.4
Horseshoe pitching	2.1	2.3	2.5	2.7	3.0	3.3	3.4	3.6	3.8	4.0	4.2	4.4	4.6	4.8	5.0	5.2	5.4	5.6	5.8	6.0	6.3	6.5
Judo, karate	7.7	8.5	9.2	10.0	10.7	11.5	12.2	13.0	13.7	14.5	15.2	16.0	16.7	17.5	18.2	19.0	19.7	20.5	21.2	22.0	22.7	23.5
Mountain climbing	6.0	6.5	7.2	7.8	8.4	9.0	9.6	10.1	10.7	11.3	11.9	12.5	13.1	13.7	14.3	14.8	15.4	16.0	16.6	17.2	17.8	18.4
Paddleball, racquetball	5.9	6.4	7.0	7.6	8.1	8.7	9.3	9.9	10.4	11.0	11.6	12.1	12.7	13.3	13.9	14.4	15.0	15.6	16.4	16.7	17.3	17.9
Pool, billiards	1.1	1.2	1.3	1.4	1.5	1.6	1.7	1.8	1.9	2.0	2.1	2.2	2.4	2.5	2.6	2.7	2.8	2.9	3.0	3.1	3.2	3.3

Body Weight in Pounds

Activity	90	99	108	117	125	134	143	152	161	170	178	187	196	205	213	222	231	240	249	257	266	275
Rowing (recreation)	3.0	3.3	3.6	3.9	4.2	4.5	4.8	5.1	5.4	5.6	6.0	6.2	6.5	6.8	7.1	7.5	7.7	8.0	8.3	8.6	8.9	9.2
Rowing (machine)	8.2	9.0	9.8	10.6	11.4	12.2	13.0	13.8	14.6	15.4	16.2	17.0	17.8	18.6	19.4	20.2	21.0	21.8	22.6	23.4	24.2	25.0
Running, 11-min. mile (5.5 mph)	6.4	7.1	7.7	8.3	9.0	9.6	10.2	10.8	11.5	12.1	12.7	13.4	14.0	14.6	15.2	15.9	16.5	17.1	17.8	18.4	19.0	19.6
Running, 8.5-min. mile (7 mph)	8.4	9.2	10.0	10.8	11.7	12.5	13.3	14.1	14.9	15.7	16.6	17.4	18.2	19.0	19.8	20.7	21.5	22.3	23.1	23.9	24.8	25.6
Running 7-min. mile (9 mph)	9.3	10.2	11.1	12.9	13.1	13.9	14.8	15.7	16.6	17.5	18.9	19.3	20.2	21.1	22.1	22.0	23.9	24.8	25.7	26.6	27.5	28.4
Running, 5-min. mile (12 mph)	11.8	13.0	14.1	15.3	16.4	17.6	18.7	19.9	21.0	22.2	23.3	24.5	25.6	26.8	27.9	29.1	30.2	31.4	32.5	33.7	34.9	36.0
Stationary running (140 counts/min.)	14.6	16.1	17.5	18.9	20.4	21.8	23.2	24.6	26.1	27.5	28.9	30.4	31.8	33.2	34.6	36.1	37.5	38.9	40.4	41.8	43.2	44.6
Sprinting	13.8	15.2	16.6	17.9	19.2	20.5	21.9	23.3	24.7	26.1	27.3	28.7	30.0	31.4	32.7	34.0	35.4	36.8	38.2	39.4	40.3	42.2
Sailing	1.8	2.0	2.1	2.3	2.4	2.7	2.8	3.0	3.2	3.4	3.6	3.8	3.9	4.1	4.3	4.4	4.6	4.8	5.0	5.1	5.3	5.5
Skating (moderate)	3.4	3.8	4.1	4.4	4.8	5.1	5.4	5.8	6.1	6.4	6.8	7.1	7.4	7.8	8.1	8.3	8.8	9.1	9.4	9.8	10.1	10.4
Skating (vigorous)	6.2	6.8	7.4	8.0	8.6	9.2	9.8	9.9	11.0	11.6	12.2	12.8	13.4	14.0	14.6	15.2	15.8	16.4	17.0	17.6	18.2	18.8
Skiing (downhill)	5.8	6.4	6.9	7.5	8.1	8.6	9.2	9.8	10.3	10.9	11.4	12.0	12.6	13.1	13.7	14.3	14.8	15.4	16.0	16.5	17.1	17.7
Skiing (level, 5 mph)	9.9	10.9	11.9	12.9	13.7	14.7	15.7	16.7	17.7	18.7	19.6	20.6	21.6	22.6	23.4	24.4	25.4	26.4	27.4	28.3	29.3	30.2

Body Weight in Pounds

Activity	90	99	108	117	125	134	143	152	161	170	178	187	196	205	213	222	231	240	249	257	266	275
Snowshoeing (2.3 mph)	3.7	4.1	4.5	4.8	5.2	5.5	5.9	6.3	6.7	7.0	7.4	7.8	8.1	8.5	8.8	9.2	9.6	9.9	10.3	10.6	11.0	11.4
Snowshoeing (2.5 mph)	5.4	5.9	6.5	7.0	7.5	8.0	8.6	9.1	9.7	10.2	10.7	11.2	11.8	12.3	12.8	13.3	13.9	14.4	14.9	15.4	16.0	16.5
Soccer	5.4	5.9	6.4	6.9	7.5	8.0	8.5	9.0	9.6	10.1	10.6	11.1	11.6	12.2	12.7	13.2	13.4	14.3	14.8	15.3	15.8	16.9
Squash	6.2	6.8	7.5	8.1	8.7	9.3	9.9	10.5	11.1	11.7	12.3	12.9	13.5	14.2	14.8	15.4	16.0	16.6	17.2	17.8	18.4	19.0
Swimming, pleasure (25 yds./min.)	3.6	4.0	4.3	4.7	5.0	5.4	5.7	6.1	6.4	6.8	7.1	7.5	7.8	8.2	8.5	8.9	9.2	9.6	10.0	10.3	10.6	11.0
Swimming, back (20 yds./min.)	2.3	2.6	2.8	3.0	3.2	3.5	3.7	3.9	4.1	4.2	4.6	4.8	5.0	5.3	5.5	5.7	6.0	6.2	6.4	6.6	6.9	7.4
Swimming, back (30 yds./min.)	3.2	3.5	3.8	4.1	4.4	4.7	5.1	5.4	5.7	6.0	6.3	6.6	6.9	7.2	7.4	7.9	8.2	8.5	8.8	9.3	9.4	9.7
Swimming, back (40 yds./min.)	5.0	5.5	5.8	6.5	7.0	7.5	7.9	8.5	8.9	9.4	9.9	10.4	10.9	11.4	11.9	12.3	12.8	13.3	13.8	14.3	14.8	15.3
Swimming, breast (20 yds./min.)	2.9	3.2	3.4	3.8	4.0	4.3	4.6	4.9	5.1	5.4	5.7	6.0	6.3	6.5	6.8	7.1	7.4	7.7	7.9	8.2	8.5	8.8
Swimming, breast (30 yds./min.)	4.3	4.8	5.2	5.7	6.0	6.4	6.9	7.3	7.7	8.1	8.6	9.0	9.4	9.9	10.3	10.8	11.1	11.5	11.9	12.4	13.0	13.3
Swimming, breast (40 yds./min.)	5.8	6.3	6.9	7.5	8.0	8.6	9.2	9.7	10.3	10.8	11.4	12.0	12.5	13.1	13.7	14.2	14.8	15.4	15.9	16.5	17.0	17.6
Swimming, butterfly (50 yds./min.)	7.0	7.7	8.4	9.1	9.8	10.5	11.1	11.9	12.5	13.2	13.9	14.6	15.2	15.9	16.6	17.3	18.0	18.7	19.4	20.0	20.7	21.4

Body Weight in Pounds

Activity	90	99	108	117	125	134	143	152	161	170	178	187	196	205	213	222	231	240	249	257	266	275
Swimming, crawl (20 yds./min.)	2.9	3.2	3.4	3.8	4.0	4.3	4.6	4.9	5.1	5.4	5.7	5.8	6.3	6.5	6.8	7.1	7.3	7.7	7.9	8.2	8.5	8.8
Swimming, crawl (45 yds./min.)	5.2	5.8	6.3	6.8	7.3	7.8	8.3	8.8	9.3	9.8	10.4	10.9	11.4	11.9	12.4	12.9	13.4	13.9	14.4	15.0	15.5	16.0
Swimming, crawl (50 yds./min.)	6.4	7.0	7.6	8.3	8.9	9.5	10.1	10.7	11.4	12.0	12.6	13.2	13.9	14.5	15.1	15.7	16.3	17.0	17.4	17.9	18.8	19.5
Table tennis	2.3	2.6	2.8	3.0	3.2	3.5	3.7	3.9	4.1	4.2	4.6	4.8	5.0	5.3	5.5	5.7	6.0	6.2	6.4	6.6	6.9	7.4
Tennis (recreation)	4.2	4.6	5.0	5.4	5.8	6.2	6.6	7.0	7.4	7.8	8.2	8.6	9.0	9.4	9.8	10.2	10.6	11.0	11.5	11.9	12.3	12.6
Tennis (competition)	5.9	6.4	7.0	7.6	8.1	8.7	9.3	9.9	10.4	11.0	11.6	12.1	12.7	13.3	13.9	14.4	15.0	15.6	16.4	16.7	17.3	17.9
Timed calisthenics	8.8	9.6	10.5	11.4	12.2	13.1	13.9	14.8	15.6	16.5	17.4	18.2	19.1	19.9	20.8	21.5	22.5	23.9	24.2	25.1	25.9	26.8
Volleyball (moderate)	3.4	3.8	4.0	4.4	4.8	5.1	5.4	5.8	6.1	6.4	6.8	7.1	7.4	7.8	8.1	8.3	8.8	9.1	9.4	9.8	10.4	10.4
Volleyball (vigorous)	5.9	6.4	7.0	7.6	8.1	8.7	9.3	9.9	10.4	11.0	11.6	12.1	12.7	13.3	13.9	14.4	15.0	15.6	16.4	16.7	17.3	17.9
Walking (2.0 mph)	2.1	2.3	2.5	2.7	2.9	3.1	3.3	3.5	3.7	4.0	4.2	4.4	4.6	4.8	5.0	5.2	5.4	5.6	5.8	6.0	6.2	6.4
Walking (4.5 mph)	4.0	4.4	4.7	5.1	5.5	5.9	6.3	6.7	7.1	7.5	7.8	8.2	8.6	9.0	9.4	9.8	10.1	10.6	10.9	11.3	11.7	12.0
Walking 110–120 steps/min.	3.1	3.4	3.7	4.0	4.3	4.7	5.0	5.3	5.6	5.9	6.2	6.5	6.8	7.1	7.4	7.7	8.0	8.3	8.6	8.9	9.2	9.5
Waterskiing	4.7	5.1	5.6	6.1	6.5	7.0	7.4	7.9	8.3	8.8	9.3	9.7	10.2	10.6	11.1	11.5	12.0	12.5	12.9	13.4	13.8	14.3
Weight training	4.7	5.1	5.7	6.2	6.7	7.0	7.5	7.9	8.4	8.9	9.4	9.9	10.3	10.8	11.1	11.7	12.2	12.6	13.4	13.5	14.0	14.4
Wrestling	7.7	8.5	9.2	10.0	10.7	11.5	12.2	13.0	13.7	14.5	15.2	16.0	16.7	17.5	18.2	19.0	19.7	20.5	21.2	22.0	22.7	23.5

Source: Adapted from Frank C. Consolazio et al. Physiological Measurements of Metabolic Functions in Man (New York: McGraw-Hill, 1963). Reprinted by permission.

Appendix B:
Physical Fitness
Information Resources

ORGANIZATIONS: PHYSICAL FITNESS AND SPORTS

Organizations for Specific Sports and Physical Fitness Activities

BASKETBALL

- Amateur Basketball Association of the United States of America (ABAUSA), 1750 East Boulder St., Colorado Springs, CO 80909. (303) 636-7687. The ABAUSA serves as the national governing body for the sport of basketball. It will respond to requests for information on its programs.

BICYCLING

- Bicycle Touring Group of America, P.O. Drawer 330976, Coconut Grove, FL 33133. (305) 661-8846. The Bicycle Touring Group is an industry-sponsored association to promote noncompetitive recreational bicycling.
- Bikecentennial, The Bicycle Travel Association, P.O. Box 8308, Missoula, MT 59807. (406) 721-1776. Bikecentennial is a national service organization for touring bicyclists. The organization's efforts are aimed at educating the public in bicycle use and safety and researching and mapping bicycle touring routes. A publications list is available and questions are answered on all aspects of bike touring.

- League of American Wheelmen, P.O. Box 988, Baltimore, MD 21203. (301) 727-2022. The League answers inquiries on topics such as where to ride, what to take along, routes, how to plan and conduct bicycle events, and safety.
- United States Cycling Federation, 1750 East Boulder St., Colorado Springs, CO 80909. (303) 632-5551. The governing body for amateur and professional cycling in the United States, and an organization concerned with the preservation, development, and administration of bicycle racing.

BOWLING

- American Bowling Congress (ABC) and Women's International Bowling Congress (WIBC), 5301 South 76th St., Greendale, WI 53129. (414) 421-6400. These two groups are the primary organizations promoting bowling for men and for women. Direct your questions on bowling to the public relations department of the appropriate organization (men should write to the ABC, and women should write to the WIBC).

DANCING

- Aerobic Dancing, Inc., 18907 Nordhoff St., Box 6600, Northridge, CA 91328. (213) 885-0032. Aerobic dancing is a fitness program originated by Jacki Sorenson, consisting of vigorous dances designed to improve physical fitness. Contact Aerobic Dancing at the address given for a location near you, or check your local telephone directory.
- Jazzercise, Inc., 2808 Roosevelt St., Carlsbad, CA 92008. (619) 434-2101. Jazzercise is a dance and fitness program of simple jazz dance movements set to a variety of music. Contact Jazzercise at the address given for classes near you.

HIKING/BACKPACKING

- Forest Service, U.S. Department of Agriculture, Information Office, P.O. Box 2417, Washington, DC 22013. (202) 447-3957. The Information Office of the Forest Service will provide a list of Forest Service field offices and addresses. It requests that inquirers contact the field offices to obtain information on recreation opportunities in the national forests.
- National Campers and Hikers Association (NCHA), 7172 Transit Rd., Buffalo, NY 14221. (716) 634-5433. The NCHA will answer questions on hiking and camping. This organization is dedicated to camping fellowships, the preservation of our natural heritage, and the strengthening of family bonds through activities in the out-of-doors.
- Sierra Club, 530 Bush St., San Francisco, CA 94108. (415) 981-8634. The Sierra Club is dedicated to the principles of wilderness conservation. The national office will answer inquiries on hiking, camping, backpacking, canoeing, and other outdoor activities.

RACQUETBALL

- American Amateur Racquetball Association (AARA), 815 North Weber St., Colorado Springs, CO 80903. (303) 635-5396. The AARA promotes the sport of racquetball and is a member of the U.S. Olympic Committee. It will respond to requests for information on racquetball.

RUNNING/JOGGING

- American Running and Fitness Association (ARFA), 2420 K St. NW, Washington, DC 20037. (202) 965-3430. The American Running and Fitness Association serves as a clearinghouse of information on running and jogging. It promotes healthful running by physically qualified people. Their Runner's Referral Service will match you with a runner of similar ability in your area. To be included in the referral service, a runner can complete an information form and file it with the ARFA.
- Road Runners Club of America (RRCA), 1226 Orchard Village, Manchester, MO 63011. (314) 391-6712. The RRCA promotes long distance running on an amateur basis. It can answer requests on organizing a running club or a running competition.

SKATING

- Ice Skating Institute of America, 1000 Skokie Blvd., Wilmette, IL 60091. (312) 256-5060. The goals of the Ice Skating Institute are to improve the ice rink business and to increase public interest in ice skating. It can respond to requests for information on ice skating.
- Roller Skating Rink Operators Association (RSROA), P.O. Box 811846, Lincoln, NE 68510. (402) 489-8811. RSROA's membership consists of almost 2,000 roller skating rinks across the country. It promotes and popularizes the sport of roller skating. Publications on skating are available, but it cannot respond to specific requests for information. These questions should be directed to your local rink.
- United States Figure Skaing Association, 20 First St., Colorado Springs, CO 80906. (303) 635-5200. The U.S. Figure Skating Association is the governing body for amateur figure skating in the United States. Information will be provided by mail on local clubs and on learning to ice skate.

SKIING

- American Water Ski Association, P.O. Box 191, Winter Haven, FL 33880. (813) 324-4341. The American Water Ski Association promotes competitive and noncompetitive water skiing in the United States. It acts as a clearinghouse for information on water skiing.

SOCCER

- United States Soccer Federation (USSF), 350 Fifth Ave., Room 4010, New York, NY 10118. (212) 736-0915. The United States Soccer Federation is the national governing body for the sport of soccer. It serves as a clearinghouse for information, publications, and audiovisuals on soccer.

SOFTBALL

- Amateur Softball Association of America, 2801 NE 50th St., Oklahoma City, OK 73111. (405) 424-5266. The Amateur Softball Association of America develops and promotes the sport of softball on an organized basis. It will answer inquiries on all aspects of softball.

SWIMMING

- International Amateur Swimming Federation (IASF), 200 Financial Center, Des Moines, IA 50309. (515) 244-1116. The IASF promotes and encourages the development of amateur swimming, diving, water polo, and synchronized swimming. It will respond to mail and telephone requests for information on swimming.
- United States Swimming, Inc. (USS), 1750 East Boulder St., Colorado Springs, CO 80909. (303) 578-4578. The USS is the national governing body for amateur competitive swimming. It offers a variety of programs geared to all levels of swimmers. It will answer requests for information on its programs.

TENNIS

- United States Tennis Association Education and Research Center, 729 Alexander Rd., Princeton, NJ 08540. (609) 452-2580. The objective of the United States Tennis Association is to develop tennis as a means of healthful recreation and physical fitness. It serves as a clearinghouse for information on recreational tennis.

VOLLEYBALL

- United States Volleyball Association, 1750 East Boulder St., Colorado Springs, CO 80909. (303) 632-5551, ext. 3331. The U.S. Volleyball Association is the national governing body for the sport of volleyball. It will refer inquirers to an appropriate regional director.

WALKING

- Walking Association, 4113 Lee Highway, Arlington, VA 22207. (703) 527-5374. The Walking Association is concerned with all matters related to walking, including its health and recreational aspects. It will respond to inquiries on walking but suggests that inquirers first check their local libraries.

Organizations for Special Groups

- American Athletic Association for the Deaf (AAAD), 3916 Lantern Dr., Silver Spring, MD 20902. (202) 224-8637. The AAAD provides physical recreation activities for members of its clubs. The group can refer a deaf person to a local club and answer inquiries on subjects pertaining to athletics for the deaf. It also promotes participation in the World Games for the Deaf.
- Blind Outdoor Leisure Development, Inc. (BOLD), 533 East Main St., Aspen, CO 81611. (303) 925-2086. BOLD is dedicated to encouraging and helping blind people engage in outdoor recreation activities such as skating, swimming, and skiing. BOLD can refer the inquirer to a local club, advise individuals interested in setting up a club, and answer questions on athletics for the blind.
- National Handicapped Sports and Recreation Association, Capitol Hill Station, P.O. Box 18664, Denver, CO 80218. (303) 978-0564. The National Handicapped Sports and Recreation Association promotes physical activities for handicapped persons as a means of enhancing physical and mental well-being and the overall quality of life. It will refer the inquirer to a local chapter for more information on becoming involved in a particular physical activity.
- National Wheelchair Athletic Association (NWAA), 2107 Templeton Gap Rd., Suite C, Colorado Springs, CO 80907. (303) 632-0698. The NWAA establishes the rules and regulations for and governs all wheelchair sports in the United States except basketball and bowling. It will answer inquiries by telephone or mail on subjects pertaining to wheelchair sports, including archery, field events, slalom, table tennis, swimming, track, and weightlifting.
- National Wheelchair Basketball Association (NWBA), 110 Seaton Bldg., University of Kentucky, Lexington, KY 40506. (606) 257-1623. The NWBA is the governing body for all teams playing in organized competition in the United States. It will respond to inquiries by telephone or mail on topics such as where a person can join a local team, rules of wheelchair basketball, and how to start a team.
- North American Riding for the Handicapped Association (NARHA), P.O. Box 100, Ashburn, VA 22011. (703) 471-1621. The NARHA promotes horsebackriding as therapeutic recreation for the handicapped and coordinates the activities of local programs. Local programs provide instruction in horseback riding and sponsor recreational events. It will direct inquiries to programs in their area.
- Special Olympics, 1701 K St. NW, Suite 203, Washington, DC 20006. (202) 331-1346. Special Olympics is the largest international program of physical fitness, sports training, and athletic competition for mentally retarded children and adults. The international headquarters, at the address given, will mail an information package that provides a general

introduction to the Special Olympics. A list of state and U.S. territory chapters is included.

- United States Association for Blind Athletes, 55 West California Ave., Beach Haven, NJ 08008. (609) 492-1017. The United States Association for Blind Athletes develops and promotes sports programs for the blind and visually impaired. The association serves as a clearinghouse of information on sports for the blind including track and field, swimming, wrestling, gymnastics, and goal ball.

Other Organizations

- American Alliance for Health, Physical Education, Recreation and Dance (AAPHERD), 1900 Association Dr., Reston, VA 22091. (703) 476-3424. AAPHERD is a voluntary education organization made up of seven national and six regional associations. Publications produced cover general physical fitness, individual sports, women's sports, safety education, recreation education, health education, and career opportunities. Materials for teaching special groups such as the handicapped and the mentally retarded are available.
- American College of Sports Medicine (ACSM), 1440 Monroe St., Madison, WI 53706. (608) 262-3632. The American College of Sports Medicine is a nonprofit multidisciplinary professional and scientific society created to generate and disseminate information concerning the responses, adaptations, and clinical aspects of the human organism engaged in exercise and in recreational and competitive sports.
- American Volkssport Association (AVA), Phoenix Square, Suite 203, 1001 Pat Booker Rd., Universal City, TX 78148. (512) 659-2112. The concept of volkssport involves walking, biking, swimming, and snow skiing events sponsored by clubs across the country. AVA-sanctioned events include noncompetitive family walks of distances between 6 and 12 miles. It will answer general questions and direct you to a club in your area.
- National Recreation and Park Association (NRPA), 3101 Park Center Dr., Alexandria, VA 22302. (703) 820-4940. The NRPA promotes the interests of the park and recreation movement. It promotes public awareness of the role of physical fitness in health, encourages recreation among the elderly, and promotes recreation services for the handicapped. It maintains an information center on park and recreation interests.
- President's Council on Physical Fitness and Sports, 450 5th St., NW, Room 7103, Washington, DC 20001. (202) 272-3430. The President's Council on Physical Fitness and Sports promotes physical fitness opportunities for Americans of all ages. It produces informational materials on exercise, school physical education programs, sports, and physical fitness for youth, adults, and the elderly.
- Women's Sport Foundation (WSF), 195 Moulton St., San Francisco, CA 94123. (415) 563-6266, (800) 227-3988, (800) 652-1455 in CA, 12:00-5:00

P.M. weekdays. The WSF was created to encourage and support the participation of women in sports; to provide opportunities, facilities, and training for women in sports; and to educate women and the public about women's athletic capabilities and the value of sports for them. It maintains an information and resource center on all women's sports and related topics.

Source: National Health Information Clearinghouse. "Selected Sources of Information on Physical Fitness and Sports," *Healthfinder*. Published by the Office of Disease Prevention and Health Promotion, U.S. Dept. of Health and Human Services, 1983.

PHYSICAL FITNESS MICROCOMPUTER SOFTWARE PROGRAMS

Body Composition
Adults, $100
Apple II, DOS 3.3; IBM-PC;
TRS-80, Model 111

Computerized Health Appraisals
13705 Southeast 142nd St.
Clackamas, OR 97015
(503) 658-5959

Determines degree of "fatness" by calculating body density and percentage of fat. Sex-specific norms and standards are shown for comparison and evaluation.

Body Composition—Skinfold
Adults, $100
Apple II, DOS 3.3;
IBM-PC; TRS-80, Model III

Computerized Health Appraisals
13705 Southeast 142nd St.
Clackamas, OR 97015
(503) 658-5959

Determines body fat through skinfold measurements, using the multiple regression equations developed by Drs. Gettman and Pollock.

Fitlog
Adults, $150
Apple II, DOS 3.3;
TRS-80, Model III

Computerized Health Appraisals
13705 Southeast 142nd St.
Clackamas, OR 97015
(503) 658-5959

Calculates the amount of exercise a person has performed, including distance and time, and then shows the number of calories expended. This program is most useful in exercise classes, where a summary of the week's or month's activities is desired.

Fitness Profile
Adults, $150-$250
Apple II, DOS 3.3; IBM-PC;
TRS-80; Model III

Computerized Health Appraisals
13705 Southeast 142nd St.
Clackamas, OR 97015
(503) 658-5959

Generates a report giving results from fitness testing, including body fat, height and weight, grip strength, dynamic muscle strength, flexibility, balance, lung function, and aerobic capacity. Gives recommended values and a personalized exercise prescription.

Healthpath
Adults, health professionals, 3,000
IBM-PC; Datapoint Minicomputer

Healthpath
68 Olive St.
Chagrin Falls,OH 44022
(216) 247-5298

Allows users to determine personal caloric requirements and fitness levels and then recommends an exercise regimen. Designed to be used by participants in fitness clubs, this system also has a program for club managers which includes components for word processing and for managing membership information.

Heart and Exercise
Junior high—adults, $30
Apple II with Applesoft, DOS 3.3

Project REACT
66 Malcolm Ave. SE
Minneapolis, MN 55414
(612) 379-0428

Instructs the student on how the heart works and how exercise affects it. A teacher utility program generates tests and worksheets.

Inshape
Adults, $95
IBM-PC with 80-column monitor,
DOS 1.0/1.1 with 64K, DOS 2.0
with 96K

DEG Software
11999 Kay Freeway, Suite 150
Houston,TX 77079
(713) 531-6100

Analyzes carbohydrate, fat, protein and calorie content of foods, using an uncoded database of over 1800 items. Calculates point values for over 24 aerobic exercises and can plot 60-day and 52-week summaries.

Physical Evaluation Program (PEP)
Senior high—adults, $98
Apple IIe, II plus; TRS-80, Model I
or III; PET or Commodore 64
with emulator; Atari

Educational Activities
P.O. Box 392
Freeport, NY 11520
(800) 645-3739; (516) 223-4666

Assesses physical condition, prescribes exercise, and monitors progress. A teacher's guide, 20 student manuals, and an audiocassette are included. (By Bob Antonacci)

Physical Fitness
Junior high—adults, $29.95
TI-99/4A

Texas Instruments
Box 10508
Lubbock, TX 79408
(800) 858-4565

Allows user to design a personal exercise program based on guidelines from the President's Council on Physical Fitness and Sports.

Response Time
Elementary—adults, $20
Apple II with Applesoft

Andent
1000 North Ave.
Waukegan, IL 60085
(312) 244-0292

Checks reaction and response time, measuring alertness and motor coordination. Can be used to determine effects of alcohol and drugs.

Step Test   Computerized Health Appraisals
Adults, $100   13705 Southeast 142nd St.
Apple II, DOS 3.3; TRS-80, Model III   Clackamas, OR 97015
                                             (503) 658-5959

Calculates maximal oxygen uptake from results of an exercise test, shows maximum levels reached and energy expended, and records pulse and blood pressure recovery rates. It then assigns a fitness category.

Source: National Health Information Clearinghouse. "Health Promotion Software," *Healthfinder*. Published by the Office of Disease Prevention and Health Promotion, U.S. Department of Health and Human Services, 1983.

Appendix C:
Preventing Heat Injuries During Distance Running

THE AMERICAN COLLEGE OF SPORTS MEDICINE POSITION STATEMENT

Based on research findings and current rules governing distance running competition, it is the position of the American College of Sports Medicine that:

1. Distance races (>16 km or 10 miles) should *not* be conducted when the wet bulb temperature—globe temperature* exceeds 28° C (82.4° F). (1, 2)
2. During periods of the year, when the daylight dry bulb temperature often exceeds 27° C (80°F), distance races should be conducted before 9:00 A.M. or after 4:00 P.M. (2, 7, 8, 9)
3. It is the responsibility of the race sponsors to provide fluids which contain small amounts of sugar (less than 2.5 g glucose per 100 ml of water) and electrolytes (less than 10 mEq sodium and 5 mEq potassium per liter of solution). (5, 6)
4. Runners should be encouraged to ingest fluids frequently during competition and to consume 400–500 ml (13–17 oz.) of fluid 10–15 minutes before competition. (5, 6, 9)
5. Rules prohibiting the administration of fluids during the first 10 kilometers (6.2 miles) of a marathon race should be amended to permit fluid ingestion at frequent intervals along the race course. In light of the

---

*Adapted from D. Minard, "Prevention of Heat Casualties in Marine Corps Recruits." *Milit. Med.* 126 (1961); 261, WB-GT = 0.7 (WBT) +0.2 (GT) +0.1 (DBT)

high sweat rates and body temperatures during distance running in the heat, race sponsors should provide "water stations" at 3–4 kilometer (2–2.5 mile) intervals for all races of 16 kilometers (10 miles) or more. (4, 8, 9)

6. Runners should be instructed in how to recognize the early warning symptoms that precede heat injury. Recognition of symptoms, cessation of running, and proper treatment can prevent heat injury. Early warning symptoms include the following: piloerection on chest and upper arms, chilling, throbbing pressure in the head, unsteadiness, nausea, and dry skin. (2, 9)

7. Race sponsors should make prior arrangements with medical personnel for the care of cases of heat injury. Responsible and informed personnel should supervise each "feeding station." Organizational personnel should reserve the right to stop runners who exhibit clear signs of heat stroke or heat exhaustion.

It is the position of the American College of Sports Medicine that policies established by local, national, and international sponsors of distance running events should adhere to these guidelines. Failure to adhere to these guidelines may jeopardize the health of competitors through heat injury.

Research Support

1. ADOLPH, E. F. *Physiology of Man in the Desert*. New York: Interscience, 1947.

2. BUSKIRK, E. R., AND W. C. GRASLEY. "Heat Injury and Conduct of Athletes." In W. R. Johnson and E. R. Buskirk (eds.), *Science and Medicine of Exercise and Sport*, 2nd ed., Ch. 16. New York: Harper & Row, 1974.

3. BUSKIRK, E. R., P. F. IAMPIETRO, AND D. E. BASS. "Work Performance After Dehydration: Effects of Physical Conditioning and Heat Acclimatization." *J. Appl. Physiol.* 12 (1958): 189–94.

4. COSTILL, D. L., W. F. KAMMER, AND A. FISHER. "Fluid Ingestion During Distance Running." *Arch. Environ. Health* 21 (1970): 520–25.

5. COSTILL, D. L., AND B. SALTIN. "Factors Limiting Gastric Emptying During Rest and Exercise." *J. Appl. Physiol.* 37 (1974): 679–83.

6. FORDTRAN, J. A., AND B. SALTIN. "Gastric Emptying and Intestinal Absorption During Prolonged Severe Exercise." *J. Appl. Physiol.* 23 (1967): 331–35.

7. MYHRE, L. G. "Shifts in Blood Volume During and Following Acute Environmental and Work Stresses in Man," Doctoral dissertation. Indiana University, Bloomington, 1967.

8. PUGH, L. G. C., J. I. CORBETT, AND R. H. JOHNSON. "Rectal Temperatures, Weight Losses, and Sweating Rates in Marathon Running." *J. Appl. Physiol.* 23 (1957): 347–53.

9. WYNDHAM, C. H., AND N. B. STRYDOM. "The Danger of an Inadequate Water Intake During Marathon Running. *S. Afr. Med. J.* 43 (1969): 893–98.

Appendix D:
The Recommended Quantity and Quality of Exercise for Developing and Maintaining Fitness in Healthy Adults

AMERICAN COLLEGE OF SPORTS MEDICINE POSITION STATEMENT

Increasing numbers of persons are becoming involved in endurance training activities and thus, the need for guidelines for exercise prescription is apparent. Based on the existing evidence concerning exercise prescription for healthy adults and the need for guidelines, the American College of Sports Medicine makes the following recommendations for the quantity and quality of training and developing and maintaining cardiorespiratory fitness and body composition in the healthy adult:

1. Frequency of training: 3 to 5 days per week.
2. Intensity of training: 60 to 90 percent of maximum heart rate reserve or, 50 to 85 percent of maximum oxygen uptake (Vo_2 max).
3. Duration of training: 15 to 60 minutes of continuous aerobic activity. Duration is dependent on the intensity of the activity, thus lower-intensity activity should be conducted over a longer period of time. Because of the importance of the "total fitness" effect and the fact that it is more readily attained in longer-duration programs, and because of the potential hazards and compliance problems associated with high-

intensity activity, lower- to moderate-intensity activity of longer duration is recommended for the nonathletic adult.

4. Mode of activity: Any activity that uses large muscle groups, that can be maintained continuously, and is rhythmical and aerobic in nature, for example, running-jogging, walking-hiking, swimming, skating, bicycling, rowing, cross-country skiing, rope skipping, and various endurance game activities.

Rationale and Research Background

The questions, "How much exercise is enough and what type of exercise is best for developing and maintaining fitness?" are frequently asked. It is recognized that the term "physical fitness" is composed of a wide variety of variables included in the broad categories of cardiovascular-respiratory fitness, physique and structure, motor function, and many histochemical and biochemical factors. It is also recognized that the adaptive response to training is complex and includes peripheral, central, structural, and functional factors. Although many such variables and their adaptive response to training have been documented, the lack of sufficient in-depth and comparative data relative to frequency, intensity, and duration of training make them inadequate to use as comparative models. Thus, in respect to the foregoing questions, fitness will be limited to changes in Vo_2 max, total body mass, fat weight (FW), and lean body weight (LBW) factors.

Exercise prescription is based upon the frequency, intensity, and duration of training, the mode of activity (aerobic in nature, for example, listed under 4), and the initial level of fitness. In evaluating these factors, the following observations have been derived from studies conducted with endurance training programs.

1. Improvement in Vo_2 max is directly related to frequency (2, 23, 32, 58, 59, 65, 77, 79), intensity (2, 10, 13, 26, 33, 37, 42, 56, 77), and duration (3, 14, 29, 49, 56, 77, 86) of training. Depending upon the quantity and quality of training, improvement in Vo_2 max ranges from 5 to 25 percent (4, 13, 27, 31, 35, 36, 43, 45, 52, 53, 62, 71, 77, 78, 82, 86). Although changes in Vo_2 max greater than 25% have been shown, they are usually associated with large total body mass and FW loss, or a low initial level of fitness. Also, as a result of leg fatigue or a lack of motivation, persons with low initial fitness may have spuriously low initial Vo_2 max values.

2. The amount of improvement in Vo_2 max tends to plateau when frequency of training is increased above 3 days per week (23, 62, 65). For the non-athlete, there is not enough information available at this time to speculate on the value of added improvement found in programs that are conducted more than 5 days per week. Participation of less than two days per week does not show an adequate change in Vo_2 max (24, 56, 62).

3. Total body mass and FW are generally reduced with endurance training programs (67), while LBW remains constant (62, 67, 87) or increases

slightly (54). Programs that are conducted at least 3 days per week (58, 59, 61, 62, 87), of at least 20 minutes duration (48, 62, 87) and of sufficient intensity and duration to expend approximately 300 kilocalories (kcal) per exercise session are suggested as a threshold level for total body mass and FW loss (12, 29, 62, 67). An expenditure of 200 kcal per session has also been shown to be useful in weight reduction if the exercise frequency is at least 4 days per week (80). Programs with less participation generally show little or no change in body composition (19, 25, 42, 62, 67, 84, 85, 87). Significant increases in V_{O2} max have been shown with 10 to 15 minutes of high-intensity training (34, 49, 56, 62, 77, 78); thus, if total body mass and FW reduction is not a consideration, then short-duration, high-intensity programs may be recommended for healthy, low-risk (cardiovascular disease) persons.

4. The minimal threshold level for improvement in V_{O2} max is approximately 60 percent of the maximum heart rate reserve (50 percent of V_{O2} max) (33, 37). Maximum heart rate reserve represents the percent difference between resting and maximum heart rate, added to the resting heart rate. The technique as described by Karvonen, Kentala, and Mustala (37) was validated by Davis and Convertino (14) and represents a heart rate of approximately 130 to 135 beats/minute for young persons. As a result of the aging curve for maximum heart rate, the absolute heart rate value (threshold level) is inversely related to age, and can be as low as 110 to 120/beats/minute for older persons. Initial level of fitness is another important consideration in prescribing exercise (10, 40, 46, 75, 77). The person with a low fitness level can get a significant training effect with a sustained training heart rate as low as 110 to 120 beats/minute, while persons of higher fitness levels need a higher threshold of stimulation (26).

5. Intensity and duration of training are interrelated with the total amount of work accomplished being an important factor in improvement in fitness (2, 7, 12, 40, 61, 62, 76, 78). Although more comprehensive inquiry is necessary, present evidence suggests that when exercise is performed above the minimal threshold of intensity, the total amount of work accomplished is the important factor in fitness development (2, 7, 12, 61, 62, 76, 79) and maintenance (68). That is, improvement will be similar for activities performed at a lower intensity–longer duration compared to higher intensity–shorter duration if the total energy cost of the activities is equal.

If frequency, intensity, and duration of training are similar (total kcal expenditure), the training result appears to be independent of the mode of aerobic activity (56, 60, 62, 64). Therefore, a variety of endurance activities, already listed, may be used to derive the same training effect.

6. To maintain the training effect exercise must be continued on a regular basis (2, 6, 11, 21, 44, 73, 74). A significant reduction in working capacity occurs after 2 weeks of detraining (73) with participants returning to near pretraining levels of fitness after 10 weeks (21) to 8 months of detraining

(44). Fifty percent reduction in improvement of cardiorespiratory fitness has been shown after 4 to 12 weeks of detraining (21, 41, 73). More investigation is necessary to evaluate the rate of increase and decrease of fitness with varying training loads and reduction in training in relation to level of fitness, age, and length of time in training. Also, more information is needed to identify better the minimal level of work necessary to maintain fitness.

7. Endurance activities that require running and jumping generally cause significantly more debilitating injuries to beginning exercisers than other nonweight-bearing activities (42, 55, 69). One study showed that beginning joggers had increased foot, leg, and knee injuries when training was performed more than 3 days per week and longer than 30 minutes duration per exercise session (69). Thus, caution should be taken when recommending the type of activity and exercise prescription for the beginning exerciser. Also, the increase of orthopedic injuries as related to overuse (marathon training) with chronic jogger-runners is apparent. Thus, there is a need for more inquiry into the effect that different types of activities and the quantity and quality of training has on short-term and long-term participation.

8. Most of the information concerning training described in this position statement has been conducted on men. The lack of information on women is apparent, but the available evidence indicates that women tend to adapt to endurance training in the same manner as men (8, 22, 89).

9. Age in itself does not appear to be a deterrent to endurance training. Although some earlier studies showed a lower training effect with middle-aged or elderly participants (4, 17, 34, 83, 86), more recent study shows the relative change in Vo_2 max to be similar to younger age groups (3, 52, 66, 75, 86). Although more investigation is necessary concerning the rate of improvement in Vo_2 max with age, at present it appears that elderly participants need longer periods of time to adapt to training (17, 66). Earlier studies showing moderate to no improvement in Vo_2 max were conducted over a short timespan (4) or exercise was conducted at a moderate to low kcal expenditure (17), thus making the interpretation of the results difficult.

   Although Vo_2 max decreases with age, and total body mass and FW increase with age, evidence suggests that this trend can be altered with endurance training (9, 12, 38, 39, 62). Also 5- to 10-year follow-up studies where participants continued their training at a similar level showed maintenance of fitness (39, 70). A study of older competitive runners showed decreases in Vo_2 max from the fourth to seventh decade of life, but also showed reductions in their training load (62). More inquiry into the relationship of long-term training (quantity and quality) for both competitors and noncompetitors and physiological function with increasing age, is necessary before more definitive statements can be made.

10. An activity such as weight training should not be considered as a means of training for developing Vo_2 max, but has significant value for increasing muscular strength and endurance, and LBW (16, 24, 47, 49, 88). Recent studies evaluating circuit weight training (weight training conducted almost continuously with moderate weights, using 10 to 15 repetitions per exercise session with 15 to 30 seconds rest between bouts of activity) showed little to no improvements in working capacity and Vo_2 max (1, 24, 90).

Despite an abundance of information available concerning the training of the human organism, the lack of standardization of testing protocols and procedures, methodology in relation to training procedures and experimental design, a preciseness in the documentation and reporting of the quantity and quality of training prescribed, make interpretation difficult (62, 67). Interpretation and comparison of results are also dependent on the initial level of fitness (18, 74–76, 81), length of time of the training experiment (20, 57, 58, 61, 62), and specificity of the testing and training (64). For example, data from training studies using subjects with varied levels of Vo_2 max, total body mass and FW have found changes to occur in relation to their initial values (5, 15, 48, 50, 51); that is the lower the initial Vo_2 max, the larger the percent of improvement found and the higher the FW the greater the reduction. Also data evaluating trainability with age, comparison of the different magnitudes and quantities of effort, and comparison of the trainability of men and women may have been influenced by the initial fitness levels.

In view of the fact that improvement in the fitness variables discussed in this position statement continue over many months of training (12, 38, 39, 62), it is reasonable to believe that short-term studies conducted over a few weeks have certain limitations. Middle-aged sedentary and older participants may take several weeks to adapt to the initial rigors of training, and thus need a longer adaptation period to get the full benefit from a program. How long a training experiment should be conducted is difficult to determine, but 15 to 20 weeks may be a good minimum standard. For example, two investigations conducted with middle-aged men who jogged either 2 or 4 days per week found both groups to improve in Vo_2 max. Midtest results of the 16- and 20-week programs showed no difference between groups, while subsequent final testing found the 4-day per week group to improve significantly more (58, 59). In a similar study with young college men, no differences in Vo_2 max were found among groups after 7 and 13 weeks of interval training (20). These latter findings and those of other investigators point to the limitations in interpreting results from investigations conducted over a short time span (62, 67).

In summary, frequency, intensity and duration of training have been found to be effective stimuli for producing a training effect. In general, the lower the stimuli, the lower the training effect (2, 12, 13, 27, 35, 46, 77, 78, 90), and the greater the stimuli, the greater the effect (2, 12, 13, 27, 58, 77, 78). It has also been shown that endurance training less than two days per week, less than 50% of maximum oxygen uptake, and less than 10 minutes per day is inadequate for developing and maintaining fitness for healthy adults.

References

1. ALLEN, T.E., R.J. BYRD AND D.P. SMITH. Hemodynamic consequences of circuit weight training. *Res. Q.*43:299-306,1976.
2. AMERICAN COLLEGE OF SPORTS MEDICINE. *Guidelines for Graded Exercise Testing and Exercise Prescription,* Philadelphia. Lea and Febiger, 1976.
3. BARRY, A.J., J.W. DALY, E.D.R. PRUETT, J.R. STEINMETZ, H.F. PAGE, N.C. BIRKHEAD AND K. RODAHL. The effects of physical conditioning on older individuals. I. Work Capacity circulatory-respiratory function, and work electrocardiogram. *J. Gerontol.* 21:182-91, 1966.
4. BENSETAD, A.M. Trainability of old men. *Acta Med. Scandinav.* 178:321-27, 1965.
5. BOILEAU, R.A., E.R. BUSKIRK, D.H. HORTSMAN, J. MENDEZ AND W.C. NICHOLAS. Body composition changes in obese and lean men during physical conditioning. *Med. Sci. Sports* 3:183-89, 1971.
6. BRYNTESON, P. AND W.E. SINNING. The effects of training frequencies on the retention of cardiovascular fitness. *Med. Sci. Sports* 5:29-33, 1973.
7. BURKE, E.J. AND B.D. FRANKS. Changes in Vo_2 max resulting from bicycle training at different intensities holding total mechanical work constant. *Res. Q.* 46:31-37, 1975.
8. BURKE, E.J. Physiological effects of similar training programs in males and females. *Res. Q.* 48-510-17, 1977.
9. CARTER, J.E.L. AND W.H. PHILLIPS. Structural changes in exercising middle-aged males during a 2-year period. *J. Appl. Physiol.* 27:787-94, 1969.
10. CREWS, T.R. AND J.A. ROBERTS. Effects of interaction of frequency and intensity of training. *Res. Q.* 47:48-55, 1976.
11. CURETON, T.K. AND E.E. PHILLIPS. Physical fitness changes in middle-aged men attributable to equal eight-week periods of training, non-training and retraining. *J. Sports Med. Phys. Fitness* 4:1-7, 1964
12. CURETON, T.K. *The Physiological Effects of Exercise Programs upon Adults.* Springfield C. Thomas Company, 1969.
13. DAVIES, C.T.M. AND A.V. KNIBBS. The training stimulus, the effects of intensity, duration and frequency of effort on maximum aerobic power output. *Int. Z. Angew. Physiol.* 29:299-305, 1971.
14. DAVIS, J.A. AND V.A. CONVERTINO. A comparison of heart rate methods for predicting endurance training intensity. *Med. Sci. Sports* 7:295-98, 1975.
15. DEMPSEY, J.A. Anthropometrical observations on obese and non-obese young men undergoing a program of vigorous physical exercise. *Res. Q.*35:275-87, 1964.
16. DELORME, T.L. Restoration of muscle power by heavy resistance exercise. *J. Bone and Joint Surgery* 27:645-67, 1945.

17. DEVRIES, H.A. Physiological effects of an exercise training regimen upon men aged 52 to 88. *J. Gerontol.* 24:325-36, 1970.
18. EKBLOM, B. P.O. Astrand, B. Saltin, J. Sternberg and B. Wallstrom. Effect of training on circulatory response to exercise. *J. Appl. Physiol.* 24:518-28, 1968.
19. FLINT, M.M. B.L. DRINKWATER AND S.M. HORVATH. Effects of training on women's response to submaximal exercise. *Med. Sci. Sports* 6:89-94, 1974.
20. FOX, E.L. R.L. BARTELS. C.E. Billings, R. O'Brien, R. Bason and D.K. Mathews. Frequency and duration of interval training programs and changes in aerobic power. *J. Appl. Physiol.* 38:481-84, 1975.
21. FRINGER, M.N. AND A.G. STULL. Changes in cardiorespiratory parameters during periods of training and detraining in young female adults. *Med. Sci. Sports* 6:20-25, 1974.
22. GETCHELL, L.H. AND J.C. MOORE. Physical training: comparative responses of middle-aged adults. *Arch. Phys. Med. Rehab.* 56:250-54, 1975.
23. GETTMAN, L.R., M.L. POLLOCK, J.L., DURSTINE, A. WARD, J. AYRES AND A. C. LINNERUD. Physiological responses of men to 1, 3, and 5 day per week training programs. *Res. Q.* 47:638-46, 1976.
24. GETTMAN, L.R., J. AYRES, M.L. POLLOCK, J.L. DURSTINE AND W. GRANTHAM. Physiological effects of circuit strength training and jogging on adult men. *Arch. Phys. Med. Rehab.* In press.
25. GIRANDOLA, R.N. Body composition changes in women. Effects of high and low exercise intensity. *Arch. Phys. Med. Rehab.* 57:297-300, 1976.
26. GLIEDHILL, N. AND R.B. EYNON. The intensity of training. In A. W. Taylor and M. L. Howell (editors). *Training Scientific Basis and Application.* Springfield: Charles C. Thomas, pp. 97-102, 1972.
27. GOLDING, L. Effects of physical training upon total serum cholesterol levels. *Res. Q.* 32:499-505, 1961.
28. GOODE, R.C., A. VIRGIN, T.T. ROMET, P. CRAWFORD, J. DUFFIN, T. PALLANDI AND Z. WOCH. Effects of a short period of physical activity in adolescent boys and girls. *Canad. J. Appl. Sports Sci.* 1:241-50, 1976.
29. GWINUP, G. Effect of exercise alone on the weight of obese women. *Arch. Int. Med.* 135:676-80, 1975.
30. HANSON, J.S., B.S. TABAKIN, A.M. LEVY AND W. NEDDE. Long-term physical training and cardiovascular dynamics in middle-aged men. *Circulation* 38:783-99, 1968.
31. HARTLEY, L.H., G. GRIMBY, A. KILBOM, N.J. NILSSON, I. ASTRAND, J. BJURE, B. EKBLOM AND B. SALTIN. Physical training in sedentary middle-aged and older men. *Scand. J. Clin. Lab. Invest.* 24:335-44, 1969.
32. HILL, J.S. The effects of frequency in exercise on cardiorespiratory fitness of adult men. M.S. Thesis, Univ. of Western Ontario, London, 1969.
33. HOLLMANN, W. AND H. VENRATH. Experimentelle Untersuchungen zur bedeutung eines trainings unterhalb und oberhalb der dauerbeltz stungsgranze. In: Korbs (editor). *Carl Diem Festschrift.* W. u.a. Frankfurt/Wein, 1962.

34. HOLLMANN, W. Changes in the capacity for maximal and continuous effort in relation to age. *Int. Res. Sport Phys. Ed.* (E. Joki and E. Simon, editors) Springfield: C.C. Thomas Co., 1964.

35. HUIBREGTSE, W.H., H.H. HARTLEY, L.R. JONES, W.D. DOOLITTLE AND T.L. CRIBLEZ. Improvement of aerobic work capacity following non-strenuous exercise. *Arch. Env. Health,* 27:12-15, 1973.

36. ISMAIL, A.H., D. CORRIGAN AND D.F. MCLEOD. Effect of an eight-month exercise program on selected physiological, biochemical, and audiological variables in adult men. *Brit. J. Sports Med.* 7:230-40, 1973.

37. KARVONEN, M., K. KENTALA AND O. MUSTALA. The effects of training heart rate: a longitudinal study. *Ann. Med. Exptl. Biol. Fenn.* 35:307-15, 1957.

38. KASCH, F.W., W.H. PHILLIPS, J.E.L. CARTER AND J.L. BOYER. Cariovascular changes in middle-aged men during two years of training. *J. Appl. Physiol.* 314:53-57, 1972.

39. KASCH, F.W. AND J. P. WALLACE. Physiological variables during 10 years of endurance exercise. *Med. Sci Sports* 8:5-8, 1976.

40. KEARNEY, J.T., A.G. STULL, J.L. EWING AND J.W. STREIN. Cardiorespiratory responses of sedentary college women as a function of training intensity. *J. Appl. Physiol.* 41:822-25, 1976.

41. KENDRICK, Z.B., M.L. POLLOCK, T.N. HICKMAN AND H.S. MILLER. Effects of training and detraining on cardiovascular efficiency. *Amer. Corr. Ther. J.* 25:79-83, 1971.

42. KILBOM, A., L. HARTLEY, B. SALTIN, J. BJURE, G. GRIMBY AND I. ASTRAND. Physical training in sedentary middle-aged and older men. *Scand. J. Clin. Lab. Invest.* 24:315-22, 1969.

43. KNEHR, C.A., D.B. DILL AND W. NEUFELD. Training and its effect on man at rest and at work. *Amer. J. Physiol.* 136:148-56, 1942.

44. KNUTTGEN, H.G., L.O. NORDESJO, B. OLLANDER AND B. SALTIN. Physical conditioning through interval training with young male adults. *Med. Sci. Sports* 5:220-26, 1973.

45. MANN, G.V., L.H. GARRETT, A. FARHI, H. MURRAY, T.F. BILLINGS, F. SHUTE AND S.E. SCHWARTEN. Exercise to prevent coronary heart disease. *Amer. J. Med.* 46:12-27, 1969.

46. MARIGOLD, E.A. The effect of training at predetermined heart rate levels for sedentary college women. *Med. Sci. Sports* 6:14-19, 1974.

47. MAYHEW, J.L. AND P.M. GROSS. Body composition changes in young women with high resistance weight training. *Res. Q.* 45:433-39, 1974.

48. MILESIS, C.A., M.L. POLLOCK, M.D. BAH, J.J. AYRES, A. WARD AND A.C. LINNERUD. Effects of different durations of training on cardiorespiratory function, body composition and serum lipids. *Res. Q.* 47:716-725, 1976.

49. MISNER, J.E., R.A. BOILEAU, B.H. MASSEY AND J.H. MAYHEW. Alterations in body composition of adult men during selected physical training programs. *J. Amer. Geriatr. Soc.* 22:33-38, 1974.

50. MOODY, D.L., J. KOLLIAS AND E.R. BUSKIRK. The effect of a moderate exercise program on body weight and skinfold thickness in overweight college women. *Med. Sci. Sports* 1:75-80, 1969.

51. MOODY, D.L., J.H. WILMORE, R.N. GIRANDOLA AND J.P. ROYCE. The effects of a jogging program on the body composition of normal and obese high school girls. *Med. Sci. Sports* 4:210-13, 1972.

52. MYRHE, L., S. ROBINSON, A. BROWN AND F. PYKE. Paper presented to the American College of Sports Medicine, Albuquerque, New Mexico, 1970.

53. NAUGHTON, J. AND F. NAGLE. Peak oxygen intake during physical fitness and program for middle-aged men. *JAMA* 191:899-901, 1965.

54. O'HARA, W., C. ALLEN AND R.J. SHEPHARD. Loss of body weight and fat during exercise in a cold chamber. *Europ. J. Appl. Physiol.* 37:205-18, 1977.

55. OJA, P., P. TERASLINNA, T. PARTANER AND R. KARAVA. Feasibility of an 18 months' physical training program for middle-aged men and its effect on physical fitness. *Am. J. Public Health* 64:459-65, 1975.

56. OLREE, H.D., B. CORBIN, J. PENROD AND C. SMITH. Methods of achieving and maintaining physical fitness for prolonged space flight. Final Progress Rep. to NASA, Grant No. NGR-04-002-004, 1969.

57. OSCAI, L.B., T. WILLIAMS AND B. HERTIG. Effects of exercise on blood volume. *J. Appl. Physiol.* 24:622-24, 1968.

58. POLLOCK, M.L., T.K. CURETON AND L. GRENINGER. Effects of frequency of training on working capacity, cardiovascular function, and body composition of adult men. *Med. Sci. Sports* 1:70-74, 1969.

59. POLLOCK, M.L., J. TIFFANY, L. GETTMAN, R. JANEWAY AND H. LOFLAND. Effects of frequency of training on serum lipids, cardiovascular function, and body composition. In: *Exercise and Fitness* (B.D. Franks, ed.). Chicago: Athletic Institute, 1969, pp. 161-78.

60. POLLOCK, M.L., H. MILLER, R. JANEWAY, A.C. LINNERUD, B. ROBERTSON AND R. VALENTINO. Effects on walking on body composition and cardiovascular function of middle-aged men. *J. Appl. Physiol.* 30: 126-30, 1971.

61. POLLOCK, M.L., J. BROIDA, Z. KENDRICK, H.S. MILLER, R. JANEWAY AND A.C. LINNERUD. Effects of training two days per week at different intensities on middle-aged men. *Med. Sci. Sports* 4:192-97, 1972.

62. POLLOCK, M.L. The quantification of endurance training program. *Exercise and Sport Sciences Reviews*. (J. Wilmore, editor). New York: Academic Press, pp. 155-88, 1973.

63. POLLOCK, M.L., H.S. MILLER, JR. AND J. WILMORE. Physiological characteristics of champion American track athletes 40 to 70 years of age. *J. Gerontol.* 29:645-49, 1974.

64. POLLOCK, M.L., J. DIMMICK, H.S. MILLER, Z. KENDRICK AND A.C. LINNERUD. Effects of mode of training on cardiovascular function and body composition of middle-aged men. *Med. Sci. Sports* 7:139-45, 1975.

65. POLLOCK, M.L., H.S. MILLER, A.C. LINNERUD AND K.H. COOPER. Frequency of training as a determinant for improvement in cardiovascular function and body composition of middle-aged men. *Arch. Phys. Med. Rehab.* 56:141-45, 1975.

66. POLLOCK, M.L., G.A. DAWSON, H.S. MILLER, JR., A. WARD, D. COOPER, W. HEADLY, A.C. LINNERUD AND M.M. NOMEIR. Physiologic response of men

49 to 65 years of age to endurance training. *J. Amer. Geriatr. Soc.* 24:97-104, 1976.

67. POLLOCK, M.L. AND A. JACKSON. Body composition: measurement and changes resulting from physical training. Proceedings of the National College Physical Education Association for Men and Women, pp. 125-37, January, 1977.

68. POLLOCK, M.L., J. AYRES AND A. WARD. Cardiorespiratory fitness: Response to differing intensities and durations of training. *Arch. Phys. Med. Rehab.* 58:467-73, 1977.

69. POLLOCK, M.L., L.R. GETTMAN, C.A. MILESIS, M.D. BAH, J.L. DURSTINE AND R.B. JOHNSON. Effects of frequency and duration of training on attrition and incidence of injury. *Med. Sci. Sports* 9:31-36, 1977.

70. POLLOCK, M.L., H.S. MILLER AND P.M. RIBISL. Body composition and cardiorespiratory fitness in former athletes. *Phys. Sports, Med.,* 1978.

71. RIBISL, P.M. Effects of training upon the maximal oxygen uptake of middle-aged men. *Int. Z. Angew. Physiol.* 26:272-78, 1969.

72. ROBINSON, S. AND P.M. HARMON. Lactic acid mechanism and certain properties of blood in relation to training. *Amer. J. Physiol.* 132:757-69, 1941.

73. ROSKAMM, H. Optimum patterns of exercise for healthy adults. *Canad. Med. Ass. J.* 96:895-99, 1967.

74. SALTIN, B., G. BLOMQVIST, J. MITCHELL, R.L. JOHNSON, K. WILDENTHAL AND C.B. CHAPMAN. Response to exercise after bed rest and after training. *Circulation* 37 and 38, Supp. 7, 1-78, 1968.

75. SALTIN. B., L. HARTLEY, A. KILBOM AND I. ASTRAND. Physical training in sedentary middle-aged and older men. *Scand. J. Clin. Lab. Invest.* 24:323-34, 1969.

76. SHARKEY, B.J. Intensity and duration of training and the development of cardiorespiratory endurance. *Med. Sci. Sports* 2:197-202, 1970.

77. SHEPHARD, R.J. Intensity, duration, and frequency of exercise as determinants of the response to a training regime. *Int. Z. Angew. Physiol.* 26:272-78, 1969.

78. SHEPHARD, R.J. Future research on the quantifying of endurance training. *J. Human Ergology* 3:163-81, 1975.

79. SIDNEY, K.H., R.B. EYNON AND D.A. CUNNINGHAM. Effect of frequency of training of exercise upon physical working performance and selected variables representative of cardiorespiratory fitness. In: *Training Scientific Basis and Application* (A.W. Taylor, ed.). Springfield: C.C. Thomas, Co., pp. 144-88, 1972.

80. SIDNEY, K.H., R.J. SHEPHARD AND J. HARRISON. Endurance training and body composition of the elderly. *Amer. J. Clin. Nutr.* 30:326-33, 1977.

81. SIEGEL, W., G. BLOMQVIST AND J.H. MITCHELL. Effects of a quantitated physical training program on middle-aged sedentary males. *Circulation* 41:19, 1970.

82. SKINNER, J., J. HOLLOSZY AND T. CURETON. Effects of a program of endurance exercise on physical work capacity and anthropometric measurements of fifteen middle-aged men. *Amer. J. Cardiol.* 14:747-52, 1964.

83. SKINNER, J. The cardiovascular system with aging and exercise. In: Brunner, D. and E. Jokl (editors). *Physical Activity and Aging*. Baltimore: University Park Press, 1970, pp. 100-108.

84. SMITH, D.P. AND F.W. STRANSKY. The effect of training and detraining on the body composition and cardiovascular response of young women to exercise. *J. Sports Med.* 16:112-20, 1976.

85. TERJUNG, R.L., K.M. BALDWIN, J. COOKSEY, B.SAMSON AND R.A. SUTTER. Cardiovascular adaptation to twelve minutes of mild daily exercise in middle-aged sedentary men. *J. Amer. Geriatr. Soc.* 21:164-68, 1973.

86. WILMORE, J.H., J. ROYCE, R.N. GIRANDOLA, F.I. KATCH AND V.L. KATCH. Physiological alterations resulting from a 10-week jogging program. *Med. Sci. Sports* 2(1):7-14, 1970.

87. WILMORE, J.H., J. ROYCE, R.N. GIRANDOLA, F.I. KATCH AND V.L. KATCH. Body composition changes with a 10-week jogging program. *Med. Sci. Sports* 2:113-17, 1970.

88. WILMORE, J.H. Alterations in strength, body composition, and anthropometric measurements consequent to a 10-week weight training program. *Med. Sci. Sports* 6:133-38, 1974.

89. WILMORE, J. Inferiority of female athletes: Myth or reality. *J. Sports Med.* 3:1-6, 1974.

90. WILMORE, J., R.B. PARR, P.A. VODAK, T.J. BARSTOW, T.V. PIPES, A. WARD AND P. LESLIE. Strength, endurance, BMR, and body composition changes with circuit weight training. *Med. Sci. Sports* 8:58-60, 1976. (Abstract)

Bibliography

ADAMS, W. C., W. M. SAVIN, AND A. E. CHRISTA. "Detection of Ozone Toxicity during Continuous Exercise via the Effective Dose Concept." *Journal of Applied Physiology* 51 (1981): 415–27.

ALLEN, R. C. "Shin Splints." *The Athletic Journal* 60 (1979): 59.

ALLEN, ROGER J., AND DAVID HYDE. *Investigations in Stress Control*. Minneapolis: Burgess, 1980.

AMERICAN COLLEGE OF SPORTS MEDICINE. *Guidelines for Graded Exercise Testing and Exercise Prescriptions*. Philadelphia: Lea and Febiger, 1980.

AMERICAN COLLEGE OF SPORTS MEDICINE. "Position Statement on Prevention of Heat Injuries during Distance Running." *Medicine and Science in Sports* 7 (1975): vii–ix.

AMERICAN COLLEGE OF SPORTS MEDICINE. "The Recommended Quantity and Quality of Exercise for Developing and Maintaining Fitness in Healthy Adults." *Medicine and Science in Sports* 10 (1978): vii.

AMERICAN HEART ASSOCIATION. *Jump for the Health of It*. Dallas, TX: American Heart Association, 1983.

AMERICAN PODIATRY ASSOCIATION. *Jogging Advice from Your Podiatrist*. Washington, DC: American Podiatry Association, undated.

ANDERSON, G. E. "College Schedule of Recent Experience." Master's thesis. North Dakota State University, 1972.

APPLE, DAVID F., AND JOHN D. CANTWELL. *Medicine for Sport*. Chicago: Year Book Medical Publishers, 1979.

AYRES, ALEX. "Will Running Change the Kind of Person You Are?" *Running Times*, September 1982, pp. 17–22.

BALOG, L. F. "The Effects of Exercise on Muscle Tension and Subsequent Muscle Relaxation Training." *Research Quarterly for Exercise and Sport* 54 (1983): 119–25.

BARTLEY, DIANNE A. R. AND FAYE Z. BELGRAVE. "Physical Fitness and Psychological Wellbeing in College Students." *Health Education* 18 (1987): 57–60.

BECKER, MARSHALL H. "The Health Belief Model and Personal Behavior." *Health Education Monographs* 2 (1974): 326–473.

BECKER, MARSHALL H., AND LAWRENCE W. GREEN. "A Family Approach to Compliance with Medical Treatment—A Selective Review of the Literature." *International Journal of Health Education* 18 (1975): 1–11.

BENSON, HERBERT. *The Relaxation Response*. New York: Avon, 1975.

BERGER, RICHARD A. *Applied Exercise Physiology*. Philadelphia: Lea and Febiger, 1982.

BLAKELAND, F. "Exercise Deprivation." *Archives of General Psychiatry* 22 (1970): 365–69.

BLOOR, C. M., S. PASYK, AND A. S. LEON. "Interaction of Age and Exercise on Organ and Cellular Development." *The American Journal of Pathology* 58 (1970): 185–99.

BORG, G. "Physical Performance and Perceived Exertion," *Studia Psychologia et Paedogogica, Series Altera, Investigatione*, Gleerup, Lund, 1962.

BOWER, SHARON ANTHONY, AND GORDON BOWER. *Asserting Yourself: A Practical Guide for Positive Change*. Reading, MA: Addison-Wesley, 1976.

BRAY, G. (ed.). *Obesity in America*. Bethesda, MD: National Institutes of Health, Publication No. 80–359, 1980.

BRENNER, M. HARVEY. "Assessing the Social Costs of National Unemployment Rates." Testimony presented before the Subcommittee on Domestic Monetary Policy of the Committee on Banking, Finance, and Urban Affairs, U.S. House of Representatives, Washington, DC, August 12, 1982.

BROUHA, LUCIEN. "The Step Test: A Simple Method of Testing the Physical Fitness of Boys." *Research Quarterly* 14 (1943): 23.

BROWNELL, K. D., et. al. "The Effects of Couples Training and Partner Cooperativeness in the Behavior Treatment of Obesity." *Behavior Therapy* 16 (1978): 323–33.

BUSKIRK, E. R., J. KOLLIAS, E. PICON-REATIQUE, R. AKERS, E. PROKOP, AND P. BAKER. "Physiology and Performance of Track Athletes at Various Altitudes in the United States and Peru." In R.F. Goddard (ed.), *The Effects of Altitude on Physical Performance*. Albuquerque: Athletic Institute, 1967, pp. 65–71.

CAIRNS, D., AND J. A. PASINO. "Comparison of Verbal Reinforcement and Feedback in the Operant Treatment of Disability due to Chronic Low Back Pain." *Behavior Therapy* 8 (1977): 621–30.

CANN, C. E., M. C. MARTIN, H. K. GENANT, AND R. B. JAFFE. "Decreased Spinal Mineral Content of Amenorrheic Women." *Journal of the American Medical Association* 251 (1984): 626–29.

CANNON, WALTER B. *The Wisdom of the Body*. New York: W. W. Norton, 1932.

CAVANAGH, PETER R., AND KEITH R. WILLIAMS. "Testing Procedure for the 1982 Runner's World Shoe Survey." *Runner's World* 16 (1981): 26–33.

COMMITTEE ON MEDICAL AND BIOLOGICAL EFFECTS OF ENVIRONMENTAL POLLUTANTS. *Carbon Monoxide*. Washington, DC: National Academy of Sciences, 1977.

COOPER, KENNETH. *The Aerobics Program for Total Well-Being*. New York: M. Evans, 1983.

CURETON, T. K. "Improvement of Psychological States by Means of Exercise-Fitness Programs." *Journal of the Association of Physical and Mental Rehabilitation* 17 (1963): 14–17.

DANIELS, J. T. "Effects of Altitude on Athletic Accomplishment." *Modern Medicine*, June 26, 1972, pp.73–76.

DAVIS, MARTHA, MATTHEW MCKAY AND ELIZABETH ROBBINS ESHELMAN. *The Relaxation and Stress Reduction Workbook*. Richmond, CA: New Harbinger, 1980.

DEAN, DWIGHT G. "Alienation: It's Meaning and Measurement." *American Sociological Review* 26 (1961): 753–58.

DEAUX, K. *The Behavior of Women and Men*. Monterey, CA: Brooks/Cole, 1976.

DINTIMAN, GEORGE B., AND JERROLD S. GREENBERG. *Health Through Discovery*. Reading, MA: Addison-Wesley, 1980.

DINTIMAN, GEORGE B. AND JERROLD S. GREENBERG. *Health Through Discovery*, 3rd ed. New York: Random House, 1986.

DRINKWATER, B. L. "Physiological Responses of Women to Exercise." In J. H. Wilmore (ed.), *Exercise and Sports Sciences Review*, Vol. I. New York: Academic Press, 1973.

DRINKWATER, B. L., et al. "Bone Mineral Content of Amenorrheic and Eumenorrheic Athletes." *The New England Journal of Medicine* 311 (1984): 277–81.

DRINKWATER, B. L., P. B. RAVEN, S. M. HORVATH, J. A. GLINER, R. D. RUHLING, N. W. BOLDRAN, AND S. TAGUCHI. "Air Pollution, Exercise and Heat Stress." *Archives of Environmental Health* 28 (1974): 177–81.

DUNBAR, JACQUELINE M., GARY D. MARSHALL, AND MEL F. HOVELL. "Behavioral Strategies for Improving Compliance." In R. B. Haynes, D.W. Taylor, and D.L. Sackett (eds.), *Compliance in Health Care*. Baltimore, MD: Johns Hopkins University Press, 1979.

"Economy Has Direct Health Effects." *The Nation's Health*, January 1977, p. 12.

EDWARDS, SALLY. "Cycling Minutes off Your Time," *Runner's World*, April 1983, pp. 61–68.

EKBLOM B., AND R. HUOT. "Responses to Submaximal and Maximal Exercise at Different Levels of Carboxyhemoglobin." *Acta Physiologica Scandinavica* 86 (1972): 474–82.

ELLIS, JOE, AND PATRICIA YAVORSKY. "Stretching Specifics: The Right Stretch Gets Directly to a Trouble Spot to Prevent Injury." *Runner's World*, July 1986, pp. 40–45.

ENGLAND, A. C., et al. "Preventing Severe Heat Injury in Runners: Suggestions from the 1979 Peachtree Road Race Experience." *Annals of Internal Medicine* 97 (1982): 196–201.

FELDMAN, ROBERT H. L. "Modifying Stressful Behaviors." In Jerrold S. Greenberg, *Comprehensive Stress Management*. pp. 223–43, Dubuque, IA: Wm. C. Brown, 1986.

FELDMAN, ROBERT H. L. "The Assessment and Enhancement of Health Compliance in the Workplace." In George S. Everly and Robert H.L. Feldman,

Occupational Health Promotion: Health Behavior in the Workplace, pp. 33–46, New York: John Wiley, 1985.

FLINT, M. M., B. L. DRINKWATER, AND S. M. HORVATH. "Effects of Training on Women's Response to Submaximal Exercise." *Medicine and Science in Sports* 6 (1974): 89–94.

FOOD AND NUTRITION BOARD, NATIONAL ACADEMY OF SCIENCES—NATIONAL RESEARCH COUNCIL. *Recommended Dietary Allowances*, 9th ed. Washington, DC: National Academy of Sciences, 1970.

FOX, E. L. *Sports Physiology*. Philadelphia: W. B. Saunders, 1979.

FRIEDMAN, MEYER AND RAY H. ROSENMAN. *Type A Behavior and Your Heart*. New York: Alfred A. Knopf, 1974.

FRIEDMAN, MEYER AND DIANE ULMER. *Treating Type A Behavior and Your Heart*. New York: Alfred A. Knopf, 1984.

GALWAY, W. TIMOTHY. *The Inner Game of Tennis*. New York: Random House, 1974.

GETCHELL, BUD. *Physical Fitness: A Way of Life*. New York: John Wiley, 1983.

GILLISON, G. "Living Theater in New Guinea Highlands." *National Geographic* 1640 (1983): 147–49.

GIRDANO, DANIEL AND GEORGE EVERLY. *Controlling Stress and Tension*. Englewood Cliffs, NJ: Prentice Hall, 1986.

GREEN, TIM. "My Favorite Routine: Chair Acrobics." *Shape*, June 1986, pp. 150–53.

GREEN, WALTER. "The Search for a Meaningful Definition of Health." In Donald A. Read (ed.), *New Directions in Health Education: Some Contemporary Issues for an Emerging Age*, p. 114. New York: Macmillan, 1974.

GREENBERG, JERROLD S. *Comprehensive Stress Management*. Dubuque, IA: Wm. C. Brown, 1986.

GREIST, J. H., M. H. KLEIN, R. R. EISCHENS, J. FARIS, A. S. GURMAN, AND W. P. MORGAN. "Running as Treatment for Depression." *Comparative Psychiatry* 20 (1979): 41–54.

GRIMBY, G., AND B. SALTIN. "Physiological Analysis of Physically Well Trained Middle-Aged and Old Athletes." *Acta Medica Scandinavica* 179 (1966): 513–26.

GUTIN, BERNARD. *The High Energy Factor*. New York: Random House, 1983.

GUYTON, ARTHUR C. *Function of the Human Body*. Philadelphia: W. B. Saunders, 1974.

HAGE, P. "Air Pollution: Adverse Effects on Athletic Performance." *The Physician and Sports Medicine* 10 (1982): 126–32.

HARRIS, D. "Research Studies on the Female Athlete—Psychosocial Considerations." *Journal of Physical Education and Recreation* 46 (1975): 33.

HAYMES, E. M., AND C. L. WELLS. *Environment and Human Performance*. Champaign, IL: Human Kinetics, 1986.

HAYMES. S. G., et al. "The Relationship of Psychosocial Factors to Coronary Heart Disease in the Framingham Study: I. Methods and Risk Factors." *American Journal of Epidemiology* 107 (1978): 362–83.

HEATH, G. W., J. M. HAGBERG, A. A. EHSANI, AND J. O. HOLLOSZY. "A Physiological Comparison of Young and Older Endurance Athletes." *Journal of Applied Physiology* 51 (1981): 634–40.

HINSON, MARILYN M. *Kinesiology*. Dubuque, IA: Wm. C. Brown, 1977.

HOLLOSZY, J. O. "Exercise, Health and Aging: A Need For More Information." *Medicine and Science in Sports and Exercise* 15 (1983): 1–5.

HOLMES, THOMAS H., AND RICHARD H. RAHE. "The Social Readjustment Rating Scale." *Journal of Psychosomatic Research* 11 (1967): 213–18.

JACKSON, D. W. "Shinsplints: An Update." *Physical Sports Medicine* 6 (1978): 10.

JACOBSON, EDMUND. *Progressive Relaxation*. Chicago: University of Chicago Press, 1938.

KATZ, J. *Swimming Through Pregnancy*. Garden City, NY: Doubleday/Dolphin, 1983.

KATZ, JANE. "The W.E.T. Workout: A Swimmer's Guide to Water Exercise Techniques." *Shape*, June 1986, pp. 82–88ff.

KLAFS, CARL E., AND DANIEL ARNHEIM. *Modern Principles of Athletic Training*. St. Louis: C.V. Mosby, 1981.

LAMB, D. R. *Physiology of Exercise*. New York: Macmillan, 1978.

LEON, A. S. "Age and Other Predictors of Coronary Heart Disease." *Medicine and Science in Sports and Exercise* 19 (1987): 159–67.

LIEBMAN, SHELLY. *Do It at Your Desk: An Office Worker's Guide to Fitness and Health*. Washington, DC: Tilden Press, 1982.

MAHONEY, M. J., AND C. E. THORESON. *Self-Control: Power to the Person*. Monterey, CA: Brooks/Cole, 1974.

MARTIN, J. E., AND P. M. DUBBERT. "Exercise Applications and Promotion in Behavioral Medicine: Current Status and Future Directions." *Journal of Consulting and Clinical Psychology* 50 (1982): 1004–17.

MCFARLAND, R. A. "Review of Experimental Findings in Sensory and Mental Functions." In A.H. Hegnauer (ed.), *Biomedicine Problems of High Terrestrial Elevations*. Natick, MA: U.S. Army Research Institute of Environmental Medicine, 1969, pp. 250–65.

MICHELI, L. J. "Sports Injuries in Children and Adolescents." In R.H. Strauss (ed.), *Sports Medicine and Physiology*. Philadelphia: W. B. Saunders, 1979.

MIKEVIC, P. "Anxiety, Depression and Exercise." *Quest* 33 (1982): 140–53.

MIRKIN, GABE, AND MARSHALL HOFFMAN. *The Sportsmedicine Book*. Boston: Little, Brown, 1978.

MONKMAN, G. R., G. ORWOLL, AND J. C. IVINS. "Trauma and Oncogenesis." *Mayo Clinic, Proceedings* 49 (1974): 157–63.

MONTOYE, H., AND D. LAMPHLEAR. "Grip and Arm Strength in Males and Females, Age 10 to 69." *The Research Quarterly* 48 (1977): 109–120.

MORGAN, W. P. "Anxiety Reduction Following Acute Physical Activity." *Psychiatric Annals* 9 (1979).

MOSS, G. E. *Illness, Immunity and Social Interaction*. New York: John Wiley, 1973.

MUCKLE, DAVID SUTHERLAND. *Injuries in Sport*. Bristol, Eng.: John Wright, 1982.

NATIONAL CENTER FOR HEALTH STATISTICS. "Births, Marriages, Divorces, And Deaths For 1981." *Monthly Vital Statistics Report* 30 (March 18, 1982).

NATIONAL CENTER FOR HEALTH STATISTICS. "Births, Marriages, Divorces, And Deaths For 1986." *Monthly Vital Statistics Report* 35 (April 1987).

NATIONAL HEART, LUNG AND BLOOD INSTITUTE. *Exercise and Your Heart*. Washington, DC: Public Health Service, 1981.

NOBLE, B. J. *Physiology of Exercise of Sport*. St. Louis: Times Mirror, 1986.

NORTHRUP, J., G. A. LOGAN AND W. C. MCKINNEY. *Introduction to Biomechanic Analysis of Sport,* 2nd ed. Dubuque, IA: Wm. C. Brown, 1979.

O'DONOGHUE, DON H. *Treatment of Injuries to Athletes*. Philadelphia: W. B. Saunders, 1976.

OFFICE OF DISEASE PREVENTION AND HEALTH PROMOTION. *The 1990 Health Objectives for the Nation: A Midcourse Review*. Washington, DC: Public Health Service, 1986.

OFFICE OF THE ASSISTANT SECRETARY FOR HEALTH AND THE SURGEON GENERAL. *Healthy People, The Surgeon General's Report on Health Promotion and Disease Prevention, 1979*. Public Health Service, DHEW Pub. No. (PHS) 70–55071, Washington, DC: U.S. Government Printing Office, July 1979.

OFFICE OF THE ASSISTANT SECRETARY FOR HEALTH AND THE SURGEON GENERAL. *Healthy People, The Surgeon General's Report on Health Promotion and Disease Prevention—Background Papers, 1979*. Public Health Service, DHEW Pub. No. (PHS) 79-55071A, Washington, DC: U.S. Government Printing Office, 1979.

PAFFENBARGER, R. S., et al. "Physical Activity, All Causes Mortality and Longevity of College Alumni." *The New England Journal of Medicine* 314 (1986): 605–13.

PARIZKOVA, J. *Body Composition and Exercise during Growth and Development*. New York: Academic Press, 1973, pp. 98–124.

PARIZKOVA, J., AND E. EISELT. "Longitudinal Changes in Body Build and Skinfolds in a Group of Old Men over a 16-Year Period." *Human Biology* 52 (1980): 803–9.

PARLEE, M. B. "The Premenstrual Syndrome." *Psychological Bulletin* 80 (1973): 454–65.

PELLETIER, KENNETH R. *Mind as Healer, Mind as Slayer*. New York: Dell, 1977.

POLLACK, M. L. "The Quantification of Endurance Training Programs." *Exercise and Sport Sciences Reviews* 1 (1973): 55–188.

POLLACK, M. L. H. S. MILLER, AND J. WILMORE. "Physiological Characteristics of Champion American Track Athletes 40–75 Years of Age." *Journal of Gerontology* 29 (1974): 645–49.

POLLOCK, MICHAEL L., JACK H. WILMORE, AND SAMUEL M. FOX. *Health and Fitness through Physical Activity*. New York: John Wiley, 1978.

PRESIDENT'S COUNCIL ON PHYSICAL FITNESS AND SPORTS. *An Introduction To Physical Fitness*. Washington, DC: President's Council on Physical Fitness and Sports, 1980.

PRESIDENT'S COUNCIL ON PHYSICAL FITNESS AND SPORTS. *An Introduction to Running*. Washington, DC: President's Council on Physical Fitness and Sports, 1980.

PRESIDENT'S COUNCIL ON PHYSICAL FITNESS AND SPORTS. *Aqua Dynamics*. Washington, DC: President's Council on Physical Fitness and Sports, 1981.

PRESIDENT'S COUNCIL ON PHYSICAL FITNESS AND SPORTS. *Physical Fitness Research Digest*, Series 9, no. 4. October 1979.

PROJECT ON EQUAL EDUCATION RIGHTS. *Summary of the Regulation for Title IX Education Amendments of 1972*. Washington, DC, 1975.

RANSFORD, CHARLES P. "A Role for Amines in the Antidepressant Effect of Exercise: A Review." *Medicine and Science in Sports and Exercise* 14 (1982): 1–10.

RASMUSSEN, W. "Shin Splints: Definition and Treatment." *Journal of Sports Medicine* 2 (1974): 112.

RATHUS, SPENCER A. "A 30–Item Schedule for Assessing Assertive Behavior." *Behavior Therapy* 4 (1973): 398–406.

REILLY, THOMAS (ed.). *Sports Fitness and Sports Injuries*. London: Faber and Faber, 1981.

RICHIE, DOUGLAS H., STEVEN F. KELSO, AND PATRICIA A. BELLUCCI. "Aerobic Dance Injuries: A Retrospective Study of Instructors and Participants." *The Physician and Sportsmedicine* 13 (1985): 130–40.

RIDENOUR, M. (ed.). *Motor Development, Issues and Applications*. Princeton, NJ: Princeton Book Company, 1978.

RILEY, D. P. *Strength Training: By the Experts*. West Point, NY: Leisure Press, 1977.

ROBINSON, S. "Experimental Studies of Physical Fitness in Relation to Age." *Arbeitsphysiologia* 10 (1938): 251–323.

ROBINTON, E. D., AND E. W. MOOD. "A Quantitative and Qualitative Appraisal of Microbia Pollution of Water by Swimmers: A Preliminary Report." *Journal of Hygiene* 64 (1966): 489–99.

RODIN, J., AND J. SLOCHOWER. "Externality in the Obese: Effects of Environmental Responsiveness on Weight." *Journal of Personality and Social Psychology* 33 (1976): 338–44.

ROGERS, TERENCE R. *Elementary Human Physiology*. New York: John Wiley, 1961.

RORST, R. *Athletics and the Heart*. Chicago: Yearbook Medical Publishers, 1987.

ROSENBAUM, JEAN. "Aerobics Without Injury." *Medical Self-Care*, Fall 1984, pp. 30–33.

RYAN, BILL. The Government's Surprising New Position: It May Be Okay to Start Exercising Without Seeing a Doctor First." *Parade*, November 15, 1981.

SALTIN, B. "Physiological Effects of Physical Conditioning." *Medicine and Science in Sports* 1 (1969): 50–56.

SALTIN, B., AND G. GRIMBY. "Physiological Analysis of Middle-Age and Old Former Athletes: Comparison with Still Active Athletes of the Same Age." *Circulation* 38 (1968): 1104–15.

SAVIN, M., AND R. H. MCCLEARY. "Clearing the Air of a Clouded Issue." *Runner's World*, July 1983, p. 55.

SCHWINN, BETH. "Burned in Pursuit of the Burn." *Washington Post, Health*, August 14, 1986, pp. 12.

SECORD, PAUL F., AND SIDNEY M. JOURARD. "The Appraisal of Body-Cathexis: Body-Cathexis and the Self." *Journal of Consulting Psychology* 17 (1953): 343–47.

SEEMAN, M. "Alienation and Social Learning in a Reformatory." *American Journal of Sociology* 69 (1963): 270–84.

SEEMAN, M., AND J. W. EVANS. "Alienation and Learning in a Hospital Setting." *American Sociological Review* 27 (1962): 772–83.

SELYE, HANS. *The Stress of Life*. New York: McGraw-Hill, 1956.

SHANGOLD, MONA. "The Woman Runner: Her Body, Her Mind, Her Spirit." *Runner's World* 16 (July 1981): 34.

SHEPHERD, R. J. *Alive Man! The Physiology of Physical Activity*. Springfield, IL: Charles C. Thomas, 1972.

SIDNEY, K. H., R. J. SHEPHERD, AND J. HARRISON. "Endurance Training and Body Composition of the Elderly." *The American Journal of Clinical Nutrition* 30 (1977): 326–33.

SIEGEL, P. "Does Bath Water Enter the Vagina?" *Obstetrics and Gynecology* 15 (1960): 660–61.

SOBOLOVA, V., V. SELIGER, D. GRUSSOVER, J. MACHOVCOCA, AND V. ZELENKA. "The Influence of Age and Sports Training in Swimming on Physical Fitness." *Acta Paediatrica Scandinavica* 217 (1971): 63–67 (supplement).

SONSTROEM, R. "Exercise and Self-Esteem: Recommendations for Expository Research." *Quest* 33 (1982): 124–34.

SORENSON, JACKI. *Aerobic Dancing*. New York: Rawson, Wade, 1979.

SPIRDUSO, W. "Exercise and the Aging Brain." *Research Quarterly for Exercise and Sport* 54 (1983): 208-18.

STEINMETZ, JENNY, ET AL. *Managing Stress Before It Manages You*. Palo Alto, CA: Bull, 1980.

STRAITS, B. C., AND L. SECHREST. "Further Support of Findings about Characteristics of Smokers and Nonsmokers." *Journal of Consulting Psychology* 27 (1963): 282.

STRAUSS, R.H. (ed.). *Sports Medicine and Physiology*. Philadelphia: W. B. Saunders, 1979.

TAYLOR, SHELLY E. *Health Psychology*. New York: Random House, 1986.

TOFFLER, ALVIN. *Future Shock*. New York: Random House, 1970.

TOFFLER, ALVIN. *The Third Wave*. New York: William Morrow, 1980.

TOM, G. AND M. RUCKER. "Fat, Full and Happy: Effects of Food Deprivation, External Cues, and Obesity on Preference Ratings, Consumption, and

Buying Intentions." *Journal of Personality and Social Psychology* 32 (1975): 761–66.

U.S. CONGRESS SELECT COMMITTEE ON NUTRITION AND HUMAN NEEDS. *Dietary Goals for the United States, Second Edition.* Washington, DC: U.S. Government Printing Office, November, 1977.

U.S. CONSUMER PRODUCTS SAFETY COMMISSION. *National Electronic Injury Surveillance System.* Bethesda, MD: National Injury Information Clearinghouse, 1976.

U.S. DEPARTMENT OF HEALTH AND HUMAN SERVICES, PUBLIC HEALTH SERVICE. *Promoting Health / Preventing Disease—Objectives for the Nation.* Washington, DC: U.S. Government Printing Office, Fall 1980.

U.S. ENVIRONMENTAL PROTECTION AGENCY. *Information Documents on Automobile Emissions: Inspection and Maintenance Programs.* EPA 400/2-78-001, February 1978.

VAZ, KATHERINE. "Shifting to Two Wheels." *Washington Post, Health,* October 7, 1986, pp. 12–14.

VICKERY, DONALD M., AND JAMES F. FRIES. *Take Care of Yourself.* Reading, MA: Addison-Wesley, 1976.

VINGER, PAUL F., AND EARL F. HOERNER (Eds.). *Sports Injuries: The Unthwarted Epidemic.* Littleton, MA: PSG Publishing, 1981.

WEIL, J. V., M. H. KRYGER, AND C. H. SCOGGIN. "Sleep and Breathing at High Altitude." In C. Guilleminault (ed.), *Sleep Apnea Syndrome.* New York: Alan R. Liss, 1978.

WELDON, GAIL. "The ABC's of Aerobics Injuries." *Shape,* September 1986, pp. 86–90ff.

WELLS, C. L. *Women Sport and Performance.* Champaign, IL: Human Kinetics, 1985.

WILLIAMS, J. G. P. *Color Atlas of Injury in Sport.* Chicago: Year Book Medical Publishers, 1980.

WILMORE, J. H., AND A. R. BEHNKE. "An Anthropometric Estimation of Body Density and Lean Body Weight in Young Men." *Journal of Applied Physiology* 27 (1969): 25–31.

WILMORE, J. H., AND A. R. BEHNKE. "An Anthropometric Estimation of Body Density and Lean Body Weight in Young Women." *American Journal of Clinical Nutrition* 23 (1970): 267–74.

WOMERSLEY, J., J. V. G. A. DURNIN, K. BODDY, AND M. MAHAFFY. "Influence of Muscular Development, Obesity, and Age on the Fat-Free Mass of Adults." *Journal of Applied Physiology* 41 (1976): 223–29.

ZOHMAN, LENORE R. *Beyond Diet . . . Exercise Your Way to Fitness and Heart Health.* Best Foods, 1979.

Index

A

Abrasions, 277, 279
Abstinence, 146, 148
Acclimatization, 166, 177
Achilles tendon:
  rupture, 273, 278
  stretch, 41, 284
ACSM (see American College
  of Sports Medicine)
ACTH (see Hormones)
Adams, W.C., et al., 168
Adenohyphosis, 24
Adenosine triphosphate (ATP),
  22, 36, 37
Adrenal cortex, 240, 241
Adrenaline (see Hormones)
Adrenal medulla, 240
Adrenocorticotrophin hormone
  (ACTH) (see Hormones)
Aerobic Center, 295
Aerobic endurance, 200, 201,
  210 (see also Car-
  diorespiratory fitness)
Aerobics:
  activities, 137, 201-5, 210
    (see also specific ac-
    tivities)
  chair, 296
  dance, 150, 294-95, 298
  endurance, 200, 201, 210
  exercise forms, 96
  injuries from, 295
  low-impact, 295, 298
  process in metabolism, 27
Aerobics and Fitness Associa-
  tion of America, 295
*Aerobics Program for Total
  Well-Being*, 258
Affect, 54
Afferent message, 24
Age, 53 (see also Aging)
Ageism, 10
Aggressive behavior, 107
Aging, 53, 144, 147, 148
  effect of exercise, 150

effect on the body, 150, 152,
  153
information about, 148
Air pollution, 167-69
Alcohol abuse, 9, 12
Alienation, 10, 107-10
  normlessness, 109, 110
  powerlessness, 109, 110
  social isolation, 109, 110
Allen, R.C., 273
Allen, Roger J., 243, 244
Altitude:
  effect on exercising body, 165-
  67, 177
Amenorrhea, 145, 275
American Aerobics Association,
  295
American College of Sports
  Medicine (ACSM), 40,
  97, 201, 295
  frequency of training, 40, 142
  guidelines for exercise testing, 66
  guidelines relative to heat injuries in distance run-
  ning, 163, 318-19
  medical examination, 65
  position statement, 97,
  320-25
American Heart Association,
  198, 221, 286
American Podiatry Association, 285
Anaerobic:
  exercises, 96
  process in metabolism, 27
Androgen serum concentration,
  59
Angina pectoris, 197
Ankle sprain (see Injuries;
  Sprained ankle)
Anorexia nervosa, 229
Anorexiants (see Appetite suppressants)
Antidepressant effects of training, 57

Anxiety, 32, 54
  state, 54
  trait, 54
Aorta, 22, 29
Appetite, 219
Appetite suppressants, 230, 302
Apple, D.F., 274
Aqua Dynamics, 291
Arnheim, Daniel, 266, 273
Arterial blood, 29
Arteries, 28
Arteriosclerosis, 197, 223
Arthritis, 152, 233
Assertive behavior, 105
Assertiveness assessment,
  105-7
Assessment:
  body composition, 77-78
  cardiorespiratory:
    Harvard steptest, 67, 69
    1.5 mile test, 67, 68
  flexibility:
    shoulder reach, 75
    trunk extension, 76
    trunk flexion, 76
  health behavior, 11, 14
  life style, 101, 102
  motor skill, 78, 79, 86
  muscle endurance:
    flexed-arm hang, 74, 75
    pullup, 74
    situp, 73, 74
  muscle strength:
    bench press, 69, 70
    curl, 71
    half-squat, 73
    leg press, 71
    standing press, 70
  psychosocial, 103-16
    alienation, 107-10
    assertiveness, 105
    locus of control, 103
    motivation, 103
    review, 116
    self-esteem, 110-12
    stress, 112-16